UNDERSTANDING NONLINEAR DYNAMICS

Springer

New York
Berlin
Heidelberg
Barcelona
Budapest
Hong Kong
London
Milan
Paris
Santa Clara
Singapore
Tokyo

Understanding Nonlinear Dynamics

□ Daniel Kaplan □

Department of Mathematics and Computer Science
Macalester College □ St. Paul, Minnesota, USA

□ Leon Glass □

Department of Physiology
McGill University □ Montréal, Québec, Canada

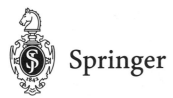

Springer

Textbooks in Mathematical Sciences

Series Editors:

Thomas F. Banchoff
Brown University

Jerrold Marsden
University of California, Berkeley

John Ewing
Indiana University

Stan Wagon
Macalester College

Gaston Gonnet
ETH Zentrum, Zürich

Library of Congress Cataloging-in-Publication Data
Kaplan, Daniel, 1959–
        Understanding nonlinear dynamics / Daniel Kaplan and Leon Glass.
        p. cm. – (Textbooks in mathematical sciences)
Includes bibliographical references and index.
ISBN 0-387-94440-0
1. Dynamics. 2. Nonlinear theories. I. Glass, Leon, 1943–. II. Title. III. Series.
QA845.K36   1995   94-43113
515'.352–dc20

Printed on acid-free paper.

Production managed by Frank Ganz; manufacturing supervised by Jeff Taub.
Photocomposed copy prepared from the author's LaTeX files.
Printed and bound by Hamilton Printing Co., Castleton on Hudson, NY.
Printed in the United States of America.

9 8 7 6 5 4 3 2 (Corrected second printing, 1998)

ISBN 0-387-94440-0 Springer-Verlag New York Berlin Heidelberg   SPIN 10645103

To Maya and Tamar. — DTK

To Kathy, Hannah, and Paul
      and in memory of Daniel. — LG

Preface

This book is about *dynamics*—the mathematics of how things change in time. The universe around us presents a kaleidoscope of quantities that vary with time, ranging from the extragalactic pulsation of quasars to the fluctuations in sunspot activity on our sun; from the changing outdoor temperature associated with the four seasons to the daily temperature fluctuations in our bodies; from the incidence of infectious diseases such as measles to the tumultuous trend of stock prices.

Since 1984, some of the vocabulary of dynamics—such as *chaos, fractals,* and *nonlinear*—has evolved from abstruse terminology to a part of common language. In addition to a large technical scientific literature, the subjects these terms cover are the focus of many popular articles, books, and even novels. These popularizations have presented "chaos theory" as a scientific revolution. While this may be journalistic hyperbole, there is little question that many of the important concepts involved in modern dynamics—global multistability, local stability, sensitive dependence on initial conditions, attractors—are highly relevant to many areas of study including biology, engineering, medicine, ecology, economics, and astronomy.

This book presents the main concepts and applications of nonlinear dynamics at an elementary level. The text is based on a one-semester undergraduate course that has been offered since 1975 at McGill University and that has been constantly updated to keep up with current developments. Most of the students enrolled in the course are studying biological sciences and have completed a year of calculus with no intention to study further mathematics. Since the main concepts of nonlinear dynamics are largely accessible using only elementary arguments, students are able to understand the mathematics and successfully carry out computations. The exciting nature and modernity of the concepts and the graphics are further stimuli that motivate students.

Mathematical developments since the mid 1970's have shown that many interesting phenomena can arise in simple finite-difference equations. These are introduced in Chapter 1, where the student is initiated into three important mathematical themes of the course: local stability analysis, global multistability, and problem solving using both an algebraic and a geometric approach. The graphical iteration of one-dimensional, finite-difference equations, combined with the analysis of the local stability of steady states, provides two complementary views of the same problem. The concept of chaos is introduced as soon as possible, after the student is able graphically to iterate a one-dimensional, finite-difference equation, and understands the concept of stability. For most students, this is the first exposure to mathematics from the twentieth century!

From the instructor's point of view, this topic offers the opportunity to refresh students' memory and skills in differential calculus. Since some students take this course several years after studying geometry and calculus, some skills have become rusty. Appendix A reviews important functions such as the Hill function, the Gaussian distribution, and the conic sections. Many exercises that can help in solidifying geometry and calculus skills are included in Appendix A.

Chapters 2 and 3 continue the study of discrete-time systems. Networks and cellular automata (Chapter 2) are important both from a conceptual and technical perspective, and because of their relevance to computers. The recent interest in neural and gene networks makes this an important area for applications and current research.

Many students are familiar with fractal images from the myriad popularizations of that topic. While the images provide a compelling motivation for studying nonlinear dynamics, the concepts of self-similarity and fractional dimension are important from a mathematical perspective. Chapter 3 discusses self-similarity and fractals in a way that is closely linked to the dynamics discussed in Chapter 1. Fractals arise from dynamics in many unexpected ways. The concept of a fractional dimension is unfamiliar initially but can be appreciated by those without advanced technical abilities. Recognizing the importance of computers in studying fractals, we use a computer-based notation in presenting some of the material.

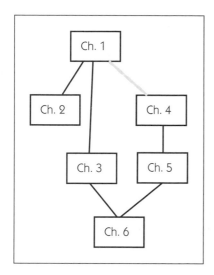

Dependencies among the chapters.

The study of continuous-time systems forms much of the second half of the book. Chapter 4 deals with one-dimensional differential equations. Because of the importance of exponential growth and decay in applications, we believe that every science student should be exposed to the linear one-dimensional differential equation, learning what it means and how to solve it. In addition, it is essential that those interested in science appreciate the limitations that nonlinearities impose on exponential ("Malthusian") growth. In Chapter 4, algebraic analysis of the linear stability of steady states of nonlinear equations is combined with the graphical analysis of the asymptotic dynamics of nonlinear equations to provide another exposure to the complementary use of algebraic and geometric methods of analysis.

Chapter 5 deals with differential equations with two variables. Such equations often appear in the context of compartmental models, which have been proposed in diverse fields including ion channel kinetics, pharmacokinetics, and ecological systems. The analysis of the stability of steady states in two-dimensional nonlinear equations and the geometric sketching of the trajectories in the phase plane provide the most challenging aspect of the course. However, the same basic conceptual approach is used here as is used in the linear stability analyses in Chapter 1 and Chapter 4, and the material can be presented using elementary methods only.

In most students' mathematical education, a chasm exists between the concepts they learn and the applications in which they are interested. To help bridge this gap, Chapter 6 discusses methods of data analysis including classical methods (mean, standard deviation, the autocorrelation function) and modern methods derived from nonlinear dynamics (time-lag embeddings, dimension and related topics). This chapter may be of particular interest to researchers interested in applying some of the concepts from nonlinear dynamics to their work.

In order to illustrate the practical use of concepts from dynamics in applications, we have punctuated the text with short essays called "Dynamics in Action." These cover a wide diversity of subjects, ranging from the random drift of molecules to the deterministic patterns underlying global climate changes.

Following each chapter is supplementary material. The notes and references provide a guide to additional references that may be fun to read and are accessible to beginning students. A set of exercises reviewing concepts and mathematical skills is also provided for each chapter. Solutions to selected exercises are provided at the end of the book. For each chapter, we also give a set of computer exercises. The computer exercises introduce students to some of the ways computers can be used in nonlinear dynamics. The computer exercises can provide many opportunities for a term project for students.

The appropriate use of this book in a course depends on the student clientele and the orientation of the instructors. In our instruction of biological science students at McGill, emphasis has been on developing analytical and geometrical skills to carry out stability analysis and analysis of asymptotic dynamics in one-dimensional finite-difference equations and in one- and two-dimensional differential equations. We also include several lectures on neural and gene networks, cellular automata, and fractals.

Although this text is written at a level appropriate to first- and second-year undergraduates, most of the material dealing with nonlinear finite-difference and differential equations and time-series analysis is not presented in standard undergraduate or graduate curricula in the physical sciences or mathematics. This book might well be used as a source for supplementary material for traditional courses in advanced calculus, differential equations, and mathematical methods in physical sciences. The link between dynamics and time series analysis can make this book useful to statisticians or signal processing engineers interested in a new perspective on their subject and in an introduction to the research literature.

Over the years, a number of teaching assistants have contributed to the development of this material and the education of the students. Particular thanks go to Carl Graves, David Larocque, Wanzhen Zeng, Marc Courtemanche, Hiroyuki Ito, and Gil Bub. We also thank Michael Broide, Scott Greenwald, Frank Witkowski, Bob Devaney, Michael Shlesinger, Jim Crutchfield, Melanie Mitchell, Michael Frame, Jerry Marsden, and the students of McGill University Biology 309 for their many corrections and suggestions. We thank André Duchastel for his careful redrawing of many of the figures reproduced from other sources. Finally, we thank Jerry Lyons, Liesl Gibson, Karen Kosztolnyik, and Kristen Cassereau for their excellent editorial assistance and help in the final stages of preparation of this book.

McGill University has provided an ideal environment to carry out research and to teach. Our colleagues and chairmen have provided encouragement in many ways. We would like to thank in particular, J. Milic-Emili, K. Krjnevic, D. Goltzman, A. Shrier, M. R. Guevara, and M. C. Mackey. The financial support of the Natural Sciences Engineering and Research Council (Canada), the Medical Research Council (Canada), the Canadian Heart and Stroke Association has enabled us to carry out research that is reflected in the text. Finally, Leon Glass thanks the John Simon Guggenheim Memorial Foundation for Fellowship support during the final stages of the preparation of this text.

We are making available various electronic extensions to this book, including additional exercises, solutions, and computer materials. For information, please contact understanding@cnd.mcgill.ca.

February 1995

Daniel Kaplan
kaplan@macalester.edu

Leon Glass
glass@cnd.mcgill.ca

About the Authors

Daniel Kaplan specializes in the analysis of data using techniques motivated by nonlinear dynamics. His primary interest is in the interpretation of irregular physiological rhythms, but the methods he has developed have been used in geophysics, economics, marine ecology, and other fields. He joined Macalester College in 1996, after receiving his Ph.D from Harvard University and working at MIT and McGill. His undergraduate studies were completed at Swarthmore College. He has worked with several instrumentation companies to develop novel types of medical monitors.

Leon Glass is one of the pioneers of what has come to be called chaos theory, specializing in applications to medicine and biology. He has worked in areas as diverse as physical chemistry, visual perception, and cardiology, and is one of the originators of the concept of "dynamical disease." He has been a professor at McGill University in Montreal since 1975, and has worked at the University of Rochester, the University of California in San Diego, and Harvard University. He earned his Ph.D. at the University of Chicago and did postdoctoral work at the University of Edinburgh and the University of Chicago.

Contents

CHAPTER 1

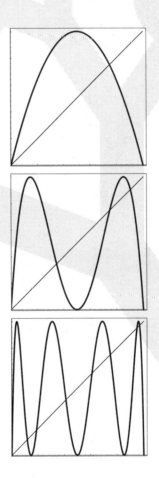

Finite-Difference Equations

1.1 A MYTHICAL FIELD

Imagine that a graduate student goes to a meadow on the first day of May, walks through the meadow waving a fly net, and counts the number of flies caught in the net. She repeats this ritual for several years, following up on the work of previous graduate students. The resulting measurements might look like the graph shown in Figure 1.1. The graduate student notes the variability in her measurements and wants to find out if they contain any important biological information.

Several different approaches could be taken to study the data. The student could do statistical analyses of the data to calculate the mean value or to detect long-term trends. She could also try to develop a detailed and realistic model of the ecosystem, taking into account such factors as weather, predators, and the fly populations in previous years. Or she could construct a simplified theoretical model for fly population density.

Sticking to what she knows, the student decides to model the population variability in terms of actual measurements. The number of flies in one summer

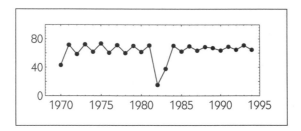

Figure 1.1 The number of flies caught during the annual fly survey.

depends on the number of eggs laid the previous year. The number of eggs laid depends on the number of flies alive during that summer. Thus, the number of flies in one summer depends on the number of flies in the previous summer. In mathematical terms, this is a relationship, or **function**,

$$N_{t+1} = f(N_t). \tag{1.1}$$

This equation says simply that the number of flies in the $t + 1$ summer is determined by (or *is a function of*) the number of flies in summer t, which is the previous summer. Equations of this form, which relate values at **discrete times** (e.g., each May), are called **finite-difference equations**. N_t is called the **state** of the system at time t. We are interested in how the state changes in time: the **dynamics** of the system.

Since the real-world ecosystem is complicated and since the measurements are imperfect, we do not expect a model like Eq. 1.1 to be able to duplicate exactly the actual fly population measurements. For example, birds eat flies, so the population of flies is influenced by the bird population, which itself depends on a complicated array of factors. The assumption behind Eq. 1.1 is that the number of flies in year $t + 1$ depends solely on the number of flies in year t. While this is not strictly true, it may serve as a working approximation. The problem now is to figure out an appropriate form for this dependence that is consistent with the data and that encapsulates the important aspects of fly population biology.

1.2 THE LINEAR FINITE-DIFFERENCE EQUATION

Let us start by making a simple assumption about the propagation of flies: For each fly in generation t there will be R flies in generation $t + 1$. The corresponding finite-difference equation is

$$N_{t+1} = RN_t. \tag{1.2}$$

Equation 1.2 is called a **linear equation** because a graph of N_{t+1} versus N_t is a straight line, with a slope of R.

The **solution** to Eq. 1.2 is a sequence of states, $N_1, N_2, N_3, \ldots$, that satisfy Eq. 1.2 for each value of t. That is, the solution satisfies $N_2 = RN_1$, and $N_3 = RN_2$, and $N_4 = RN_3$, and so on.

One way to find a solution to the equation is by the process of **iteration**. Given the number of flies N_0 in the initial generation, we can calculate the number of flies in the next generation, N_1. Then, having calculated N_1, we can apply Eq. 1.2 to find N_2. We can repeat the process for as long as we care to. The state N_0 is called the **initial condition**.

For the linear equation, it is possible to carry out the iteration process using simple algebra. By iterating Eq. 1.2 we can find N_1, N_2, N_3, and so forth.

$$N_1 = RN_0,$$

$$N_2 = RN_1 = R^2 N_0,$$

$$N_3 = RN_2 = R^2 N_1 = R^3 N_0,$$

$$\vdots$$

There is a simple pattern here: It suggests that the solution to the equation might be written as

$$N_t = R^t N_0. \tag{1.3}$$

We can verify that Eq. 1.3 is indeed the solution to Eq. 1.2 by **substitution**. Since Eq. 1.3 is valid for all values of time t, it is also valid for time $t + 1$. By replacing the variable t in Eq. 1.3 with $t + 1$, we can see that $N_{t+1} = R^{t+1} N_0$. Expanding this, we get

$$N_{t+1} = R^{t+1} N_0 = RR^t N_0 = RN_t,$$

which shows that the solution implies the finite-difference equation in Eq. 1.2.

BEHAVIOR OF THE LINEAR EQUATION

Equation 1.3 can produce several different types of solution, depending on the value of the parameter R:

Decay   When $0 < R < 1$, the number of flies in each generation is smaller than that in the previous generation. Eventually, the number falls

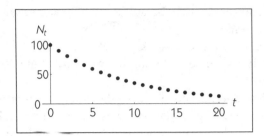

Figure 1.2
The solution to
$N_{t+1} = 0.90N_t$.

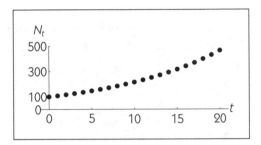

Figure 1.3
The solution to
$N_{t+1} = 1.08N_t$.

to zero and the flies become extinct (see Figure 1.2). Since the solution is an exponential function of time (see Appendix A), this behavior is called **exponential decay**.

Growth   When $R > 1$, the population of flies increases from generation to generation without bound. The solution is said to "explode" to ∞ (see Figure 1.3). Again the solution is an exponential function, and this behavior is thus called **exponential growth.**

Steady-state behavior   When R is exactly 1, the population stays at the same level (see Figure 1.4). This is clearly an extraordinary solution, because it only happens for a single, exact value of R, whereas the other types of solutions occur for a range of R values.

The behaviors in the fly population study involve $R > 0$. It doesn't make biological sense to consider cases where $R < 0$ in Eq. 1.2. After all, how can flies

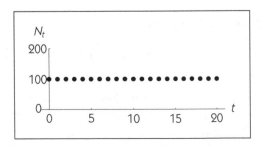

Figure 1.4
The solution to
$N_{t+1} = 1.00N_t$.

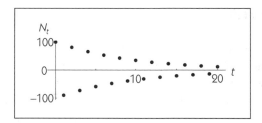

Figure 1.5
The solution to
$N_{t+1} = -0.90N_t$.

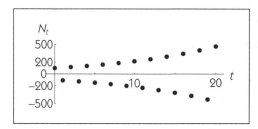

Figure 1.6
The solution to
$N_{t+1} = -1.08N_t$.

lay negative eggs? Later, in Section 1.5, we shall see cases where it makes sense to talk about $R < 0$. Such cases produce different types of behavior:

Alternating decay When $-1 < R < 0$, the solution to Eq. 1.2 alternates between positive and negative values. At the same time, the amplitude of the solution decays to zero in the same exponential fashion seen for $0 < R < 1$ (see Figure 1.5).

Alternating growth When $R < -1$, the solution still alternates between positive and negative values. However, the amplitude of the solution grows exponentially and explodes to $\pm\infty$ (see Figure 1.6).

Periodic cycle When R is exactly -1, the solution alternates between N_0 and $-N_0$ and neither grows nor decays in amplitude. A periodic cycle occurs when the solution repeats itself. In this case, the solution repeats every two time steps, $\ldots, N_0, -N_0, N_0, -N_0, \ldots$, and so the duration of the period is two time steps (see Figure 1.7).

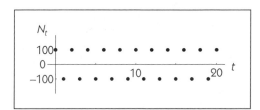

Figure 1.7
The solution to
$N_{t+1} = -1.00N_t$.

1.3 METHODS OF ITERATION

We have seen how the solution to Eq. 1.2 could be found using algebra. Later we will encounter finite-difference equations in which an algebraic solution cannot be found. Here, we introduce two other methods for iterating finite-difference equations, the cobweb method and the method of numerical iteration.

THE COBWEB METHOD

The **cobweb method** is a graphical method for iterating a finite-difference equation like Eq. 1.1. No algebra is required in order to perform the iteration; one only needs to graph the function $f(N_t)$ on a piece of paper.

To illustrate the cobweb method, we will start with the linear system of Eq. 1.2. To perform the iteration using the cobweb method, we do the following:

1. Graph the function. In this case, $f(N_t) = RN_t$. In order to make a plot of the function RN_t, we need to pick a specific value for R. (Note that the algebraic method for finding solutions did not require this.) As an example, we will set $R = 1.9$ so that the finite-difference equation is $N_{t+1} = 1.9N_t$. The resulting function is shown by the dark line in Figure 1.8.

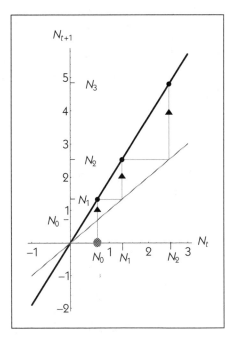

Figure 1.8
The cobweb method applied to the linear dynamical system $N_{t+1} = 1.9N_t$ with initial condition $N_0 = 0.7$.

2. Pick a numerical value for the initial condition. In this case, as an example, we will select $N_0 = 0.7$, shown as the gray dot on the x-axis in Figure 1.8. (In the algebraic method, we did not need to select a specific numerical value. Instead we were able to use the symbol N_0 to stand for any initial condition.)

3. Draw a vertical line from N_0 on the x-axis up to the function. The position where this vertical line hits the function (shown as a solid dot at the end of the arrow) tells us the value of N_1.

4. Take this value of N_1, plot it again on the x-axis, and again draw a vertical line to find the value of N_2. There is a simple shortcut in order to avoid plotting N_1 on the x-axis: Draw a horizontal line to the $N_{t+1} = N_t$ line (shown in gray—it's the 45-degree line on the plot). The place where the horizontal line intersects the 45-degree line is the point from which to draw the next vertical line to find N_2.

5. In order to find N_3, N_4, and so on, repeat the process of drawing vertical lines to the function and horizontal lines to the line of $N_{t+1} = N_t$.

As Figure 1.8 shows, the result of iterating $N_{t+1} = 1.9N_t$ is growth toward ∞. This is consistent with the algebraic solution we found in Eq. 1.3 for $R > 1$.

NUMERICAL ITERATION

Since the cobweb method is a graphical method, it may not be very precise. In order to acheive more precision, we can use **numerical iteration**. This is a simple procedure, easily implemented on a computer or even a hand calculator. To illustrate, suppose we want to find a numerical solution to $N_{t+1} = RN_t$ with $R = 0.9$ and $N_0 = 100$.

$$N_0 = 100,$$
$$N_1 = f(N_0) = 0.9 \times 100 = 90,$$
$$N_2 = f(N_1) = 0.9 \times 90 = 81, \qquad (1.4)$$
$$N_3 = f(N_2) = 0.9 \times 81 = 72.9,$$
$$\vdots$$

When applied to the linear finite-difference equation in Eq. 1.2, the cobweb method and the method of numerical iteration merely allow us to confirm the existence of the types of behavior we found algebraically. Since the cobweb and numerical iteration methods require that specific numerical values be specified for the parameter R and the initial condition N_0, it might seem that they are inferior to the algebraic method. However, when we consider nonlinear equations, algebraic methods are often impossible and numerical iteration and the cobweb method may provide the only means to find solutions.

1.4   NONLINEAR FINITE-DIFFERENCE EQUATIONS

The measurements of the fly population shown in Figure 1.1 don't suggest explosion or extinction, nor do they remain steady. This suggests that the model of Eq. 1.2 is not good. It does not take much of an ecologist to see where a mistake was made in formulating Eq. 1.2. Although it is all right to have rapid growth in populations for low densities, when the fly population is high, competition for food limits growth and starvation may cause a decrease in fertility. The larger population may also increase predation, as predators focus their attention on an abundant food supply.

A simple way to modify the model is to add a new term that lowers the number of surviving offspring when the population is large. In the linear equation, R was the number of offspring of each fly in generation t. In order to make the number of offspring per fly decrease as N_t gets larger, we can make the growth rate a function of N_t. For simplicity, we will chose the function $(R - bN_t)$. The positive number b governs how the growth rate decreases as the population gets bigger. R is the growth rate when the population is very, very small.

This assumption that the number of offspring per fly is $(R - bN_t)$ gives us a new finite-difference equation,

$$N_{t+1} = (R - bN_t)N_t = RN_t - bN_t^2. \tag{1.5}$$

Equation 1.5 is a **nonlinear equation** since the rightmost side is *not* the equation of a straight line. Nonlinear equations arise commonly in mathematical models of biological systems, and the study of such equations is the focus of this book.

In Eq. 1.5 there are two parameters, R and b, that can vary independently. However, a simple change of variables shows that there is only one parameter that affects the dynamics. We define a new variable $x_t = \frac{bN_t}{R}$, which is just a way of scaling the number of flies by the number $\frac{b}{R}$. Substituting x_t and x_{t+1} in Eq. 1.5, we find the equation

$$x_{t+1} = Rx_t(1 - x_t). \tag{1.6}$$

Although Eq. 1.6 (called the **quadratic map**) may not seem much more complicated than Eq. 1.2, the solution cannot generally be found using algebra. Numerical iteration and the cobweb method, however, can be used to find solutions. In order to apply the cobweb method to Eq. 1.6, we first must draw a

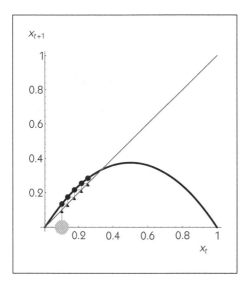

Figure 1.9
Cobweb iteration of
$x_{t+1} = 1.5(1 - x_t)x_t$.

graph of the function. (Anyone who has not practiced calculus recently may find sketching the graph of an equation intimidating. If you are in this category, go over the material in Appendix A and pay particular attention to the section on quadratic functions since this is what we have here.) In this case, the graph is a parabola, with intercepts at $x_t = 0$ and $x_t = 1$, as Figure 1.9 shows.

Next, we need to pick specific values for the parameter R in Eq. 1.6. Since we don't yet know what the behavior of this equation will be, we will have to study a range of parameter values. Doing so reveals a number of different behaviors:

Steady state The nonlinear equation can have a solution that approaches a certain state and remains fixed there. This is shown in Figure 1.10 for $R = 1.5$, where the solution creeps up on the steady state from one side; this is called a **monotonic** approach.

As shown for $R = 2.9$ in Figure 1.11, the approach to a steady state can also **alternate** from one side to the other.

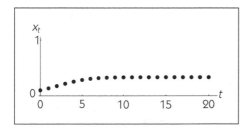

Figure 1.10
The solution to
$x_{t+1} = 1.5(1 - x_t)x_t$.

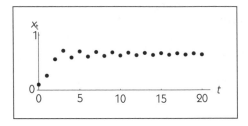

Figure 1.11
The solution to
$x_{t+1} = 2.9(1 - x_t)x_t$.

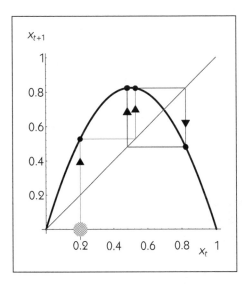

Figure 1.12
Cobweb iteration of
$x_{t+1} = 3.3(1 - x_t)x_t$.

Periodic cycles   The solution to the nonlinear equation can have cycles. This is shown for $R = 3.3$ in Figures 1.12 and 1.13, where the cycle has duration 2. When carrying out the cobweb iteration, a cycle of period two looks like a square that is repeatedly traced out (see Figure 1.12). The cycle in this case follows the sequence $x_t = 0.48, x_{t+1} = 0.82, x_{t+2} = 0.48$, and so on.

For $R = b = 3.52$ (see Figure 1.14), the cycle has duration 4 and follows the sequence $x_t = 0.88, x_{t+1} = 0.37, x_{t+2} = 0.82, x_{t+3} = 0.51, x_{t+4} = 0.88$, and so forth.

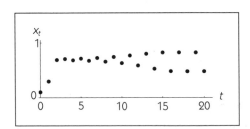

Figure 1.13
The solution to
$x_{t+1} = 3.3(1 - x_t)x_t$.

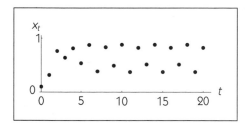

Figure 1.14
The solution to
$x_{t+1} = 3.52(1 - x_t)x_t$.

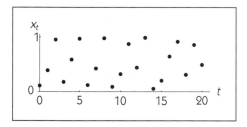

Figure 1.15
The solution to
$x_{t+1} = 4(1 - x_t)x_t$.

Aperiodic behavior The solution to the nonlinear equation may oscillate, but not in a periodic manner. Setting $R = 4$, we find the behavior shown in Figures 1.15 and 1.16—a kind of irregular oscillation that is neither exponential growth or decay, nor a steady state. The cobweb iteration shows how the irregular iteration arises from the shape of the function (see Figure 1.15). This behavior is called **chaos**, and we will investigate it in greater detail in later sections in the book.

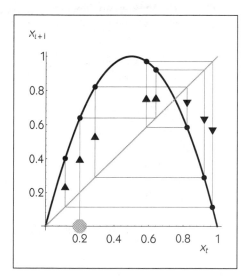

Figure 1.16
Cobweb iteration of
$x_{t+1} = 4(1 - x_t)x_t$.

1.5 STEADY STATES AND THEIR STABILITY

A simple, but important, type of dynamical behavior is when the system stays at a **steady state**. A steady state is a state of the system that remains fixed, that is, where

$$x_{t+1} = x_t.$$

Steady states in finite-difference equations are associated with the mathematical concept of a **fixed point**. A fixed point of a function $f(x_t)$ is a value x_t^* that satisfies $x_t^* = f(x_t^*)$. Later on, we shall see how fixed points can also be associated with periodic cycles.

There are three important questions to ask about fixed points in a finite-difference equation:

- Are there any fixed points—in other words, are there any values of x_t^* that satisfy $x_t^* = f(x_t^*)$?
- If the initial condition happens to be near a fixed point, will the subsequent iterates approach the fixed point? If subsequent iterates approach the fixed point, we say the fixed point is **locally stable**. (Mathematicians call this "locally asymptotic stability.")
- Will the system approach a given fixed point regardless of the initial condition? If the fixed point is approached for all initial conditions, we say that the fixed point is **globally stable**.

FINDING FIXED POINTS

From the graph of $x_{t+1} = f(x_t)$ it is easy to locate fixed points: They are simply those points where the graph intersects the line $x_{t+1} = x_t$. Or, we can use algebra to solve the equation $x_t = f(x_t)$.

For the linear finite-difference equation, x_t^* is a fixed point if it satisfies the equation $x_t^* = Rx_t^*$. One solution to this equation is always $x_t^* = 0$. This means that the origin is a fixed point for a linear system. This has an obvious biological interpretation: If there are no flies in one year, there can't be any the next year (unless, of course, they migrate from distant parts or evolve again, both of which are beyond the scope of our simple model).

The solution $x_t = 0$ is the only fixed point, unless $R = 1$. If R is exactly 1, then all points are fixed points. Clearly, this is an exceptional case, because any change in R, no matter how small, will eliminate all of the fixed points except the one at the origin.

Nonlinear finite-difference equations can have more than one fixed point. Figures 1.17 and 1.18 show the location of the fixed points for Eq. 1.6 for $R = 2.9$

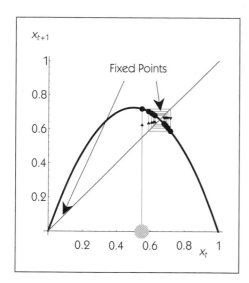

Figure 1.17
$x_{t+1} = 2.9(1 - x_t)x_t$

and $R = 3.52$, respectively. For the quadratic map of Eq. 1.6, the fixed points can also be found using algebra from the **roots** of the quadratic equation

$$x_t = Rx_t(1 - x_t) \quad \text{or,} \quad x_t(R - Rx_t - 1) = 0.$$

The roots of this equation are

$$x_t = 0 \quad \text{and} \quad x_t = \frac{R - 1}{R}.$$

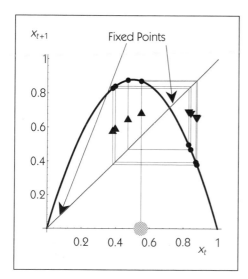

Figure 1.18
$x_{t+1} = 3.52(1 - x_t)x_t$

Again, in our model the biological meaning of the root $x_t = 0$ is that flies don't appear from nowhere. The biological interpretation of the fixed point at $x_t = \frac{R-1}{R}$ is that this is a self-sustaining level of the population, with neither a decrease nor an increase.

Clearly, it is impossible for the fly population to be at both these fixed points at the same time. So now we have to address the question of which of these fixed points will be reached by iterating from the initial condition, if indeed either of them will be.

LOCAL STABILITY OF FIXED POINTS

Figures 1.17 and 1.18 both have two fixed points, but in Figure 1.17 the iterates approach the nonzero fixed point while in Figure 1.18 the iterates do not. The difference between these cases is the *local stability* of the fixed points.

We say that a fixed point is **locally stable** if, given an initial condition sufficiently close to the fixed point, subsequent iterates eventually approach the fixed point.

How do we tell if a fixed point is locally stable? For a linear finite-difference equation, $x_{t+1} = Rx_t$, we already know the answer: The stability of the fixed point at the origin depends on the slope R of the line. If $|R| < 1$, future iterates are successively closer to the fixed point at the origin—this is exponential decay to zero. If $|R| > 1$, future iterates are successively farther away from the fixed point at the origin.

How does one determine the stability of a fixed point in a nonlinear finite-difference equation? In calculus classes, one discusses the notion that over limited regions a curve can be approximated by a straight line of the appropriate slope. In the neighborhood of the intersection of the straight line $x_{t+1} = x_t$ with the curve $x_{t+1} = f(x_t)$, it is therefore possible to approximate the curve by a straight line.

Figures 1.19 through 1.22 illustrate four separate cases that show the region of intersection. Let $x^\star$ be a fixed point of $f(\cdot)$, that is a state for which $x^\star = f(x^\star)$. The slope of the curve at the fixed point, $\frac{df}{dx_t}\big|_{x^\star}$, establishes the stability of the fixed point. We will designate this slope by m. Figures 1.19 through 1.22 plot y_{t+1} versus y_t, where $y_t = x_t - x^\star$. This means that in the figures the fixed point appears at the origin, whereas in the original variable, x_t, the fixed point is at $x^\star$. Observe that

- If $|m| < 1$, the fixed point is *stable* so that nearby points approach the fixed point under iteration.
- If $|m| > 1$, the fixed point is *unstable* and points leave the neighborhood of the fixed point.

Also, note that

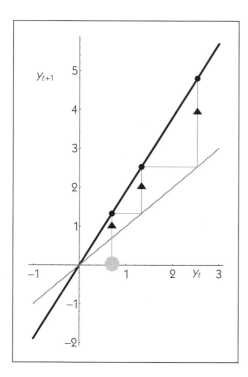

Figure 1.19
The dynamics of $y_{t+1} = my_t$. $m > 1$ produces monotonic growth as shown here with $m = 1.9$.

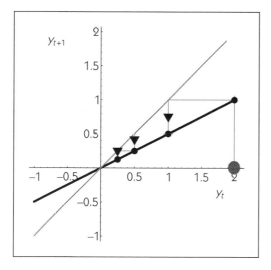

Figure 1.20
The dynamics of $y_{t+1} = my_t$. $0 < m < 1$ produces monotonic decay to $y_t = 0$. Here, $m = 0.5$.

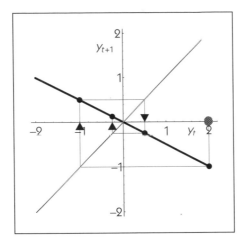

Figure 1.21
The dynamics of $y_{t+1} = my_t$.
$-1 < m < 0$ produces
alternating decay as shown here
with $m = -0.5$.

- If $m > 0$, the points approach or leave the fixed point in a *monotonic* fashion.

- If $m < 0$, the points approach or leave the fixed point in an *oscillatory* fashion.

From the above considerations, a general method can be given for determining the stability of a fixed point in finite-difference equations with one variable. The steps are as follows:

1. Solve for the fixed points. This involves solving the equation

$$x_t = f(x_t).$$

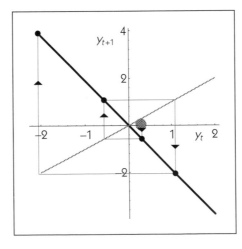

Figure 1.22
The dynamics of $y_{t+1} = my_t$.
$m < -1$ produces alternating
growth. Here, $m = -1.9$.

Linear equations always have only one fixed point—the one at $x_t = 0$. Nonlinear equations may have more than one fixed point. Steps 2 and 3 can be applied to each of the fixed points, one at a time. Call the fixed point we are studying $x^\star$. Like all fixed points, this satisfies $x^\star = f(x^\star)$.

2. Calculate the slope m of $f(x_t)$, evaluating x_t at the fixed point $x^\star$. That is, compute

$$m = \left. \frac{df}{dx_t} \right|_{x_t = x^\star}.$$

3. The slope m at the fixed point determines its stability.

$1 < m$	Unstable, exponential growth.
$0 < m < 1$	Stable, monotonic approach to $y_t = 0$ (i.e., approach to $x_t = x^\star$).
$-1 < m < 0$	Stable, oscillatory approach to $y_t = 0$ (i.e., approach to $x_t = x^\star$).
$m < -1$	Unstable, oscillatory exponential growth.

TRANSIENT AND ASYMPTOTIC BEHAVIOR

If a fixed point is locally stable, then once the state is very near to the fixed point, it will stay near throughout the future. Before the state reaches the fixed point, it may show different behavior. For example, in Figure 1.10, the state is far enough away from the fixed point for the first five or six iterations that we can see it change from iteration to iteration. After that, the state appears to have reached the fixed point. In Figure 1.11, the movement toward the fixed point is visible for approximately twenty iterations. The term **asymptotic dynamics** refers to the dynamics as time goes to infinity. Behavior before the asymptotic dynamics is called **transient**.

STABILITY AND NUMERICAL ITERATION

Suppose that we want to use numerical iteration to find fixed points. One strategy would be to pick a large number of initial conditions and iterate numerically each of these initial conditions. If the iterates converge to a fixed value, then we have identified a fixed point at that value. (Figure 1.10 shows an example of this.)

If a fixed point is locally stable, then this strategy may well succeed, since the fixed point will eventually be approached if any of the initial conditions is close to the fixed point. Once the state is close to the fixed point, it will remain near the fixed point.

If a fixed point is unstable, however, then we will find it only if one of the iterates happens to land on the fixed point *exactly*, and this is extremely unlikely. In general, we can use numerical iteration only to find stable fixed points. If we want to find unstable fixed points, another approach is needed, namely solving the equation $x_t = f(x_t)$.

❏ EXAMPLE 1.1

Cells reproduce by division; the process by which the cell nucleus divides is called **mitosis**. One way to regulate the rate of reproduction of cells is by regulating mitosis. There is (controversial!) biochemical evidence that there are compounds, called **chalones**, that are tissue-specific inhibitors of mitosis (see Bullough and Laurence, 1968).

For simplicity, assume that the generations of cells are distinct and that the number of cells in each generation is given by N_t. Following the same logic as in Eq. 1.2, assume that for each cell in generation t, there are R cells in generation $t+1$. (If every cell divided in half every time step, then R would equal 2.) The finite-difference equation describing this situation is the linear equation $N_{t+1} = R N_t$, which leads either to exponential growth or to decay to zero.

A possible role of chalones is to make R depend on the number of cells. Assume that the amount of chalone produced is proportional to the number of cells. The more chalone there is, the greater the inhibitory effect on mitosis.

The biochemical action of chalones is to bind to a protein involved in mitosis, rendering the protein inactive. Binding of molecules to proteins is often modeled by a Hill function (see Section A.5), which suggests that an appropriate equation for the hypothetical chalone control mechanism is

$$N_{t+1} = f(N_t) = \frac{R N_t}{1 + \left(\frac{N_t}{\theta}\right)^n},$$

where θ and n are parameters. We will assume that $n \geq 2$. Figure 1.23 shows this finite difference equation when $R = 2$, $\theta = 5$, and $n = 3$.

Find the fixed points of this system and determine their stability.

1. To determine the fixed points we solve the equation

$$N^\star = \frac{R N^\star}{1 + \left(\frac{N^\star}{\theta}\right)^n}.$$

There are two real solutions: $N^\star = 0$ and $N^\star = \theta (R - 1)^{\frac{1}{n}}$. These are the only fixed points. There are also imaginary solutions that can be ignored in this case because we are only concerned with biologically

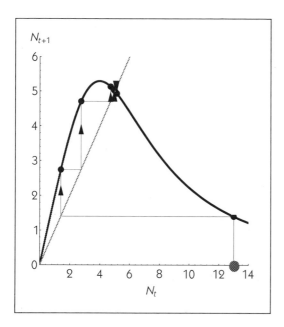

Figure 1.23 A cobweb analysis of chalone production for the parameters $R = 2$, $\theta = 5, n = 3$.

meaningful solutions, and the number of cells in each generation must be a real number.

2. To determine the stability of the fixed points it is necessary to compute the slope at the fixed points. Differentiating the right-hand side of the finite-difference equation, we find

$$\frac{df}{dN_t} = \frac{R + R\left(\frac{N_t}{\theta}\right)^n(1-n)}{\left(1 + \left(\frac{N_t}{\theta}\right)^n\right)^2}.$$

3. From the above equation we find that the slope at the fixed point $N^\star = 0$ is just R. If $R > 1$, the fixed point at the origin is always unstable. (To be a plausible model of the regulation of cell reproduction, we must have $R > 1$. Otherwise, the population would always fall to zero even in the complete absence of the mitosis-inhibiting chalones.)

The slope at the fixed point $N^\star = \theta(R-1)^{\frac{1}{n}}$ is

$$\frac{df}{dN_t}\bigg|_{N^\star} = 1 + n\left(\frac{1}{R} - 1\right).$$

For $R = 2$, the fixed point will be unstable when $n > 4$ and stable otherwise.

$\square$

GLOBAL STABILITY OF FIXED POINTS

In this section we've studied local stability. Local stability tells us whether the fixed point is approached if the initial condition is sufficiently close to the fixed point. The local stability can be assessed simply by looking at the slope of the function at the fixed point.

A slightly different—and often much more difficult—question is whether a locally stable fixed point is **globally stable**.

For linear finite-difference equations, the answer is straightforward. A locally stable fixed point is also globally stable: Regardless of the initial condition, the iterates will eventually reach the locally stable point (i.e., the origin) from any initial condition.

For nonlinear finite-difference equations, there can be more than one fixed point. When multiple fixed points are present, none of the fixed points can be globally stable.

The set of initial conditions that eventually leads to a fixed point is called the **basin of attraction** of the fixed point. Often, the basin of attraction for fixed points in nonlinear systems can have a very complicated geometry (see Chapter 3). If multiple fixed points are locally stable we say there is **multistability**.

1.6   CYCLES AND THEIR STABILITY

In Figures 1.7, 1.13, and 1.14 we can see that periodic cycles are one form of behavior for finite-difference equations. In everyday language, a **cycle** is a pattern that repeats itself, and the **period** of the cycle is the length of time between repetitions. In finite-difference equations like Eq. 1.1, a cycle arises when

$$x_{t+n} = x_t, \quad \text{but} \quad x_{t+j} \neq x_t \quad \text{for } j = 1, 2, \ldots, n - 1. \tag{1.7}$$

There is a useful correspondence between fixed points and periodic cycles which helps in understanding how to find cycles and assess their stability. A simple case is a cycle of period 2. Consider the finite-difference equation

$$x_{t+1} = f(x_t) = 3.3(1 - x_t)x_t. \tag{1.8}$$

As shown in Figure 1.13, the solution is a cycle of period 2. The definition of a cycle of period 2 is that

$$x_{t+2} = x_t \quad \text{while } x_{t+1} \neq x_t. \tag{1.9}$$

By substitution into $x_{t+1} = f(x_t)$, we can write the value of x_{t+2} as

$$x_{t+2} = f(x_{t+1}) = f(f(x_t)). \tag{1.10}$$

If there is a cycle of period 2, then $x_t = f(f(x_t))$. For the quadratic map (Eq. 1.6), we can find $f(f(x_t))$ with a bit of algebra:

$$\begin{aligned}
f(f(x_t)) = f(x_{t+1}) &= Rx_{t+1} - Rx_{t+1}^2 \\
&= R(Rx_t - Rx_t^2) - R(Rx_t - Rx_t^2)^2 \tag{1.11} \\
&= R^2 x_t - (R^2 + R^3)x_t^2 + 2R^3 x_t^3 - R^3 x_t^4.
\end{aligned}$$

The equation may seem a little formidable, but the M-shaped graph, shown in the lower graph in Figure 1.24, is quite simple.

We can see from Eq. 1.10 that there is an analogy between fixed points and cycles: If a system $x_{t+1} = f(x_t)$ has a cycle of period 2, then the function $f(f(x_t))$ has at least two fixed points. Thus, we can find the cycles of period 2 by solving the equation $x_t = f(f(x_t))$. This can be done graphically, algebraically, or numerically.

One trivial type of solution to $x_t = f(f(x_t))$ is a solution to $x_t = f(x_t)$. These solutions correspond to the fixed points of $f(x_t)$ and hence are not cycles of period 2—they are "cycles of period 1," that is, steady states. In the graph of Eq. 1.11 shown in Figure 1.24, we can see four fixed points of $f(f(x_t))$: at $x_t = 0$, at $x_t = 0.479$, at $x_t = 0.697$, and at $x_t = 0.823$. Two of these values are also fixed points of $f(x_t)$ and therefore correspond to cycles of period 1.

Longer cycles can be found in the same way. A cycle of period n is found by solving the equation

$$x_t = \underbrace{f(f(\cdots f(x_t))}_{n \text{ times}},$$

avoiding solutions that correspond to periods less than n. In practice, this problem can be very hard to solve algebraically.

STABILITY OF CYCLES

Just as a fixed point can be locally stable or unstable, a cycle can be stable or unstable. We say that a cycle is **locally stable** if, given that the initial condition is

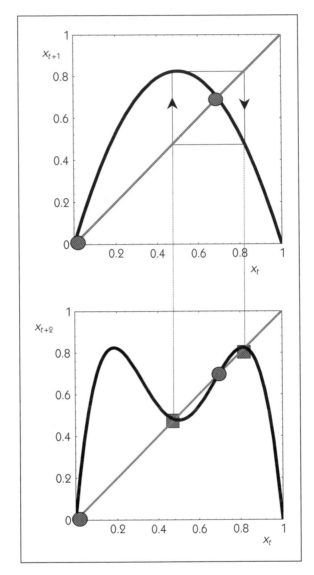

Figure 1.24 A cycle of period 2 in the system $x_{t+1} = R(1 - x_t)x_t = f(x_t)$ for $R = 3.3$. The graph of x_{t+1} versus x_t has two fixed points, marked as gray dots, but neither of them is stable. When plotted as x_{t+2} versus x_t, the cycle of period two looks like 2 fixed points in the finite-difference equation $x_{t+2} = f(f(x_t))$. Altogether, this system has four fixed points—the two corresponding to the cycle of period 2 (marked as small gray squares) and the two fixed points from the system $x_{t+1} = f(x_t)$.

close to a point on the cycle, subsequent iterates approach the cycle. (Again, this is what mathematicans call "local asymptotic stability").

We can now consider the computation of the stability of the fixed point of the finite-difference equation $x_{t+2} = f(f(x_t))$. We will use $x^\star$ to denote a solution to the equation $x_t = f(f(x_t))$ that is not also a fixed point of $x_t = f(x_t)$. Referring to Section 1.5, we can see that the stability of the fixed point of $x_{t+2} = f(f(x_t))$ depends on the value of

$$\frac{df(f(x_t))}{dx_t}\bigg|_{x^\star}.$$

Using the chain rule for derivatives, we have

$$\frac{df(f(x_t))}{dx_t}\bigg|_{x^\star} = \frac{df}{dx_t}\bigg|_{f(x^\star)} \frac{df}{dx_t}\bigg|_{x^\star}.$$

Thus, the stability of a fixed point of period 2 depends on the slope of the function $f(x_t)$ at both of the two points $x^\star$ and $f(x^\star)$.

A method for finding cycles by numerical iteration is quite easy in principle: Start at some initial condition and at each iteration, see if the value has been produced previously. Once the same value is encountered twice, the intervening values will cycle over and over again.

When cycles are found by numerical iteration, it is important to realize that unstable cycles will tend not to be found. This is exactly analogous to the situation when using numerical iteration to look for fixed points. When a cycle is stable, any initial condition in the cycle's basin of attraction will eventually lead to the cycle. For unstable cycles, the cycle will not be approached unless some iterate of the initial condition lands exactly on a point on the cycle.

❏ EXAMPLE 1.2

Consider the finite-difference equation

$$x_{t+1} = \frac{1 - x_t}{3x_t + 1}.$$

a. Sketch x_{t+1} as a function of x_t.

b. Determine the fixed point(s), if any, and test algebraically for stability.

c. Algebraically determine x_{t+2} as a function of x_t and determine if there are any cycles of period 2. If so, are they stable? Based on the analysis above, determine the dynamics starting from any initial condition.

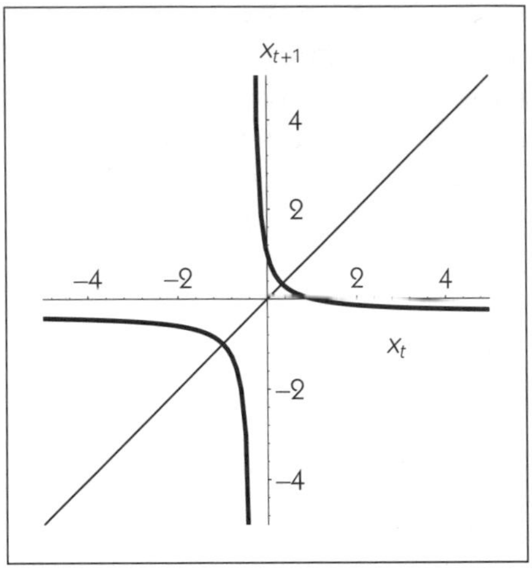

Figure 1.25
The graph of $x_{t+1} = \frac{1-x_t}{3x_t+1}$.

Solution:

a. This is the graph of a hyperbola, see Figure 1.25. There are no local maxima or minima, but there are asymptotes at $x_t = -\frac{1}{3}$ and at $x_{t+1} = -\frac{1}{3}$.

b. The fixed points are determined by setting $x_{t+1} = x_t$ to give the quadratic equation

$$3x_t^2 + 2x_t - 1 = 0.$$

This equation can be factored to yield two solutions, $x_t = \frac{1}{3}$ and $x_t = -1$. To determine stability, we compute

$$\frac{dx_{t+1}}{dx_t} = \frac{-4}{(3x_t + 1)^2}.$$

When this is evaluated at the fixed points, the slope is -1. Note that a slope of -1 does not fall into the classification scheme presented in Section 1.5—if the slope were slightly steeper than -1, the fixed point would be unstable; if the slope were slightly less steep than -1, the fixed point would be stable. We cannot determine the stability of the steady states from this computation: The steady state is neither stable nor unstable.

c. Iterating directly we find that

$$x_{t+2} = \frac{1 - x_{t+1}}{3x_{t+1} + 1}$$

$$= \frac{1 - \left(\frac{1-x_t}{3x_{t+1}}\right)}{3\left(\frac{1-x_t}{3x_t+1}\right) + 1}$$

$$= x_t.$$

Amazingly, all initial conditions are on a cycle of period 2. The cycles are neither locally stable nor unstable, since initial conditions neither approach nor diverge from any given cycle.

◻

The preceding discussion shows that if there are stable cycles, then an examination of the graph of x_{t+n} as a function of x_t will show certain definite features. If there is a stable cycle of period n, there must be at least n fixed points associated with the stable cycle, where the slope at each of the fixed points is equal and the absolute value of the slope at each of the fixed points is less than 1.

Now let's consider a specific situation, the quadratic map

$$x_{t+1} = f(x_t) = 4(1 - x_t)x_t. \tag{1.12}$$

This now-familiar parabola is plotted again in Figure 1.26. We can see that there are two fixed points, both of which are unstable because the slope of the function at these fixed points is steeper than 1.

To look for cycles of period 2, we can plot x_{t+2} versus x_t as shown in Figure 1.27. The four places where this graph intersects the line $x_{t+2} = x_t$ (i.e., the 45-degree line) are the possible points on the cycle of period 2—recall that two of the intersection points correspond to cycles of period 1. Since the slope of

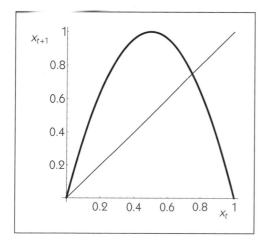

Figure 1.26
x_{t+1} versus x_t for Eq. 1.12.

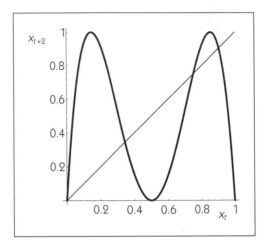

Figure 1.27
x_{t+2} versus x_t for Eq. 1.12.

the function at all these points is steeper than 1, we can conclude that there are no stable cycles of period 2 in Eq. 1.12.

We can continue looking for longer cycles. Figure 1.28 shows the graph of $x_{t+3} = f(f(f(x_t)))$. This graph intersects the line $x_{t+3} = x_t$ in eight places. (Of these, two correspond to cycles of period 1.) At all of these places the slope of the function is steeper than 1, so all of the possible cycles of period 3 are unstable. Similarly, Figure 1.29 shows that the cycles of period four are also unstable.

In fact, there are no stable cycles of *any* length, no matter how long, in Eq. 1.12, although we will not prove this here. What are the dynamics in Eq. 1.12? The next section will explore the answer to this question.

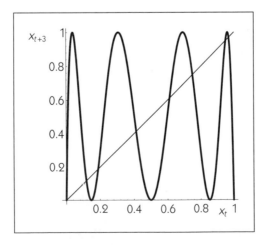

Figure 1.28
x_{t+3} versus x_t for Eq. 1.12.

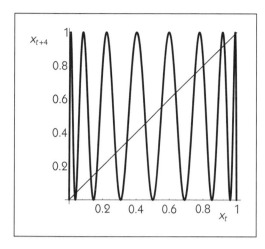

Figure 1.29
x_{t+4} versus x_t for Eq. 1.12.

1.7 CHAOS

DEFINITION OF CHAOS

Let's do a numerical experiment to investigate the properties of Eq. 1.12. Pick an initial condition, say $x_0 = 0.523423$, and iterate. Now start over, but change the initial condition by just a little bit, to $x_0 = 0.523424$. The results are shown in Figure 1.30.

There are several important features of the dynamics illustrated in Figure 1.30. In fact, based on the figure we have strong evidence that this equation displays **chaos**—which is defined to be aperiodic bounded dynamics in a deterministic system with sensitive dependence on initial conditions.

Each of these terms has a specific meaning. We define the terms and explain why each of these properties appears to be satisfied by the dynamics in Figure 1.30.

Aperiodic   means that the same state is never repeated twice. Examination of the numerical values used in this graph shows this to be the case. However, in practice, by either graphically iterating or using a computer with finite precision, we eventually may return to the same value. Although a computer simulation or graphical iteration always leaves some doubt about whether behavior is periodic, the presence of very long cycles or of aperiodic dynamics in computer simulations is partial evidence for chaos.

Bounded   means that on successive iterations the state stays in a finite range and does not approach $\pm\infty$. In the present case, as long as the initial condition x_0 is in the range $0 \leq x_0 \leq 1$, then all future iterates will also fall in this range. This is because for $0 \leq x_t \leq 1$, the minimum value of $4(1 - x_t)x_t$ is 0 and the maximum value is 1. Recall that in the linear

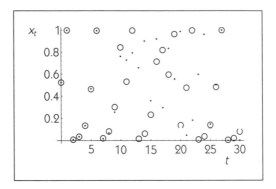

Figure 1.30 Two solutions to $x_{t+1} = (4 - 4x_t)x_t$. The solution marked with a dot has the initial condition $x_0 = 0.523423$, while the solution marked with a circle has $x_0 = 0.523424$. The solutions are almost exactly the same for the first seven iterations, and then move apart.

finite-difference equation, Eq. 1.2, we have already seen a system where the dynamics are not bounded and there is explosive growth.

Deterministic   means that there is a definite rule with no random terms governing the dynamics. The finite-difference equation 1.12 is an example of a deterministic system. For one-dimensional, finite-difference equations, "deterministic" means that for each possible value of x_t, there is only a single possible value for $x_{t+1} = f(x_t)$. In principal, for a deterministic system x_0 can be used to calculate all future values of x_t.

Sensitive dependence on initial conditions   means that two points that are initially close will drift apart as time proceeds. This is an essential aspect of chaos. It means that we may be able to predict what happens for short times, but that over long times prediction will be impossible since we can never be certain of the exact value of the initial condition in any realistic system. In contrast, for finite-difference equations with stable fixed points or cycles, two slightly different initial conditions may often lead to the same fixed point or cycle. (But this is not always the case; see Chapter 3.)

Although the possibility for chaos in dynamical systems was already known to the French mathematician Henri Poincaré in the nineteenth century, the concept did not gain broad recognition amongst scientists until T.-Y. Li and J. Yorke introduced the term "chaos" in 1975 in their analysis of the quadratic map, Eq. 1.12. The search for chaotic dynamics in diverse physical and biological fields, and the mathematical analysis of chaotic dynamics in nonlinear equations, have sparked research in recent years.

THE PERIOD-DOUBLING ROUTE TO CHAOS

We have seen that the simple finite-difference equation

$$x_{t+1} = R(1 - x_t)x_t$$

can display various qualitative types of behavior for different values of R: steady states, periodic cycles of different lengths, and chaos. The change from one form of qualitative behavior to another as a parameter is changed is called a **bifurcation**. An important goal in studying nonlinear finite-difference equations is to understand the bifurcations that can occur as a parameter is changed.

There are many different types of bifurcations. For example, in the linear finite-difference equation $x_{t+1} = Rx_t$, there is decay to zero when $-1 < R < 1$. For $R > 1$, however, the behavior changes to exponential growth. The bifurcation point, or the point at which a change in R causes the behavior to change, is at $R = 1$. Nonlinear systems can show many other types of bifurcations. For example, changing a parameter can cause a stable fixed point to become unstable and can lead to a change of behavior from a steady state to a periodic cycle.

The finite-difference equation in Eq. 1.6 and many other nonlinear systems displays a sequence of bifurcations in which the period of the oscillation doubles as a parameter is changed slightly. This type of behavior is called a **period-doubling bifurcation**.

We can derive an algebraic criterion for a period-doubling bifurcation. In a nonlinear finite-difference equation there are n fixed points of the function

$$x_t = \underbrace{f(f(\cdots f(x_t)))}_{n \text{ times}}$$

that are associated with a period-n cycle. The slope at each of these fixed points is the same. As a parameter is changed in the system, the slope at each of these fixed points also changes. When the slope for some parameter value is equal to -1, it is typical to find that at that parameter value the periodic cycle of period n loses stability and a periodic cycle of period $2n$ gains stability. In other words, there is a period-doubling bifurcation. Unfortunately, application of this algebraic criterion can be very difficult in nonlinear equations since iteration of nonlinear equations such as Eq. 1.6 can lead to complex algebraic expressions that are not handled easily. Consequently, people have turned to numerical studies.

Using a programmable pocket calculator in a numerical investigation of period-doubling bifurcations in Eq. 1.6 led Mitchell J. Feigenbaum to one of the major discoveries in nonlinear dynamics. Feigenbaum observed that as the parameter R varies in Eq. 1.6, there are successive doublings of the period of oscillation. Numerical estimation of the values of R at the successive bifurcations lead to the following approximate values:

- For $3.0000 < R < 3.4495$, there is a stable cycle of period 2.
- For $3.4495 < R < 3.5441$, there is a stable cycle of period 4.
- For $3.5441 < R < 3.5644$, there is a stable cycle of period 8.
- For $3.5644 < R < 3.5688$, there is a stable cycle of period 16.
- As R is increased closer to 3.570, there are stable cycles of period 2^n, where the period of the cycles increases as 3.570 is approached.
- For values of $R > 3.570$, there are narrow ranges of periodic solutions as well as aperiodic behavior.

These results illustrate a sequence of period-doubling bifurcations at $R = 3.0000$, $R = 3.4495$, $R = 3.5441$, $R = 3.5644$, with additional period-doubling bifurcations as R increases. This transition from the stable periodic cycles to the chaotic behavior at $R = 3.570$ is called the **period-doubling route to chaos**.

Notice that the range of values for each successive periodic cycle gets narrower and narrower. Call Δ_n the range of R values that give a period-n cycle. For example, since $3.4495 < R < 3.5441$ gives a period-4 cycle, we have $\Delta_4 = 3.5441 - 3.4495 = 0.0946$. Similarly, $\Delta_8 = 3.5644 - 3.5441 = 0.0203$.

The ratio $\frac{\Delta_4}{\Delta_8}$ is $\frac{0.0946}{0.0203} = 4.6601$. By considering successive period doublings, Feigenbaum discovered that

$$\lim_{n \to \infty} \frac{\Delta_n}{\Delta_{2n}} = 4.6692 \ldots.$$

The constant, 4.6692 . . . is now called **Feigenbaum's number**. This number appears not only in the simple theoretical model that we have discussed here but also in other theoretical models and in experimental systems in which there is a period-doubling route to chaos.

One way to represent graphically complex bifurcations in finite-difference equations is to plot the asymptotic values of the variable as a function of a parameter that varies. This type of plot is called a **bifurcation diagram**. Figure 1.31 shows a bifurcation diagram of Eq. 1.6. This figure is constructed by scanning many values of R in the range $3 \le R \le 4$. For each value of R, 1.6 is iterated many times. After allowing enough time for transients to decay, several of the values x_t, x_{t+1}, x_{t+2}, and so on are plotted. For example, when $R = 3.2$, Eq. 1.6 approaches a cycle of period 2, so there are two values plotted. The period-doubling bifurcations appear as "forks" in this diagram.

A summary of the dynamic behaviors discussed in Eq. 1.6 is contained in Figure 1.32. As the parameter R changes, different behaviors are observed. If you

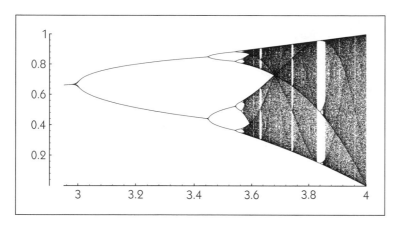

Figure 1.31 A bifurcation diagram of Eq. 1.6. The asymptotic values of x_t are plotted as a function of R using the method described in the text.

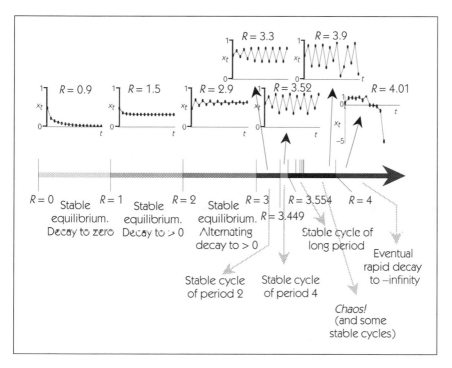

Figure 1.32 The various types of qualitative dynamics seen in $x_{t+1} = Rx_t(1 - x_t)$ for different values of the parameter R.

understand the origin of each of these behaviors, you have mastered the material in this chapter!

❑ EXAMPLE 1.3

The following equation, called the **tent map**, is often used as a very simple equation that gives chaotic dynamics.

Consider the finite-difference equation

$$x_{t+1} = f(x_t), \qquad 0 \le x_t \le 1,$$

where $f(x_t)$ is given as

$$f(x_t) = \begin{cases} 2x_t & \text{for } 0 \le x_t \le \dfrac{1}{2}, \\[2mm] 2 - 2x_t & \text{for } \dfrac{1}{2} \le x_t \le 1. \end{cases} \tag{1.13}$$

Draw a graph of x_{t+1} as a function of x_t. Graphically iterate this equation and determine if the dynamics are chaotic.

Solution: The graph of this equation looks like an old-fashioned pup tent (see Figure 1.33). Starting at two points chosen randomly near to each other we find that both points lead to aperiodic dynamics, where the distance between subsequent iterates of the points initially increases on subsequent iterations. Therefore, this system gives chaotic dynamics. This problem is tricky, however, since many people will start at a point such as 0.1, find that the subsequent iterates are $0.2, 0.4, 0.8, 0.4, 0.8, \ldots$, and then conclude that since they have found a cycle

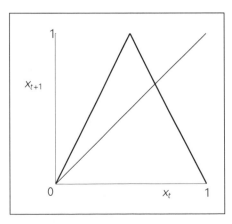

Figure 1.33
The graph of Eq. 1.13.

the dynamics in this equation are not chaotic. However, although there are many other such cycles in this equation, "almost all" values between 0 and 1 give rise to aperiodic chaotic dynamics. This is because the cycles are all unstable, as was defined in Section 1.6. Most equations that display chaotic dynamics also exhibit unstable cycles for some initial conditions, and thus this example is typical of what is found in other circumstances.

If you use a computer to iterate this map, watch out! You will probably find that the map rapidly converges to the fixed point at $x_t = 0$, even though this is an unstable fixed point. The reason involves the fact that numbers are represented in computers in base 2—all of the numbers that a computer can store in finite precision will be attracted to $x_t = 0$. To eliminate this problem, you can approximate the 2 in Eq. 1.13 by 1.9999999.

1.8   QUASIPERIODICITY

In chaotic dynamics there is an aperiodic behavior in which two points that are initially close will diverge over time. There is another type of aperiodic behavior in which two points that are initially close will remain close over time. This type of behavior is called **quasiperiodicity**. In quasiperiodic dynamics there are no fixed points, cycles, or chaos.

To see how this type of dynamics can arise, consider the equation

$$x_{t+1} = f(x_t) = x_t + b \quad (\text{mod } 1), \tag{1.14}$$

where (mod 1) is the "modulus" operator that takes the fractional part of a number (e.g., 3.67 (mod 1) − 0.67). To iterate this equation, we calculate $x_t + b$ and then take the fractional remainder. For example, if $x_t = 0.9$ and the parameter $b = 0.3$, then $x_t + b = 1.2$ and $x_t + b(\text{mod } 1) = 0.2$. Now consider the second iterate. We can do the iteration algebraically:

$$x_{t+2} = x_{t+1} + b \quad (\text{mod } 1) = (x_t + b \quad (\text{mod } 1) + b) \quad (\text{mod } 1)$$

$$= x_t + 2b \quad (\text{mod } 1).$$

In similar fashion, we can find that

$$x_{t+n} = f^n(x_t) = x_t + nb \quad (\text{mod } 1).$$

Consequently, if $nb(\text{mod } 1) = 0$, then all values are on a cycle of period n; otherwise no values will be.

One way to think of this is by analogy to the odometer of a car, that shows the total mileage driven. Imagine that the odometer has a decimal point in front of it so that it shows a number between zero and one, for instance .07325. Every day the car goes b miles. After reaching .99999 the odometer resets to zero. x_t is the odometer value at the end of the trip on day t.

An example illustrates these ideas. In Figure 1.34 we show a graph of Eq. 1.14 for the particular case where $b = \frac{1}{\pi}$. This graph shows that the function has no fixed points, because there are no intersections of the function with the line $x_{t+1} = x_t$. The cobweb diagram for several iterations shows that there does not appear to be a cycle but that nearby points stay close together under subsequent iterations. Therefore, the dynamics appear to be quasiperiodic.

Can we know that there are never any periodic points no matter how many iterations we take? Here's where a bit of advanced mathematics can help. Recall the definition of a **rational number**: A number that can be written as the ratio of two integers $\frac{p}{q}$. **Irrational numbers** cannot be written as a ratio of two integers. π is an irrational number and $\frac{1}{\pi}$ is therefore also an irrational number. It follows immediately that $\frac{n}{\pi}$ (mod 1) can never be equal to 0 for any integer n. Therefore, there can never be any periodic cycles for Eq. 1.14 with $b = \frac{1}{\pi}$. Also, from the algebraic iteration, we see that the iterates of two initial conditions that are very close will remain very close. Therefore, the dynamics are quasiperiodic.

Though the concept of quasiperiodicity depends on abstract concepts in number theory, quasiperiodic dynamics can be observed in a large number of different settings. Consider the following odd sleep habits exhibited by one of our colleagues when he was in graduate school. The first day of graduate school the graduate student fell asleep exactly at midnight. Each day thereafter, the graduate student got up, worked, and went to sleep. However, this graduate student did

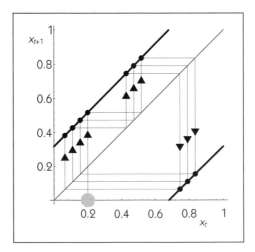

Figure 1.34
Iteration of
$x_{t+1} = x_t + \frac{1}{\pi}$ (mod 1). The dynamics are an example of quasiperiodicity.

not do this at the regular rhythms but rather with a rhythm of *about* 25 hours. The graduate student came into work about an hour later each day. Eventually, after 24 days, the graduate student goes to sleep again at about midnight. If the student's sleep cycle were exactly 25 hours, then there would be a cycle: 25 calendar days would equal 24 graduate student days exactly. However, it would be very unlikely that the graduate student's day would be exactly 25 hours. For example, suppose the graduate student days were $25 + 0.001\pi$ hours. Then, using the same arguments above, the graduate student would never again go to sleep exactly at midnight (independent of the length of time needed to complete graduate school!).

Another area in which quasiperiodic dynamics are often observed is in cardiology. There can be several different pacemakers in one heart. Normally one is in charge and sets the rhythm of the entire heart by interactions with other pacemakers (we will turn to this just ahead). However, in some pathological circumstances, pacemakers carry on their own rhythm—they are not directly coupled to each other. Typically one sees variable time intervals between the firing times of one pacemaker and the other. Cardiologists generally invent esoteric names to describe reasonably simple dynamic phenomena and have classification schemes for naming rhythms that are not based on nonlinear dynamics. Thus, two different rhythms that can be considered as quasiperiodic (to a first approximation) are *parasystole* and *third-degree atrioventricular heart block*. The analysis of these cardiac arrhythmias leads naturally into problems in number theory.

❏ EXAMPLE 1.4

The finite-difference equation, sometimes called the sine map,

$$x_{t+1} = f(x_t) = x_t + b\sin(2\pi x_t),$$

where $0 \le x_t \le 1$, has been considered as a mathematical model for the interaction of two nonlinear oscillators (Glass and Perez, 1982). See *Dynamics in Action* 1 for a typical experiment.

This system displays period-doubling bifurcations as the parameter b is varied.

a. Find the fixed points of this equation.

b. Algebraically determine the stability of all fixed points for $0 < b \le 1$. What are the dynamics in the neighborhood of each fixed point?

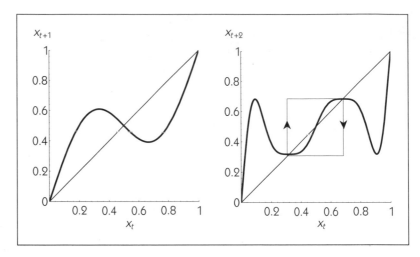

Figure 1.35 (left) The graph of $x_{t+1} = x_t + b\sin(2\pi x_t)$ for $b = 0.4$; (right) x_{t+2} versus x_t, showing the cycle of period 2 when $b = 0.4$.

Solution:

a. There are fixed points, $x^\star$, when

$$x^\star = x^\star + b\sin 2\pi x^\star.$$

This will be true when $b\sin 2\pi x^\star = 0$ which occurs when $x^\star = 0, \frac{1}{2}$, 1.

b. To evaluate the stability we must first determine the slope at the steady states. The slope evaluated at the steady state is given by

$$\frac{dx_{t+1}}{dx_t} = 1 + 2\pi b\cos 2\pi x^\star.$$

Therefore, when $x_t = 0$ or $x_t = 1$, the slope at the steady state is $1 + 2\pi b > 1$, which indicates that the steady state is unstable. For $x_t = \frac{1}{2}$ the slope at the steady state is $1 - 2\pi b$. For $0 < b < \frac{1}{\pi}$ this is a stable steady state, which is approached in an oscillatory fashion for $\frac{1}{2\pi} < b < \frac{1}{\pi}$; and for $b > \frac{1}{\pi}$ this is an unstable steady state, which is left in an oscillatory fashion (see Figure 1.35). The slope is -1 at $b = \frac{1}{\pi}$, so this value of b gives a period-doubling bifurcation. ∎

DYNAMICS IN ACTION

1 CHAOS IN PERIODICALLY STIMULATED HEART CELLS

We are all familiar with bodily functions such as sleep, breathing, locomotion, heartbeat, and reproduction, which depend in a fundamental way on rhythmic behaviors. Such rhythmic behaviors occur throughout the animal kingdom, and a vast literature analyzes the mechanisms of the oscillations and how they interact with one another and the external environment. Anyone interested in obtaining an idea of the scope of the inquiry should consult the classic book by A. T. Winfree, *The Geometry of Biological Time* (1980).

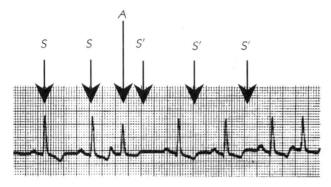

Phase resetting in the human heart. The wavey black line is an electrocardio-gram—each sharp Λ-shaped spike corresponds to one beat. Those labeled S originate in the sinus node as normal. The beat labeled A originates elsewhere in the atria. In the absence of beat A, beats would have occurred at the times labeled S', however A resets the phase of the sinus node. Adapted from Chou (1991).

It turns out that the mathematical formulation of finite-difference equations has direct applications to the study of the effects of periodic stimulation on biological oscilla-tors. The examination of periodic stimulation of biological oscillators involves many difficult issues, both in the biological and mathematical domains, and scientific investigation of these matters is still a research question under active investigation. However, compelling examples of chaotic dynamics in biological systems are found in the periodic stimulation of biological oscillations. Appreciation of the origin of the chaotic dynamics is possible using the material presented so far in this chapter.

Understanding the basics of the periodic stimulation of biological oscillators in-volves two related concepts: **phase** and **phase resetting**. The phase of an oscillation is a measure of the stage of the oscillation cycle. Because of the cyclicity of oscillations, it is common to represent the phases of the cycle as a point on the circle. For example a phase of 120° can represent a time that is one third of the way through a cycle. Alternatively, we can also represent a phase of 120° as .333. . . .

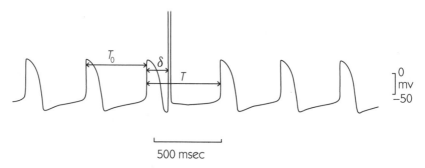

500 msec

Recording of transmembrane voltage from spontaneously beating aggregates of embryonic chick heart cells. The intrinsic cycle length is T_0. A stimulus delivered at a time δ following the start of the third action potential leads to a phase resetting so that the subsequent action potential occurs after time T. After this, the aggregate returns to its intrinsic cycle length. Adapted from Guevara et al. (1981). Copyright 1981 by the AAAS.

The term "phase resetting" refers to a change of phase that is induced by a stimulus. One example of phase resetting that many people experience is a consequence of jet travel. If you think about travel through different time zones, you will realize that the phenomenon of **jet lag** is associated with a discordance between the phase of your sleep–wake oscillator and the current local time. Staying in the new time zone for several days will lead to a phase resetting of your sleep–wake cycle. In this case the phase resetting takes place in a gradual fashion due to the different light–dark cycles and social stimuli in the new environment.

More abrupt phase resetting can be induced in many biological systems by appropriately chosen stimuli. For example, the rhythm of the human heart is normally set by a specialized region of the atria called the sinus node. However, in some people's hearts there are extra beats that can interfere with the normal sinus rhythm. Sometimes these extra beats can reset the rhythm. The figure on page 37 shows an example of an electrocardiographic (ECG) record. The normal sinus beats are labeled S and an atrial premature contraction is labeled A. If the atrial premature contraction had not occurred, the following sinus beat would have been expected at times labeled S'. However, the sinus firing is reset by the atrial premature stimulus, leading to a sinus beat at a different time than would presumably have occurred without the atrial premature contraction.

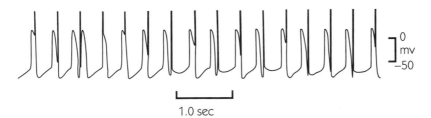

1.0 sec

Periodic stimulation of spontaneously beating chick heart cell aggregates at a period slightly longer than the intrinsic period. The interaction of the intrinsic cycle and the periodic stimulation results in chaotic dynamics. Adapted from Guevara et al. (1981). Copyright 1981 by the AAAS.

Since it is difficult to study the effects that electrical stimuli have on the heart, experimental preparations have been developed that enable detailed analysis (Guevara et al., 1981; Glass et al., 1984). The figure on page 38 shows phase resetting of spontaneously oscillating cardiac tissue derived from embryonic chick hearts. The upward deflections are called **action potentials** and are associated with the contraction cycle of the chick heart cells. The intrinsic length of the heart cycle is T_0. The sharp spike delivered after a time interval of δ after the onset of an action potential is an electrical stimulus delivered to the aggregate. The stimulus phase resets the rhythm so that following the stimulus the new cycle length is T (rather than T_0). Experimental studies show that the magnitude of phase resetting depends on both the amplitude of the stimulus and the phase of the cycle at which the stimulus is delivered.

What happens when periodic stimulation is delivered to the oscillating heart cells? Each stimulus phase resets the rhythm. In fact, to a first approximation the amount of phase resetting during periodic stimulation depends on the phase of the stimulus in the cycle. The consequence of this is that the effects of periodic stimulation can be approximated by the finite-difference equation

$$\phi_{i+1} = g(\phi_i) + \tau \quad (\mathrm{mod}\, 1), \tag{1.15}$$

where ϕ_i is the phase of the oscillation when the ith stimulus is delivered, $g(\phi_i)$ is the new phase resulting from the ith stimulus, and τ is the time interval between stimuli (measured in units of the intrinsic cycle length). Here we take ϕ to lie between 0 and 1. As explained before, the expression (mod 1) means take the fractional part of the number.

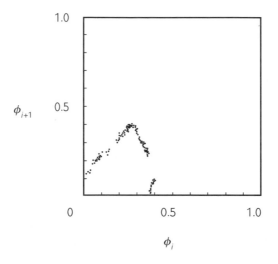

ϕ_{i+1}

ϕ_i

Each stimulus in the preceding figure occurs at a specific phase of the intrinsic cycle. Here, we plot the phase of each stimulus as a function of the phase of the preceeding stimulus, calculated for the experiment shown in the previous figure. The points suggest a function similar to the quadratic map. Adapted from Glass et al. (1984). Reprinted with permission. Copyright 1984 by the American Physical Society.

Does the theory work? M. R. Guevara, L. Glass, and A. Shrier (1981) measured $g(\phi)$ by carrying out phase resetting experiments. They used the resulting finite-difference equation to predict the dynamics. For a moderate stimulation strength, they computed that chaotic dynamics should result, provided that the stimulation period was 15 percent larger ($\tau = 1.15$) than the intrinsic cycle length. The effects of periodic stimulation with $\tau = 1.15$ are shown in the figure on page 39. Note the irregular rhythm. On this record, the phase of each stimulus can be measured and successive phases can be plotted as a function of the preceding phase; see the figure on this page. The phases fall on a one-dimensional curve that is very similar to functions that give chaotic dynamics, as we have seen earlier. This observation, combined with the more extensive analyses of Glass et al. (1984), gives convincing evidence for chaotic dynamics in this experimental system.

SOURCES AND NOTES

There are now a number of elementary texts on chaos. A fine introduction to these topics from a noncalculus perspective is in Peak and Frame (1994). Those who have a good background in calculus and are interested in a presentation from a mathematical perspective should consult Devaney (1992). Elementary texts from the perspectives of physics (Baker and Gollub, 1990) and engineering (Moon, 1992) have also appeared. The application of chaos and nonlinear dynamics to physiology and human disease is discussed by Glass and Mackey (1988).

Edward N. Lorenz realized the practical implications of the sensitive dependence to initial conditions in his famous essay on deducing the climate from the governing fluid-dynamical equations (Lorenz, 1964a). Another influential paper (May, 1976) introduced many to the concept of chaos, with an ecological twist, and contained extensive references to early experimental and mathematical work. Descriptions of the occurrence of chaos in many different contexts can be found in assorted collections of papers (Hao, 1984; Holden, 1986; Cvitanovic, 1989). The popularization by James Gleick (1987) provides an enjoyable account of some of the recent discoveries concerning chaos and description of many of the scientists, such as Mitchell Feigenbaum, who have played a role. Another good read, by Thomas Bass, recounts how a group of physics graduate students in Santa Cruz (dubbed the "Santa Cruz collective" by Gleick) in the late 1970s tried to use their knowledge of nonlinear dynamics and physics to make a fortune playing roulette (Bass, 1985). Curiously, some of the same people are trying to predict the fluctuations of the currency market and have started a company, The Prediction Company in Santa Fe, New Mexico. The Santa Cruz collective presents a brief introduction to chaos in Crutchfield et al. (1986). Feigenbaum (1980) gives a memorable description of how he discovered his number.

Those scholars interested in the history of chaos will want to look through the many volumes of Poincaré's (1954) collected works trying to find the earliest reference to the concept of chaos—most cite "New Methods of Celestial Mechanics" as the earliest source, but we have not tried to check out if there are earlier citations. Li and Yorke (1975) first used "chaos" in its current meaning, but their paper is not for the faint-hearted.

✏ **EXERCISES**

✏ **1.1** Assume that the density of flies in a swamp is described by the equation

$$x_{t+1} = Rx_t - \frac{R}{2000} x_t^2.$$

Consider three values of R, where one value of R comes from each of the following ranges:

    a. $1 \leq R < 3.00$

    b. $3.00 \leq R \leq 3.449$

    c. $3.570 \leq R \leq 4.00$.

For each value of R graph x_{t+1} as a function of x_t. Using the cobweb method follow x_t for several generations. Describe the qualitative behavior found for each case.

✏ **1.2** Not every finite-difference equation has fixed points that can be found algebraically. For example, the system

$$x_{t+1} = \cos(x_t)$$

involves a transcendental function and cannot be solved algebraically. Use a graph to find the approximate location and number of the fixed points. If you enter an initial condition into a pocket calculator and press the cosine key repeatedly, you are in effect iterating the finite-difference equation. Does the calculator approach a fixed point? Does the existence, location, or stability of the fixed point depend on whether x_t is measured in radians or in degrees?

✏ **1.3** Find a function for a nonlinear finite-difference equation with four fixed points, all of which are unstable. Find a function with eleven fixed points, three of which are stable. Find a function with no fixed points, stable or unstable. (HINT: Just give a graph of the function without worrying about specifying the algebraic form.)

✏ **1.4** In a remote region in the Northwest Territories of Canada, the dynamics of fly populations have been studied. The population satisfies the finite-difference equation

$$x_{t+1} = 11 - 0.01x_t^2,$$

where x_t is the population density (x_t must be positive).

a. Sketch x_{t+1} as a function of x_t.

b. Determine the fixed-point population densities and determine the stability of every fixed point algebraically.

c. Assume that the initial density is less than $(1100)^{\frac{1}{2}}$. Discuss the dynamics as $t \to \infty$.

✎   **1.5** A population of flies in a mangrove swamp is described by the finite-difference equation

$$x_{t+1} = \begin{cases} 0.01x_t^2, & \text{for } x_t < K; \\ 0.01K^2 \exp[-r(x_t - K)], & \text{for } x_t \geq K. \end{cases}$$

Assume that $K = 10^3$ and $r = 1.75 \times 10^4$.

a. Draw a graph of x_{t+1} as a function of x_t.

b. From this graph determine the fixed points of the fly population.

c. Determine the local stability of the fly population at each fixed point.

d. Determine the dynamics for future times if the initial population of fly is (i) 60; (ii) 600; (iii) 6000; (iv) 60,000. For each case graphically iterate the equation for several generations and guess the dynamics as $t \to \infty$.

✎   **1.6** Consider the finite-difference equation

$$x_{t+1} = x_t^2 + c, \qquad -\infty < x_t < \infty,$$

where c is a real number that can be positive or negative.

a. Sketch this function for $c = 0$. Be sure to show any maxima, minima, and inflection points (these should be determined algebraically). Show the location of all steady states.

b. For what value(s) of c are there zero steady states? one steady state? two steady states?

c. For what value of c is there a period-doubling bifurcation?

d. Consider the sequence $x_0, x_1, x_2, \ldots, x_n$. For what range of c will x_n be finite given the initial condition $x_0 = 0$?

✎   **1.7** The following equation plays a role in the analysis of nonlinear models of gene and neural networks (Glass and Pasternack, 1978):

$$x_{t+1} = \frac{\alpha x_t}{1 + \beta x_t},$$

where α and β are positive numbers and $x_t \geq 0$.

a. Algebraically determine the fixed points. For each fixed point give the range of α and β for which it exists, indicate whether the fixed point is stable or unstable, and state whether the dynamics in the neighborhood of the fixed point are monotonic or oscillatory.

For parts b and c assume $\alpha = 1, \beta = 1$.

b. Sketch the graph of x_{t+1} as a function of x_t. Graphically iterate the equation starting from the initial condition $x_0 = 10$. What happens as the number of iterates approaches ∞?

c. Algebraically determine x_{t+2} as a function of x_t, and x_{t+3} as a function of x_t. Based on these computations what is the algebraic expression for x_{t+n} as a function of x_t? What is the behavior of x_{t+n} as $n \to \infty$? This should agree with what you found in part b.

✎   **1.8** In cardiac electrophysiology, many phenomena occur in which two behaviors alternate on a beat-to-beat basis. For example, there may be an alternation in the conduction time of excitation from one region of the heart to another, or there may be an alternation of the morphology of the electrical complexes associated with each beat. A natural hypothesis is that these phenomena in electrophysiology are associated with period-doubling bifurcations in appropriate mathematical models of these phenomena. Both this problem and Problem 1.9 are motivated by possible connections between period-doubling bifurcations and cardiac electrophysiology.

During rapid electrical stimulation of cardiac tissues there is sometimes a beat-to-beat alternation of the action-potential duration.

Consider the equation

$$x_{t+1} = f(x_t),$$

where x_t is the duration of the action potential of beat t and

$$f(x_t) = 200 - 20 \exp(x_t/62) \quad \text{for } 0 \le x_t < 128;$$

$$f(x_t) = 40 \quad\quad\quad\quad\quad\quad \text{for } 128 < x_t \le 200.$$

All quantities are measured in milliseconds (msec).

a. State the conditions (using calculus) for maxima, minima, and inflection points and say if any such points satisfy these conditions for the function defined above.

b. Sketch $f(x_t)$ for $0 \leq x_t \leq 200$.

c. Determine the fixed points (an approximation is adequate).

d. In the neighborhood of each fixed point determine the stability of the dynamics and indicate if the dynamics are oscillatory or monotonic.

e. Starting from a point near the fixed point, graphically iterate the equation and say what the behavior will be in the limit $t \to \infty$. A rough picture is adequate.

✎ **1.9** In the heart, excitation generated by the normal pacemaker in the atria travels to the ventricles, causing contraction of the heart and the pumping of blood to the body and the lungs. The excitation must pass through the atrioventricular node, which electrically connects the atria and the ventricles. The following problem is based on a mathematical model for atrioventricular (AV) conduction in mammals (Simson et al., 1981).

Assume that subsequent values of AV conduction time, designated x_t, are given by the finite-difference equation

$$x_{t+1} = \frac{375}{x_t - 90} + 100, \qquad x_t \geq 90.$$

The units of all quantities are msec.

a. Sketch x_{t+1} as a function of x_t. Indicate whether there are any maxima, minima, and inflection points.

b. Determine the fixed point(s) of this equation in the range $x_t \geq 90$ msec.

c. Determine the stability of the fixed point(s) found in part b.

d. Based on your analysis, how will the dynamics evolve starting from an initial condition of $x_0 = 200$ msec?

✎ **1.10** The following equation was proposed as a model for population densities of insects in successive years:

$$x_{t+1} = \alpha x_t \exp(-\beta x_t^3),$$

where α and β are positive numbers and $x_t \geq 0$.

a. Sketch the graph of x_{t+1} as a function of x_t. Determine any maxima or minima, but it is not necessary to compute the values of any inflection points.

b. For $\alpha = 2.72$ and $\beta = 0.33$, determine the fixed point(s) and determine their stability. (HINT: The natural logarithm, designated as ln, is the logarithm to the base e. Since $e \approx 2.72$, you can assume that $\ln \alpha \approx 1$, to simplify the algebra.)

c. Starting from an initial value of $x_0 = 137$, what are the possible dynamics in the limit $t \to \infty$?

✐ **1.11** The following equation has been proposed to describe the population dynamics of flies:

$$N_{t+1} = g(N_t), \qquad N_t \geq 0,$$

where the fly density in generation t is N_t and

$$g(N_t) = N_t \exp\left[r\left(1 - \frac{pN_t^2}{1 + N_t^2}\right)\right],$$

where $r > 0$ and $p > 1$.

a. For $0 < N_t \ll 1$, N_{t+1} is approximately given by

$$N_{t+1} = N_t e^r.$$

In this case will N_1 be greater than, less than, or equal to N_0?

b. For $N_t \gg 1$ show that N_{t+1} can be approximately computed from the formula

$$N_{t+1} = K N_t,$$

where K does not depend on N_t. Compute K for $N_0 \gg 1$; will N_1 be greater than, less than, or equal to N_0?

c. Determine all fixed-point values of N_t ($N_t \geq 0$). (HINT: If $A = B$, then $\log A = \log B$.)

d. Compute $\dfrac{dg(N_t)}{dN_t}$.

e. Assume that $p = 2$ and $r = 1.2$. Use the result from part d to compute all values of N_t, $N_t > 0$ for which $g(N_t)$ is either a maximum or minimum. (HINT: Let $z = N_t^2$.)

f. Assume that $p = 2$ and $r = 1.2$. Use the result from part d to compute the stability of all fixed points found in part c.

g. Sketch the graph of N_{t+1} versus N_t for $p = 2, r = 1.2$.

✐   **1.12** Assume an ecological system is described by the finite-difference equation

$$x_{t+1} = Cx_t^2(2 - x_t), \qquad 0 \leq x_t \leq 2,$$

where x_t is the population density in year t and C is a positive constant that we assume is equal to $\frac{25}{16}$.

   a. Sketch the graph of the right-hand side of this equation. Indicate the maxima, minima, and inflection points.

   b. Determine the fixed points of this system.

   c. Determine the stability at each fixed point and describe the dynamics in the neighborhood of the fixed points.

   d. In a brief sentence or two describe the expected dynamics starting from initial values of $x_0 = \frac{1}{3}$ and also $x_0 = 1$ in the limit as $t \to \infty$. In particular, comment on the possibility that the population may go to extinction or to chaotic dynamics in the limit $t \to \infty$.

✐   **1.13** In this problem P_t represents the fraction of neurons of a large neural network that fire at time t. As a simple model of epilepsy, the dynamics of the network can be described by the finite-difference equation

$$P_{t+1} = 4C P_t^3 - 6C P_t^2 + (1 + 2C)P_t,$$

where C is a positive number, and $0 \leq P_t \leq 1$.

   a. Compute the fixed points.

   b. Determine the stability at each fixed point and describe the dynamics in the neighborhood of the fixed points as a function of C.

   c. Sketch P_{t+1} as a function of P_t for $C = 4$. Show all maxima, minima, and inflection points.

   d. On the basis of the preceding work discuss the dynamics as $t \to \infty$ starting from an initial condition of $P_0 = 0.45$ with $C = 4$. Try to do this graphically and, if possible, on a computer.

✐   **1.14** This problem deals with the equation

$$x_{t+1} = f(x_t) = 3.3x_t - 3.3x_t^2.$$

   a. Determine the fixed points of $x_{t+2} = f(f(x_t))$. Which of these points are also fixed points of $x_{t+1} = f(x_t)$?

b. Are there any cycles of period 3?

📖 **1.15** Show that if there is one solution to $x_t = g(g(x_t))$, where $x_t \neq g(x_t)$, then there must also be another, different solution.

📖 **1.16** The dependence of the stability of a fixed point on the derivative can be shown algebraically using **Taylor series**. The Taylor series gives a polynomial expansion of a function in the neighborhood of a point. The Taylor series expansion of $f(x)$ at a point a is

$$f(x) = f(a) + (x - a) \left. \frac{df}{dx} \right|_a + \frac{(x-a)^2}{2!} \left. \frac{d^2 f}{dx^2} \right|_a + \cdots. \qquad (1.16)$$

This problem is aimed at using the Taylor series to derive analytically the local stability criteria for a fixed point in the finite-difference equation

$$x_{t+1} = f(x_t).$$

Assume that there is a fixed point defined by $x_t = f(x_t) = x^*$. Define

$$m = \left. \frac{df}{dx} \right|_{x^*}$$

Derive the stability criteria for the fixed point at x^* using the Taylor series. (HINT: Define $y_t = x_t - x^*$ and consider the linear terms in the resulting equation.)

📖 **1.17** Periodically stimulated oscillators can often be described by one-dimensional finite-difference equations (see the *Dynamics in Action* 1 box). The variable ϕ_t refers to the phase of stimulus t during the cycle. The phase of the subsequent stimulus ϕ_{t+1} is a function of ϕ_t. The next three problems are all motivated by theoretical models that have been proposed for periodically stimulated oscillators.

The following finite-difference equation has been considered as a mathematical model for a periodically stimulated biological oscillator (Bélair and Glass, 1983):

$$\phi_{t+1} = \begin{cases} 6\phi_t - 12\phi_t^2, & 0 \leq \phi_t < 0.5; \\ 12\phi_t^2 - 18\phi_t + 7, & 0.5 \leq \phi_t \leq 1. \end{cases}$$

a. Sketch ϕ_{t+1} as a function of ϕ_t for $0 \leq \phi_t \leq 1$. Be sure to show all maxima and minima and to compute the values of ϕ_{t+1} at these extremal points.

b. Compute all fixed points. What are the qualitative dynamics in the neighborhood of each fixed point?

c. If you have done part (a) correctly, you should be able to find a cycle of period 2. What is this cycle? Show it on your sketch.

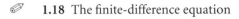 **1.18** The finite-difference equation

$$\phi_{t+1} = 0.5 + \alpha \sin 2\pi \phi_t, \qquad 0 \le \phi_t < 1,$$

where $0 \le \alpha < 0.5$, has been used as a mathematical model for periodic stimulation of biological oscillators.

a. There is one steady state. Determine this steady state and its stability as a function of α.

b. For what value of α is there a period-doubling bifurcation?

c. Sketch ϕ_{t+1} as a function of ϕ_t for $\alpha = 0.25$. Be sure to indicate all maxima, minima, and inflection points.

d. For $\alpha = 0.25$ there is a stable period-2 orbit. What is it?

1.19 The following equation arose in the study of two independent oscillators competing for control of the heart. The resulting cardiac arrhythmia is called **parasystole**. Theoretical analysis of parasystole shows interesting rhythms obeying rules derived from number theory. The following example illustrates typical dynamics found when the ratio between the two frequencies is a rational number. For more details on the mathematical modeling of this cardiac arrhythmia, see Glass et al. (1986).

A mathematical model for a periodically forced biological oscillator can be written as

$$\phi_{t+1} = \begin{cases} \phi_t + 0.4, & \text{for } 0 \le \phi_i < 0.6; \\ \phi_t - 0.2, & \text{for } 0.6 \le \phi_i < 0.7; \\ \phi_t - 0.6, & \text{for } 0.7 \le \phi_t < 1.0, \end{cases}$$

where ϕ_t is the phase in the cycle of the forced oscillator at which the tth periodic stimulus falls, $0 < \phi_t < 1$.

a. Accurately plot on graph paper ϕ_{t+1} as a function of ϕ_t.

b. Determine the fixed points, if any, and determine their stability.

c. Take an initial condition $\phi_0 = 0.65$ and determine the dynamics (both algebraically and graphically) until a periodic orbit is reached. Do the same for an initial condition of $\phi_0 = 0.95$. An accurate graph is essential here.

d. Are the periodic orbits in part c stable?

✏ **1.20** The population of a species is described by the finite-difference equation

$$x_{t+1} = ax_t \exp(-x_t), \qquad x_t \geq 0,$$

where a is a positive constant.

a. Determine the fixed points.

b. Evaluate the stability of the fixed points.

c. For what value of a is there a period-doubling bifurcation?

d. For what values of a will the population go extinct starting from any initial condition?

e. On a computer, generate the bifurcation diagram as a function of a. Even though you might not be able to do this computation, do you expect that the bifurcation diagram will display the period-doubling route to chaos similar to that shown in Figure 1.31?

✏ **1.21** If you are tired about problems concerning flies, consider the following model about bird populations. Birds eat flies. Milton and Bélair (1990) proposed this equation as a model for bird densities in successive years:

$$x_{t+1} = \begin{cases} 3.22x_t & \text{for } 0 \leq x_t \leq 1 \\ 0.5x_t & \text{for } 1 < x_t. \end{cases} \qquad (1.17)$$

Draw a graph of x_{t+1} as a function of x_t. Graphically iterate this equation and determine if the dynamics are chaotic.

✏ **1.22** Print your last name. Count the number of letters and multiply the number by 0.1. Your **magic number**, m, is 1 plus the number that you just computed. If your last name has nine or more letters, assume that $m = 1.9$.

Consider the finite-difference equation given by the following equations:

$$x_{t+1} = mx_t, \qquad \text{for } 0 \leq x_t \leq \frac{1}{m};$$

$$x_{t+1} = mx_t - 1, \qquad \text{for } \frac{1}{m} < x_t \leq 1.$$

a. Draw a graph of x_{t+1} as a function of x_t.

b. Determine the fixed point(s) and determine their stability.

c. Graphically iterate this equation.

d. Are the dynamics chaotic?

1.23 In Example 1.4 in the text, we looked for period-doubling bifurcations in the finite-difference equation:

$$x_{t+1} = f(x_t) = x_t + b \sin(2\pi x_t).$$

We found that fixed points became unstable when $b = \frac{1}{\pi}$. At these bifurcation points, a stable period-2 cycle emerges. Here, we are interested in studying the stability of these cycles of period 2. In particular, we want to know when the cycles are "superstable," meaning that a nearby point is immediately moved onto the cycle rather than approaching it exponentially. Such superstability occurs when the graph has slope zero at the fixed points of the cycle, which will occur when the graph is at a maximum or a minimum on the cycle.

a. Sketch the graph of the equation for $b = \frac{1}{\pi}$. Determine the values of all maxima, minima, and inflection points.

b. For a particular value of b the maximum and minimum of $f(x_t)$ are on a cycle of period 2. Sketch the function for this case showing the cycle of period 2. It is not necessary to determine the value of b that leads to this behavior. However, will b be greater than or less than $\frac{1}{\pi}$?

COMPUTER PROJECTS

Consider the two following one-dimensional finite-difference equations.

$$x_{t+1} = 4\lambda x_t(1 - x_t), \qquad \text{Equation A}$$

$$x_{t+1} = \lambda \sin \pi x_t, \qquad \text{Equation B}$$

where $0 \le x_t \le 1$, $0 \le \lambda \le 1$.

For both Equation A and Equation B carry out Projects 1–5.

Project 1 Write a computer program that can be used to iterate these equations.

Project 2 Compute a bifurcation diagram such as shown in Fig. 1.31. To compute this first set a value for λ. Then iterate the equation equation 200 times, but only save the values of the last 100 iterates. Plot these 100 values on a graph above the corresponding value of λ. Increment λ in small steps. In doing this you may wish to experiment with the step size in λ, the length of the transient and the number of plotted points. Getting a nice looking picture depends on taking fine steps in λ, taking a sufficiently long transient, and plotting a sufficiently large number of points.

Project 3 Write a program that can determine if a sequence of values generated from iteration of the equations is periodic. If it is periodic, what is the period of the cycle? In doing this, it is best for you to set a specific value for convergence to a periodic orbit. This means that if the distance between 2 points is closer than some value, for example $\epsilon = 10^{-5}$, you would declare that a periodic orbit had been found.

The next two projects make use of the techniques developed above. Carrying them out successfully requires some skill and careful numerical work. If you get stuck you might wish to look back at original sources. Project 4 is based on Metropolis et al. (1973), and Project 5 is based on Feigenbaum (1980).

Project 4 Determine the sequence of periodic orbits that are encountered as a function of λ. In doing this there are 3 parameters that you will have to adjust: the number of iterates, the increment in λ, and the convergence criterion. Although it probably seems like it should be trivial to decide what the period is for any value of λ you may surprised to find that different sets of the 3 parameters will give different answers. The situation can be particularly delicate when you are near values of λ that lead to bifurcations in the dynamics. The sequences of periodic orbits for the 2 different maps should be the same. Are they?

Project 5 Locate sequences of period doubling bifurcations. Write a program that can compute automatically the value of Feigenbaum's number for the two functions given above. Do you obtain the same value that has been found by Feigenbaum? Is the value the same for both of the functions? Is the value the same for the sequences of periodic orbits 2, 4, 8, . . . and 3, 6, 12, . . . ?

Project 6 Now that you have mastered functions with one parameter you are ready to explore functions with 2 parameters. Consider the function (often called the sine circle map)

$$x_{t+1} = x_t + a + b \sin(2\pi x_t) \pmod 1,$$

where $0 \leq a \leq 1, 0 \leq x_t \leq 1$, and $b \geq 0$. Your task is to study the periodic orbits as a function of a and b. Since there are 2 parameters now, you will make a plot of the behavior with a on the horizontal axis and b on the vertical. At each value of a and b, plot a dot whose color depends on the length of the period found. You will have to consider what to do if you do not find any period. An additional complication comes from the fact that the cycle that you find in some regions of parameter space will depend on the initial condition.

CHAPTER 2

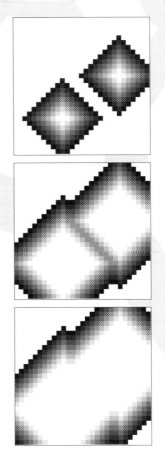

Boolean Networks and Cellular Automata

In Chapter 1 we studied dynamical systems of the form

$$x_{t+1} = f(x_t).$$

In this equation there is a single dynamical variable, x_t. If we know the value of x at time t, we can calculate the value at time $t + 1$ and at future times. In this chapter, we shall study systems in which there is more than one dynamical variable. Most complex systems that are found in biology—such as the genetic regulatory system, the nervous system, the immune system, and ecosystems—are composed of multiple interacting elements. In a living organism it is impossible to consider the dynamics of a single neuron, or gene, or immune cell, without considering the interactions with other elements of the network. However, because of the complexity of these systems, accurate mathematical descriptions are usually impossible, and one thus resorts to simplifications. One simplification is that time is discrete, and that the behavior of a system at one time depends on the state of the system at a preceding time. A second assumption is that the elements of the network have only a limited number of different values. For example, at

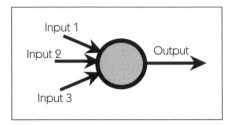

Figure 2.1
An element has inputs and a single output. The output may be connected as an input to more than one element.

any given time a gene might be "turned on" or "turned off," or a neuron might be firing or not firing. Despite the rather gross simplifying assumptions, you should realize at the outset that the resulting networks can nevertheless be extraordinarily complex, and there remain many outstanding issues that are not yet well understood.

2.1 ELEMENTS AND NETWORKS

A **network** is a collection of connected elements. Each **element** can be thought of as having a single output and possibly many inputs (see Figure 2.1). Each element also has a rule to tell what the output should be given the inputs. For example, an element might have a rule that says that the output should be the sum of the inputs. In a network, the output of an element can be the input of some other element, or can even be an input to itself. An element may send its output to more than one element.

As Figures 2.2 and 2.3 show, the connectivity of a network can be visualized as a set of **nodes** (which are drawn as gray circles), and a set of **edges** (drawn as black arrows) connecting pairs of nodes. The nodes correspond to the elements, and the edges correspond to the inputs and outputs. Whether an edge is an input or output for a given node is indicated by an arrowhead.

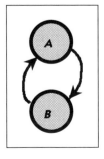

Figure 2.2
A simple network consisting of two elements.

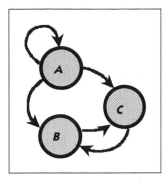

Figure 2.3
A network with three elements.

In order to complete the description of the network, it is necessary to specify the rule that governs how the output of each node is related to the inputs. One can imagine any number of rules. In this chapter, we will consider several different types of rules that produce interesting dynamical behavior.

Since there is only one output for each node, we can identify the output with the name of the node. The rule for node A in the two-element network shown in Figure 2.2 can be written as

$$A_{t+1} = f_A(B_t),$$

which says simply that the output of A at time $t + 1$ is a function of the input at time t. Similarly, the rule for node B is $B_{t+1} = f_B(A_t)$. (This notation is similar to that used in Chapter 1. The only difference here is that the function f has a subscript that identifies to which node the function applies.)

For the three-element network shown in Figure 2.3, the rule for node B is

$$B_{t+1} = f_B(A_t, C_t).$$

This says that the value of output B at time $t + 1$ depends on the values of both A and C at time t. In general, the order of the arguments to a function is important, so that $f_B(A_t, C_t)$ may not be equal to $f_B(C_t, A_t)$. The graphs, however, do not specify the order of arguments to the rule. A complete description of a network is given by a list of functions and arguments. For example, a description for the three-element network in Figure 2.3 is

$$A_{t+1} = f_A(A_t),$$

$$B_{t+1} = f_B(A_t, C_t),$$

$$C_{t+1} = f_C(A_t, B_t).$$

Once we specify the forms of the functions $f_A()$, $f_B()$, and $f_C()$, we have a complete description of the network. We will see some ways to do this in the following sections.

In this chapter we are going to consider networks where the output of each node can have only a finite set of discrete values—for example, 0, 1, 2, 3—as opposed to the continuum of values for the dynamical systems studied in Chapter 1.

2.2 BOOLEAN VARIABLES, FUNCTIONS, AND NETWORKS

An extreme limiting case for the input/output rules for elements is where the output can have only a single value. This is obviously not a case of much interest—if the output of each element can have only one value, then nothing can change in the network.

As soon as we allow each output to have two values, however, interesting things can start to happen. By convention, the two allowed values are usually written as 1 or 0 (or, alternatively, ON or OFF). A variable that can have only the values 1 or 0 is called a **Boolean variable**, and a rule that tells how a Boolean output is determined by a Boolean input is called a **Boolean function**. The foundations for this analysis were laid by George Boole (1815–1864). One area of application of the study of Boolean variables is in computer science—Boolean variables and functions are central to digital circuit design and computer architecture.

A basic concept is the **state** of a network, which specifies whether each element is ON or OFF. For example, a possible state for a three-element network at time i is $A_i = 0$, $B_i = 1$, $C_i = 1$. As a shorthand notation, we will sometimes write this as (011). For a Boolean network with two elements, there are four possible states:

$$(00), \quad (01), \quad (10), \quad (11).$$

For a network with three elements, there are eight possible states:

$$(000), \quad (001), \quad (010), \quad (011), \quad (100), \quad (101), \quad (110), \quad (111).$$

You should see the relationship between the number of elements and the number of possible states. For a network with N elements, there are 2^N possible states. This number can be very large—for a network with 100 elements, there are $\approx 1.27 \times 10^{30}$ possible states. The state at time $t = 0$ is called the **initial condition** of the network.

NETWORKS OF SINGLE-INPUT BOOLEAN ELEMENTS

Networks can be constructed out of Boolean elements with a single input. These networks can be readily studied and produce some interesting types of dynamical behavior: **fixed points**, **cycles**, and **multistability**. These behaviors are easy to understand with the simple connectivities that are possible in single-input networks.

Only four Boolean rules are possible for relating a single input to an output. They are explained in the following table.

Name	Input	
	(0)	(1)
IDENTITY	0	1
INVERSE	1	0
ZERO	0	0
ONE	1	1

For example, if an element has the IDENTITY rule and its input is (0), then its output will also be 0. On the other hand, an element whose rule is INVERSE will produce a 0 output only when its input is (1), and will produce a 1 when its input is (0). For both ZERO and ONE, the output is not influenced by the input.

The first thing to realize about single-input networks is that to analyze the dynamics we have to understand the dynamics generated by only three different classes of connectivities: unclosed strings, simple closed loops and loops to which strings are attached. It is impossible for single-input networks to have two or more connected loops (for example, a figure-eight structure).

STRINGS

The dynamics of networks with a string connectivity are very simple. Consider a string network with four elements A, B, C, and D in which element A has no input, and the inputs to the other elements follow the scheme $A \rightarrow B \rightarrow C \rightarrow D$. Since A has no input, it is constant in value. The dynamical equations for the other elements are

$$B_{t+1} = f_B(A_t); \qquad C_{t+1} = f_C(B_t); \qquad D_{t+1} = f_D(C_t).$$

By substitution, we have

$$B_{t+1} = f_B(A_t); \qquad C_{t+2} = f_C(f_B(A_t)); \qquad D_{t+3} = f_D(f_C(f_B(A_t))).$$

This says that, independent of the value B_0, after one "startup" or transient iteration, B will assume a constant value, $B_{t \geq 1} = f_B(A_0)$. Similarly, after two iterations, C will have a value that remains constant, $C_{t \geq 2} = f_C(f_B(A_0))$. After three iterations, D also remains constant; $D_{t \geq 3} = f_D(f_C(f_B(A_0)))$.

We can generalize to strings of length N and find that after $N - 1$ iterations, all the elements of the string will reach a constant value that depends only on the value of the first element in the string. All strings reach a fixed point after a transient that lasts $N - 1$ time steps. Figure 2.4 depicts an open string network.

CLOSED LOOPS—THE BUCKET BRIGADE

The dynamics of closed loops is much more interesting.

If a loop has a node whose rule is ZERO or ONE, then it is effectively cut open into a string. The rules ZERO and ONE disregard their input, and so in drawing the graph of a network including ZERO or ONE nodes, we can erase the inputs to those nodes; this clearly turns a loop into a string. (Similarly, a string is effectively cut into two parts by a ZERO or ONE node.) Since we have already seen the dynamical behavior of strings, we will consider only loops that have IDENTITY or INVERSE nodes exclusively.

A helpful way to think about loops is as a kind of "bucket brigade" (see Figure 2.5). Bucket brigades are an old-fashioned way of fighting fires using a ring of people, each person with a bucket. The ring is stretched lengthwise like a rubber band; at one end is a well or other source of water, at the other end the fire. At each call by a pacemaster, every person in the ring passes his or her bucket to his or her neighbor and takes a bucket from the neighbor on the other side. The buckets move around the ring, with the person at the water source filling the empty buckets, and the person at the fire emptying the full buckets. (In some towns in colonial America, each adult male was required to own a bucket with his name on it so that he could participate in bucket brigades.)

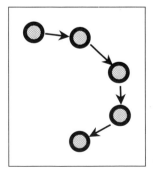

Figure 2.4
An open string network.

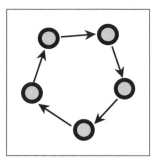

Figure 2.5
A closed loop network.

To apply the analogy of the bucket brigade to single-input Boolean networks, imagine that people in the loop can have either an IDENTITY or INVERSE rule. Those with the IDENTITY rule will simply pass along the bucket without changing its contents. Those with the INVERSE rule will empty out any full bucket that arrives, or fill any empty bucket, before passing it to his or her neighbor.

In terms of our notation for networks, a full bucket corresponds to an output value 1 and an empty bucket to value 0. Every node in the bucket brigade has the IDENTITY rule (which means that the bucket is passed on unchanged), except for the nodes at the water source and the fire, which have the ONE and ZERO rules, respectively. The initial condition is that everyone is holding an empty bucket, that is, initially the state is $000 \cdots 000$. Also, each person starts holding a bucket with his or her own name on it.

If there are N nodes in the loop, then after N time steps every bucket is returned to its original owner. It's easy to see that if every node has the IDENTITY rule, then each bucket would arrive back at its owner in the same full or empty state whence it started out. Thus, the network would return to its initial condition after N time steps. The same is true if there is an even number of INVERSE nodes in the loop. On the other hand, if there is an odd number of INVERSE nodes, then a bucket will arive back at its owner in the inverse condition to how it started the loop. After two cycles, though, each bucket will be restored to its original condition, and the network will return to its initial condition after $2N$ time steps. Loops with an odd number of INVERSE nodes are said to be **frustrated**. Loops with an even number of INVERSE nodes are called **unfrustrated**.

Whatever the initial condition, a loop provides a guarantee that it will be returned to after N time steps for unfrustrated loops or $2N$ time steps for frustrated loops. Thus, *every possible initial condition is part of a cycle*. For a cycle of period N, the network as a whole will have N different states reached in turn.

In the Boolean networks, as opposed to the colonial bucket brigades, the "buckets" do not belong to anyone and do not have names written on them. It is possible, therefore, to have a return to the initial condition after fewer than N or $2N$ time steps and therefore to have a cycle of period m less than N.

Given a network, how many different cycles are there? This is an important question, since it addresses the issue of how many different types of behavior are possible in a given network. We can put a lower bound on the number of different cycles by assuming that all cycles are of maximum length N for unfrustrated networks or $2N$ for frustrated networks. There are 2^N possible states for the network, but only N different states are reached within a given cycle, and the minimum number of distinct cycles is $\frac{2^N}{N}$ for unfrustrated networks and $\frac{2^{N-1}}{N}$ for frustrated networks. The actual number of cycles depends on the symmetry of the network and is an advanced topic. We will see some examples ahead.

Since every possible initial condition is part of a cycle, there are no transients or attractors in a loop.

LOOPS WITH STRINGS

If you look carefully at the topology of networks that consist of loops with strings coming off the loop, you will see that there is an element of the loop at the head of each string (see Figure 2.6). Since no element of the loop has an input from any string, the dynamics of the elements in the loop are unaffected by the strings. The strings simply pass along the output the loop sends them; they are in a sense passive recipients of the dynamics of the loop and will have the same period as the loop to which they are attached.

❏ EXAMPLE 2.1

A loop network with N elements can have cycles of length up to N if the network is unfrustrated, and up to $2N$ if the network is frustrated. What periodic cycles can appear in the two networks shown in Figures 2.7 and 2.8? Are the networks frustrated or unfrustrated?

Solution: The network shown in Figure 2.7 is unfrustrated, because there is an even number of INVERSE nodes in the loop. To find the cycles, pick one of the

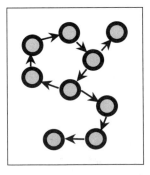

Figure 2.6
A closed loop with strings.

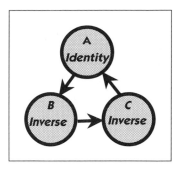

Figure 2.7
An unfrustrated network with three nodes.

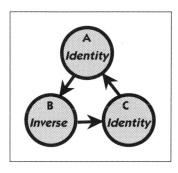

Figure 2.8
A frustrated network with three nodes.

possible states of the network, for example (111), use this as an initial condition, and follow the evolution of the state in time. For example, since B inverts its input, if $A_t = 1$, then $B_{t+1} = 0$. Similarly, since C also has INVERSE as a rule, $B_t = 1$ gives $C_{t+1} = 0$. $C_t = 1$ leads to $A_{t+1} = 1$, since A has IDENTITY as a rule. The state at time $t + 2$ can be found in a similar fashion and the process can iterate indefinitely. When the state returns back to its initial condition, the complete cycle has been traced out. Then, pick some other state that is not on the cycle to use as another initial condition, and trace out the evolution of this state until it returns back to the initial condition. Repeat this using all possible states. Following this procedure for the network in Figure 2.7, we find that the network has two cycles of period 3 and two cycles of period 1 (i.e., fixed points):

$$(111) \rightarrow (100) \rightarrow (001) \rightarrow (111) \rightarrow \cdots$$

$$(000) \rightarrow (011) \rightarrow (110) \rightarrow (000) \rightarrow \cdots$$

$$(101) \rightarrow (101) \rightarrow \cdots$$

$$(010) \rightarrow (010) \rightarrow \cdots .$$

This network in Figure 2.8 is frustrated, because there is an odd number of INVERSE nodes in the loop. The network has one cycle of period 6 and one cycle of period 2:

$$(111) \rightarrow (101) \rightarrow (100) \rightarrow (000) \rightarrow (010) \rightarrow (011) \rightarrow (111) \rightarrow \cdots$$

$$(110) \rightarrow (001) \rightarrow (110) \rightarrow \cdots .$$

DYNAMICS IN ACTION

2   A LAMBDA BACTERIOPHAGE MODEL

The **lambda bacteriophage** is a virus that invades *E. coli* bacteria. The lambda bacteriophage has two distinct modes of operation: It can become integrated into the host cell DNA and be replicated automatically each time the bacterium divides; or it can multiply in the cytoplasm of the bacterium, eventually killing its host. Once one of these modes is established, it is maintained. The mechanism for this involves two proteins: The *lambda repressor* blocks expression of the gene for the *cro* protein, and the *cro* protein blocks expression of the gene for the *lambda repressor*. When *cro* is expressed, the bacteriophage multiplies in the cytoplasm; otherwise the bacteriophage is integrated into the host cell DNA.

A simple model for this system is provided by a one-input Boolean network. Imagine that there are two nodes as the figure here shows, one for the *lambda repressor* gene and one for the *cro* gene. The node has output 1 if the gene is being expressed, and output 0 if it is not being expressed. (Expression of a gene means that the corresponding protein is being produced.) Since *cro* blocks expression of *lambda repressor* and vice versa, both of the nodes are INVERSE.

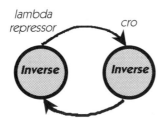

A Boolean model of gene expression in the lambda bacteriophage.

There are two nodes, so the network has $2^2 = 4$ possible states. There are two fixed points: (10) corresponds to the exclusive expression of *lambda repressor*;

(01) corresponds to the expression of *cro*. These are the two observed modes of the lambda bacteriophage.

Although this simple model shows how the lambda bacteriophage can stay locked into one of two possible modes, it does not match other aspects of gene expression in the bacteriophage. In the model network, there is also a cycle of period 2, (11) → (00) → (11), which is not a behavior observed in the lambda bacteriophage. This shows that the simple model is not a complete description of the lambda bacteriophage system. In the model, which of the two fixed points is reached depends only on the initial condition of the system; however, a real lambda bacteriophage can switch between the two if it finds itself in unfavorable conditions. The model gives a simple way to think of the control circuit, but it also shows that to understand the dynamics of the lambda bacteriophage we need more information about the gene regulation network than simply "*lambda repressor* blocks *cro* expression and vice versa." (For more discussion of the lambda bacteriophage and logical models, see Thomas, et al. (1976) and Thieffry and Thomas (1994).)

NETWORKS OF MULTIPLE-INPUT BOOLEAN ELEMENTS

As we have seen, the behavior of networks of single-input Boolean elements is quite simple: fixed points and cycles, where the length of the cycle is no more than twice the number of nodes in the loop generating the cycle.

When elements have more than one input, there can be much more complicated dynamics. There are two reasons for this:

- The connectivity of the network can become much more complicated. In single-input networks, the only geometries are strings, simple loops, and loops with strings. When some nodes have more than one input, there can be multiple, connected loops.

- The Boolean functions of multiple inputs are much more complicated than the functions of a single input.

See Figure 2.9 for a schematic of a network where some elements have two inputs.

BOOLEAN FUNCTIONS AND NETWORKS OF TWO OR MORE INPUTS

In order to count the number of Boolean functions of two inputs, you should recognize that two inputs can take on $2^2 = 4$ possible states altogether:

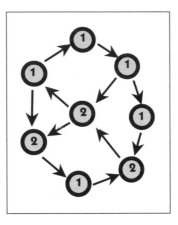

Figure 2.9
A network where some elements have two inputs (the number of inputs to each node is marked).

(00), (01), (10), (11). Each rule assigns a single Boolean value to each possible input state. Since there are four input states, the number of functions equals the number of distinct ways of combining the four zeros or ones that can be the output. Thus, there are $2^4 = 16$ distinct Boolean functions of two inputs, which are shown in Table 2.1.

If you look carefully at the table, you will notice certain patterns. For example, the output of most functions (e.g., AND, OR) depends on both of the inputs, while other functions (**3, 5, 10, 12**) depend on only one input. Two of the functions (CONTRADICTION and TAUTOLOGY) are constant regardless of their inputs.

Following the same type of procedure, we can devise a Boolean function of any number of inputs. Calling K the number of inputs, a function can be constructed in the following way:

1. Write down all the different ways of writing K zeros and ones. These are all the possible input states to a Boolean function of K inputs. For example, for $K = 3$ there are eight possible input states. These are (000), (001), (010), (011), (100), (101), (110), and (111). There are, altogether, 2^K different ways of writing K zeros and ones.

2. Assign a 0 or 1 to each of the 2^K possible input states. These are the outputs that correspond to each of the inputs.

This procedure generates a single Boolean function of K inputs. How many such Boolean functions are there? Since there are 2^K different possible input states, a single function corresponds to one way of writing 2^K zeros and ones. There are 2^{2^K} possible distinct ways of writing 2^K zeros and ones.

The number of possible Boolean functions increases enormously as the number of inputs increases, and a significant body of mathematical and engineering expertise has been developed to classify these networks and to design and build switching circuits that can compute some desired Boolean function. For

Table 2.1 The sixteen Boolean functions of two inputs

	Name	Input States			
		(00)	**(01)**	**(10)**	**(11)**
		Output			
0	CONTRADICTION	0	0	0	0
1	AND	0	0	0	1
2	INHIBITION	0	0	1	0
3	TRANSFER	0	0	1	1
4	INHIBITION	0	1	0	0
5	TRANSFER	0	1	0	1
6	XOR	0	1	1	0
7	OR	0	1	1	1
8	NOR	1	0	0	0
9	XNOR	1	0	0	1
10	COMPLEMENT	1	0	1	0
11	IMPLICATION	1	0	1	1
12	COMPLEMENT	1	1	0	0
13	IMPLICATION	1	1	0	1
14	NAND	1	1	1	0
15	TAUTOLOGY	1	1	1	1

example, a series circuit can be used to calculate the AND function, and a parallel circuit can be used to calculate the OR function. It is more difficult to figure out circuits that compute other functions such as the XOR function.

In Chapter 1 we used the cobweb method to trace the dynamics of a one-dimensional map starting from a specified initial condition. The dynamics of a Boolean network can also be traced from an initial condition. To do this, we make use of the concept of the state of the network, which was introduced at the beginning of Section 2.2.

As an example of a simple, two-input Boolean network, consider the five-node, two-input network shown in Figure 2.10, where each of the nodes applies the NOR rule to its two inputs. The "state of the network" at time t describes the

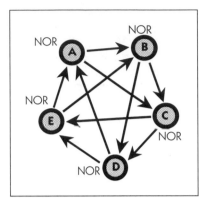

Figure 2.10
A network with five nodes with two inputs per node.

state of each of the individual nodes at that time. For example, if the state at time 0 is (10000), then $A_0 = 1$, $B_0 = C_0 = D_0 = E_0 = 0$. Applying the appropriate Boolean rule to each of the nodes individually, we can easily see that $A_1 = 1$, $B_1 = 0$, $C_1 = 0$, $D_1 = 1$, and $E_1 = 1$, giving a state at time 1 of (10011). More generally, we can create a table that relates every possible state at time t to the successor state at time $t + 1$. We call such a table a **lookup table** or a **truth table**. For the network shown here, the table has 32 rows, because there are $2^5 = 32$ possible states.

The truth table allows us to determine the dynamics. Given the state at time t, we can simply look up the state at time $t + 1$, and iterate the process to find future states. For example, we can see from the table that there is a cycle of period 2: $(00000) \rightarrow (11111) \rightarrow (00000)$.

One useful way to visualize the dynamics of a Boolean network is to do so graphically. We can represent the state at each time as a sequence of black and white dots, where a black dot stands for a 1, and a very small point stands for a

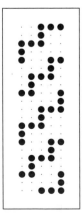

Figure 2.11
A schematic representation of the dynamics in the Boolean network with five elements shown in Fig. 2.10. The state of each element is either 1 (●) or 0 (·). Time 0 is at the top line. Each successive iteration corresponds to a new line.

Table 2.2 Truth table for the network in Figure 2.10.

$(ABCDE)_t \rightarrow (ABCDE)_{t+1}$	$(ABCDE)_t \rightarrow (ABCDE)_{t+1}$
$(00000) \rightarrow (11111)$	$(00001) \rightarrow (00111)$
$(00010) \rightarrow (01110)$	$(00011) \rightarrow (00110)$
$(00100) \rightarrow (11100)$	$(00101) \rightarrow (00100)$
$(00110) \rightarrow (01100)$	$(00111) \rightarrow (00100)$
$(01000) \rightarrow (11001)$	$(01001) \rightarrow (00001)$
$(01010) \rightarrow (01000)$	$(01011) \rightarrow (00000)$
$(01100) \rightarrow (11000)$	$(01101) \rightarrow (00000)$
$(01110) \rightarrow (01000)$	$(01111) \rightarrow (00000)$
$(10000) \rightarrow (10011)$	$(10001) \rightarrow (00011)$
$(10010) \rightarrow (00010)$	$(10011) \rightarrow (00010)$
$(10100) \rightarrow (10000)$	$(10101) \rightarrow (00000)$
$(10110) \rightarrow (00000)$	$(10111) \rightarrow (00000)$
$(11000) \rightarrow (10001)$	$(11001) \rightarrow (00001)$
$(11010) \rightarrow (00000)$	$(11011) \rightarrow (00000)$
$(11100) \rightarrow (10000)$	$(11101) \rightarrow (00000)$
$(11110) \rightarrow (00000)$	$(11111) \rightarrow (00000)$

0. For example, the state (11101) is represented as ● ● ● · ●. Then, we can make a "movie" of the dynamics by plotting the state at time $t + 1$ below the state at time t. Such a movie made from an initial condition of (00111) is shown in Figure 2.11. It should be clear that as the numbers of elements of multi-input networks increase, the possibility arises for enormously long cycles. Surprisingly, there are still many mathematical questions that have not been studied about the dynamics in multi-input networks. However, guided in part by biological and physical questions, a number of surprising properties have been found for Boolean networks and networks in which there are a few states per element.

DYNAMICS IN ACTION

3 LOCOMOTION IN SALAMANDERS

Networks of neurons are believed to underlie important biological functions such as respiration and locomotion. The earliest suggestion that logical models might be useful in providing a simplified description of the structure of neural networks was provided by G. Székely (1965), who was studying locomotion in salamanders. Székely hypothesized that a neural network generated a rhythm that innervated four different muscle pools: extensors of the elbow (A), adductors of the shoulder (B), flexors of the elbow (C), and abductors of the shoulder (D). A simplified diagram indicating the contraction sequence of the limb muscles during stepping is shown in the upper figure here.

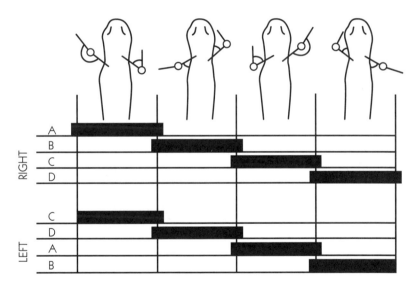

The sequence of contraction of muscles during locomotion in the salamander. On each side the four muscle groves fire sequentially. Adapted from Székely (1965).

Translating Székely's original work into the current notation, we show in the bottom diagram a simplified logical organization that can generate the sequential contraction pattern in one limb. It is assumed that each neuron pool responsible for driving a muscle pool receives tonic excitation and will fire unless inhibited. The inhibition is provided by other neuron pools. The inhibitory connections lead to a sequential pattern of activation that is similar to what is experimentally observed.

In order to appreciate how this network leads to the correct sequential patterns of muscle activation, we break the analysis into a series of steps. We first write down the truth table for this network showing the state at time $t + 1$ given the state at time t. The truth table can be calculated immediately from the knowledge of the input functions to each element. On the left hand of the table we write down all the states of the system. The elements on the right side are filled in sequentially, column by column, until completed. For example, notice that A receives input from B and C. If either B or C is 1 at t, A will be 0 at $t + 1$. Otherwise A is 1 at $t + 1$. Thus, we obtain the truth table below.

$(ABCD)_t$	$(ABCD)_{t+1}$	$(ABCD)_t$	$(ABCD)_{t+1}$
(0000) → (1111)		(0001) → (1001)	
(0010) → (0011)		(0011) → (0001)	
(0100) → (0110)		(0101) → (0000)	
(0110) → (0010)		(0111) → (0000)	
(1000) → (1100)		(1001) → (1000)	
(1010) → (0000)		(1011) → (0000)	
(1100) → (0100)		(1101) → (0000)	
(1110) → (0000)		(1111) → (0000)	

Now assume that at time $t = 0$, the state of the network is $A_0 = 1$, $B_0 = C_0 = D_0 = 0$. We can compute all subsequent states until a cycle is reached simply by using the truth table. Starting at the state (1000) we undergo a transition to the state (1100). By using the table the following cycle is confirmed:

$$1000 \rightarrow 1100 \rightarrow 0100 \rightarrow 0110 \rightarrow 0010 \rightarrow 0011$$

$$\rightarrow 0001 \rightarrow 1001 \rightarrow 1000 \rightarrow \cdots .$$

The removal of the inhibition lets each cell fire in turn. This pattern of activity mimics the activity shown in the figure on the facing page.

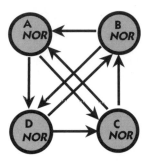

A neural network that generates the sequence observed in the salamander.

For more discussion of this sort of simplified approach to the study of neural networks, see Glass and Young (1979) and Thomas and D'Ari (1990).

☐ EXAMPLE 2.2

Suppose that we have measured a given pattern of oscillatory activity, and we want to construct a network that will produce this behavior. For example, assume that we want to design a network of four logical units with no self-input to generate the same sequence of states seen in locomotion in the salamander model:

$$1000 \rightarrow 1100 \rightarrow 0100 \rightarrow 0110 \rightarrow 0010 \rightarrow 0011$$

$$\rightarrow 0001 \rightarrow 1001 \rightarrow 1000 \rightarrow \cdots.$$

How many different logical switching networks can generate this cyclic activity? What are they?

Solution: Call the elements $w, x, y,$ and z. Start by filling in the truth table based on the transitions that have been given. This will give rise to a table with $2^4 = 16$ entries, only eight of which can be filled in from the measurements.

Since by assumption there is no self-input, the truth table for each of the individual elements can be written only in terms of the other three elements. This means that we can extract the truth table into the following four sets of rules, one for each of $w, x, y,$ and z.

Since eight different places in the truth tables are not filled in, there are a total of $2^8 = 256$ different possible ways to fill in these places. Therefore, there are 256 different networks with no self-input that all have the same cycle.

$(wxyz)_t$	$(wxyz)_{t+1}$	$(wxyz)_t$	$(wxyz)_{t+1}$
(0000)	?	(0001)	(1001)
(0010)	(0011)	(0011)	(0001)
(0100)	(0110)	(0101)	?
(0110)	(0010)	(0111)	?
(1000)	(1100)	(1001)	(1000)
(1010)	?	(1011)	?
(1100)	(0100)	(1101)	?
(1110)	?	(1111)	?

$(xyz)_t$	$(w)_{t+1}$	$(yzw)_t$	$(x)_{t+1}$	$(zwx)_t$	$(y)_{t+1}$	$(wxy)_t$	$(z)_{t+1}$
(000)	1	(000)	1	(000)	1	(000)	1
(001)	1	(001)	1	(001)	1	(001)	1
(010)	0	(010)	0	(010)	0	(010)	0
(011)	0	(011)	0	(011)	0	(011)	0
(100)	0	(100)	0	(100)	0	(100)	0
(101)	?	(101)	?	(101)	?	(101)	?
(110)	0	(110)	0	(110)	0	(110)	0
(111)	?	(111)	?	(111)	?	(111)	?

The simplest way to fill in these places is for them all to be 0. In this case, each element only depends on the state of two inputs and we recover the network proposed for salamander locomotion.

2.3 BOOLEAN FUNCTIONS AND BIOCHEMISTRY

In many enzyme and gene control systems the synthetic rates or the activity of key compounds display a **sigmoidal** (see Appendix A) dependence on the concentration of regulatory molecules, as in Figure 2.12.

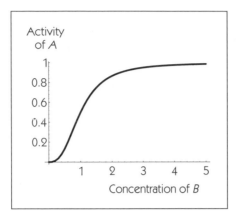

Figure 2.12
Activity of enzyme A as a function of the concentration of B for activation of A by B. $A = \frac{B^{2.7}}{1+B^{2.7}}$. This is an example of a sigmoidal function.

Although the details of how these control systems function are still the subject of active research, many of the mechanisms for the regulation of the synthesis and activities of enzymes and genes have been worked out. The sigmoidal functions that are experimentally found have suggested to theoreticians that biological control systems can be approximated by Boolean switching networks. See the following table.

B_t	A_{t+1}
1	1
0	0

The truth table approximating activation as a Boolean function.

B_t	A_{t+1}
1	0
0	1

The approximating truth table for inhibition.

The activity of some enzymes is controlled by compounds that are not the substrate of the enzyme, but which are believed to alter the configuration of the enzyme and thereby modify the activity of the enzyme. Examples of such **allosteric** activation and inhibition abound in biochemistry. If the activity of the enzyme is plotted as a function of the controllers, the kinetics are as shown in Figure 2.12. An idealization of these kinetics is that the activity of the enzyme can be modeled by a Boolean function—the IDENTITY function for activation, and the INVERSE function for inhibition.

Regulatory mechanisms also exist for the control of gene transcription. Recall that a **gene** is a segment of the DNA that carries the code for a specific protein. The gene is composed of sections called **exons** which carry the code for specific amino acid sequences in a protein, and of intervening sequences called **introns** which do not code for amino acid sequences.

Although all cells of the body carry the DNA instructions to code for all the proteins in the body, in any given cell only a subset of the proteins in the body will be made. Thus, in a given cell certain genes are expressed ("turned on") while others are not. Brilliant advances in molecular biology in recent years have reduced the problem of determining the sequence of the DNA problem to a technical matter. Given enough time and money it is possible to determine the genetic code for any organism. However, even after the genetic code in a given organism is known, the mechanisms that govern the ways in which the genes are expressed are still not completely known.

F. Jacob and J. Monod (1961) provided a major advance in our understanding of the expression of genes. They demonstrated the existence of control networks that could serve to provide flexible regulation of the synthesis of proteins in prokaryotes. Their work has led to much fruitful experimental work about enzyme systems in *E. coli*, and has now been largely substantiated for a number of individual cases.

In addition to structural genes, which specify the sequence of amino acids in the structural and enzyme proteins that are produced, Jacob and Monod showed that there are also regulatory genes that produce **repressors**. The repressor can be chemically bound to a portion of the DNA, called the **operator**, adjacent to the structural genes. If the repressor is bound, transcription of the structural genes is prevented. If the repressor is unbound, transcription is allowed.

The binding of repressor molecules to the DNA can be modulated by additional molecules in the cellular medium, which are thought to cause a conformational change in the repressor. Different mechanisms have been envisaged. For example, in **inducible** systems, a molecule called an inducer combines with the repressor, thereby preventing the repressor from binding to the operator. In

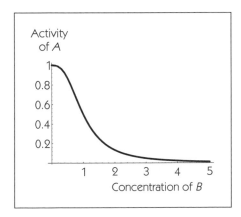

Figure 2.13
Activity of enzyme A as a function of the concentration of B for inhibition of A by B.
$A = \frac{1}{1+B^{2.7}}$.

E. coli the sugar lactose induces the production of β-galactosidase, an enzyme used to metabolize lactose.

A_t	R_t	E_{t+1}
1	1	1
1	0	1
0	1	0
0	0	1

Truth table for the induction of enzyme E by inducer A with the repressor R.

This example shows how biochemicals can conspire to produce a two-input Boolean rule for their generation (here Rule **11** from Table 2.1).

A different type of control can arise if the repressor is able to bind to the operator only after a third substance, called a **corepressor**, combines with the repressor. For example, tryptophan is a corepressor for the synthesis of tryptophan synthetase. This is the the NAND function, Rule **14** from Table 2.1.

R_t	I_t	E_{t+1}
1	1	0
1	0	1
0	1	1
0	0	1

R is a repressor. I is a corepressor of the synthesis of E.

The preceding discussion demonstrates that the control mechanisms, in which activities of proteins and genes are regulated by circulating molecules, can be modeled by Boolean functions. Thus, it has seemed to some that it may be feasible to build chemical computers, but this has not yet been carried out by humans. However, it has been conjectured that the dynamics of Boolean networks provide a framework for understanding complex dynamics and organization in the regulatory gene networks that are found in living organisms.

2.4 RANDOM BOOLEAN NETWORKS

Although nobody thinks that the gene control networks in living organisms are random, Stuart Kauffman (1969, 1993) has hypothesized that the connectivity of gene networks in living organisms might appear indistinguishable from a random network with the same number of nodes. The analogy between gene expression and Boolean networks led to the study of **random Boolean networks**. A random Boolean network is a perfectly ordinary Boolean network, where the choice of connections and Boolean functions is made randomly when the network is designed. There is nothing random about the process of iterating the dynamics of the network once it is designed—that process is the same for random Boolean networks as it is for any other "nonrandom" type of network.

To set up a random Boolean network, we select the number of nodes N and the number of inputs K to each node. Then, we use a random-number generator to select the inputs to each node. For example, for $N = 10$ and $K = 4$, the inputs to node 1 might be nodes 2, 5, 9, and 10. Next, for each node we randomly assign a Boolean function. Since there are 2^{2^K} Boolean functions of K inputs, picking a random Boolean function of K inputs can be accomplished by randomly selecting a number in the range 0 to $2^{2^K} - 1$, as in Table 2.1. Alternatively, we could set up the truth table for each element and then generate ones and zeros to populate it.

Kauffman was the first person to investigate the possible relationship between random Boolean networks and gene expression. In the 1960s he programmed a computer to iterate the dynamics of random Boolean networks and examined many different random Boolean networks for values of N between 15 and 8181.

He found the following types of behavior in networks with $K = 2$:

- A given network can have more than one fixed point or cycle. Typically, the number of fixed points or cycles increases approximately as $\sqrt{N}$ (see Figure 2.14).

- Starting in a randomly choosen initial condition, there is a startup transient before reaching the asymptotic behavior. (Of course, once a fixed point or cycle is reached, it is never left.) The length of the startup transient varies but is roughly the same as the longest cycle found in a network.

- The different cycles in a given network can have different lengths. The median length of a cycle scales roughly as $N^{0.3}$. Some cycles are much longer than this, though (see Figure 2.15).

- By perturbing the state of the network (i.e., "manually" flipping a node from 0 to 1 or vice versa), the dynamics may move from one asymptotic cycle to another. In the networks Kauffman studied there can be a

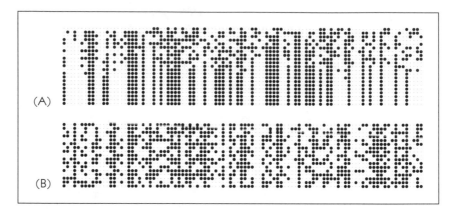

Figure 2.14 (A) A fixed point in a random Boolean network with $N = 100$ and $K = 2$. The transient lasts for twelve time steps. (B) A cycle of length 16. $N = 100$ and $K = 2$. Seventeen time steps are shown; note that the state in the first time step is identical to the state in the last one shown—once the network returns to its initial state, the network will cycle indefinitely.

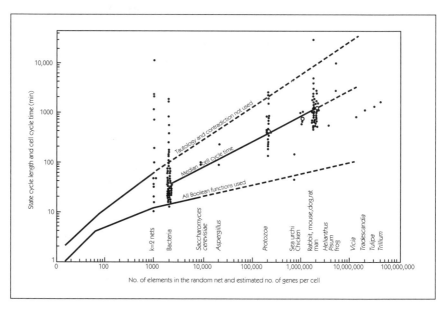

Figure 2.15 Typical cycle times versus number of Boolean elements for random Boolean networks, compared to the cell cycle time versus genome size for different organisms. Adapted from Kauffman (1969).

transition from a given asymptotic cycle to only a few other asymptotic cycles when one node is flipped.

Kauffman argues that in real cells, similar global behavior is observed (see Figure 2.15.) For a given organism, there are only a limited number of cell types, generally fewer than one hundred. Also, cell cycles are short, of the order of several hours. This corresponds roughly to the cycle lengths found by Kauffman, if one assumes that the time between iterates is the time it takes to turn a gene on or off—roughly one minute. Further, in many organisms, cells have only a limited ability to differentiate. They can only differentiate into a limited number of cell types, and these transitions will occur only if the cell is in the "right" place at the "right" time.

The "short" cycles observed by Kauffman correspond to a huge amount of dynamical order being generated by the random Boolean network. For Kauffman's networks with $K = 2$, the typical cycle has a length of roughly six time steps when $N = 200$. On the other hand, it has been found that for random Boolean networks where $K = N$, the cycle times are huge, roughly $2^{\frac{N}{2}}$. For $N = 200$ this is ten million times the estimated age of the universe (assuming 10^{-6} sec per transition). Thus, it seems that the specific N-input Boolean functions that arise from networks with $K = 2$ inputs produce much shorter cycles than randomly selected Boolean functions.

2.5 CELLULAR AUTOMATA

Gene networks consist of many different genes, each of which may have its own distinct regulatory mechanism. In contrast, some systems consist of many copies of the same thing, each regulated by exactly the same mechanism. For example, this is the case of the cells in living organisms, each of which contains the same set of genetic instructions. It might be thought that in a network of similar elements, all elements will behave similarly. This is often far from the case, however.

Motivated by the examples of living organisms, scientists have formulated the concept of a **cellular automaton**. In a cellular automaton, there are identical elements, usually located in a regular array that can be one-dimensional, two-dimensional, or even higher-dimensional. The update rule for each "cell" depends on that cell and some of its nearest neighbors as shown in Figures 2.16 and 2.17.

For the geometries drawn in these figures, the nodes on the edge of the automaton do not have as many neighbors as the nodes in the center. In order to make all nodes the same, it is conventional to connect the nodes on the edge to one another, so that one-dimensional cellular automata have the topology of a ring, and two-dimensional cellular automata have the topology of a torus.

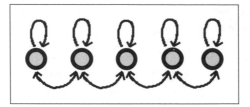

Figure 2.16 A geometry of a one dimensional cellular automaton in which each cell has two neighbors. In some cases, a connection is made between the two cells on the ends in order to form a ring.

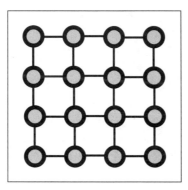

Figure 2.17
A geometry of a two-dimensional cellular automaton in which each cells has four neighbors. The cells on the edges can be connected to each other, forming a torus.

BOOLEAN CELLULAR AUTOMATA

In **Boolean cellular automata**, the state of each of the nodes is 0 or 1 and the nodes have a Boolean rule. One type of geometry for a one-dimensional cellular automaton has each node take input from itself and from its nearest neighbors on either side. Since there are three inputs, there are $2^{2^3} = 256$ possible Boolean rules. These cellular automata can produce varied types of behavior, depending on the rule and the initial condition. For example, the rule $(111) \rightarrow 0$, $(110) \rightarrow 0$, $(101) \rightarrow 0$, $(100) \rightarrow 0$, $(011) \rightarrow 1$, $(010) \rightarrow 0$, $(001) \rightarrow 1$, $(000) \rightarrow 0$ (which is conventionally named rule 10 because the binary digit 00001010 equals ten) produces left drifting stripes. In a "movie" of the automaton's activity, which Figure 2.18 depicts, these lines wrap around from one side to the other, as a result of the ring geometry. (The stripes can be either one or two nodes wide. Why?)

Not all rules produce such simple behavior. For example, rule 45 $((111) \rightarrow 0, (110) \rightarrow 0, (101) \rightarrow 1, (100) \rightarrow 0, (011) \rightarrow 1, (010) \rightarrow 1, (001) \rightarrow 0, (000) \rightarrow 1)$ produces a much more complicated pattern, as Figure 2.19 displays.

Another one-dimensional cellular automaton that produces interesting patterns is rule 90: $(111) \rightarrow 0, (110) \rightarrow 1, (101) \rightarrow 0, (100) \rightarrow 1, (011) \rightarrow 1, (010) \rightarrow 0, (001) \rightarrow 1, (000) \rightarrow 0$. Figure 2.20 shows the pattern gener-

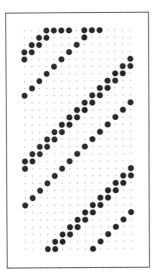

Figure 2.18
Activity of rule 10 in a cellular automaton with fifteen cells in a ring topology.

ated using rule 90 from a randomly selected initial condition. Such patterns can also be found in nature: A photo of a *conus* sea shell shows a strikingly similar pigmentation (see Figure 2.21).

Although one should not presume that this superficial resemblance implies anything controlling pattern formation in seashells, it is remarkable that such subtle patterns can be generated using simple algorithms. We will return to this subject further in Chapter 3.

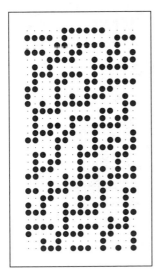

Figure 2.19
Activity of rule 45 for fifteen cells in a ring topology.

Figure 2.20
Activity of rule 90.

It is possible, of course, to have Boolean cellular automata with more than three inputs to each node. An early cellular automaton was the **game of "Life"** invented by the British mathematician John Conway in the 1970s. Conway imagined a two-dimensional geometry where each node is connected to itself and to its eight nearest neighbors. There are $2^{2^9} = 1.34 \times 10^{154}$ possible Boolean cellular automata with nine inputs, but Conway chose a particular rule inspired by interactions of living organisms with one another. Conway imagined that at any

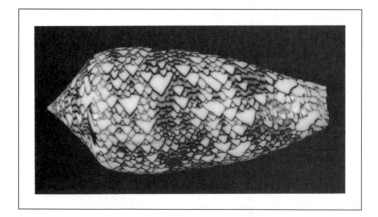

Figure 2.21   A conus sea shell.

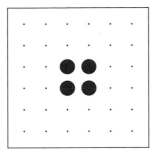

Figure 2.22
A fixed point in the "game of Life."

time each node was either "alive" (1) or "dead" (0). In order for a living cell to stay alive at time $t + 1$, either two or three of its neighbors have to be alive at time t. The rationale for this is that if fewer than two neighbors are alive, then life cannot sustain itself. If more than three neighbors are alive, then there is overcrowding and once again the conditions for staying alive are not met. On the other hand, if a node is dead and exactly three of its neighbors are alive, the node is "born" and becomes alive.

As whimsical as these rules may be, they do provide for a rich evolution starting from arbitrary initial conditions. Various forms of fixed points, cycles, and transients are possible. For example, an isolated square island of four living nodes is a fixed point (Figure 2.22), as is an isolated arrangement of eight living nodes surrounding a dead node. Periodic cycles are also possible: There is a cycle of period 2 involving a cluster of four and five cells (Figure 2.23).

NON-BOOLEAN CELLULAR AUTOMATA

Although we have just considered cellular automata in which the rules in each cell were Boolean functions, it is easy to imagine extending this concept so that variables may assume more than two values and other rules besides Boolean functions are allowed. For example, numerical schemes to solve partial differential

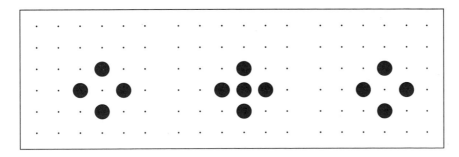

Figure 2.23 A cycle of period 2 in the "game of Life."

equations that represent dynamics in space can be thought of in terms of cellular automata. Consider the problem of diffusion. If we allow the state of each element to be any real number, we can make a cellular automaton model of diffusion along a line. If $c_t[m]$ is the concentration of the substance at site m at time t, then we can write $c_{t+1}[m]$ as a function of $c_t[m-1]$, $c_t[m]$, and $c_t[m+1]$:

$$c_{t+1}[m] - D(c_t[m-1] + c_t[m+1]) + (1-2D)c_t[m].$$

D is the diffusion coefficient, which describes how fast the substance diffuses. The activity of this cellular automaton is shown in Figure 2.24, where the initial condition is that a single node has a nonzero concentration of the substance. As time progresses, the substance diffuses out to other nodes.

There are many other physical and biological phenomena that have been modeled with cellular automata, including the patterns of coloration in animals, the immune system, interaction of predators and prey, aggregation of particles, fluid flow, structure of the visual cortex, organization of ant trails, and growth of bacteria.

EXCITABLE MEDIA

One important application of cellular automata relates to **excitable media**. There are many systems in which a wave of some sort can pass through a medium, after which the medium cannot support another wave until a suitable length of time, called the **refractory time**, has passed. For example, if a wave of fire burns through a forest, there cannot be another forest fire until enough vegetation has grown to support a new fire. Media that display the joint properties of wave propagation and refractoriness are called **excitable media**. Other examples

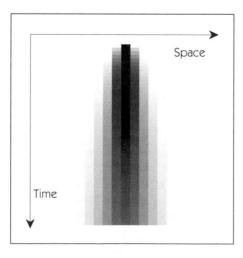

Space

Time

Figure 2.24
Diffusion in a cellular automaton.

include certain chemical media, such as the Belousov-Zhabotinsky reaction (see Figure 2.25) in which autocatalytic oxidation reactions take place, as well as neural and cardiac tissue.

If an excitable medium is two-dimensional (i.e., a sheet of medium, or a very thin layer), there are several fundamentally different geometries of waves that can be observed. In one, waves originate from a point source (e.g., the place where lightning started a forest fire) and spread in concentric circles. The effect is similar to ripples on a pond, except that two waves that meet will annihilate each other due to the refractory properties of the medium. Once the wave has moved off the edge of the medium, another wave will not occur unless it is started anew. An excitable medium—which is nonlinear—is fundamentally different than a linear medium. Waves in a linear medium, such as small waves on the surface of a pond, pass through one another, rather than annihilating each other.

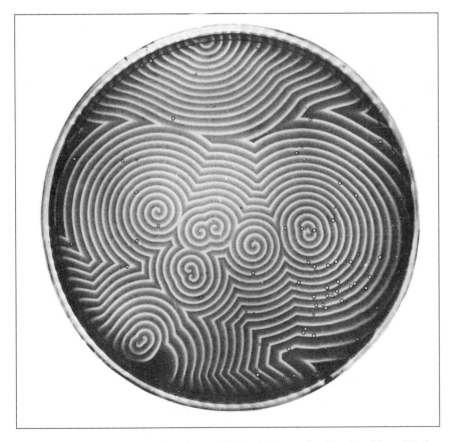

Figure 2.25 Waves in the Belousov-Zhabotinsky reaction. Reprinted from Winfree (1975). Copyright 1975 by the AAAS.

For an appropriate geometry of an excitable medium, waves can also move in closed circuits. Imagine an excitable medium arranged in the form of a ring. If a wave that propagates in one direction is started, it will eventually come back to its starting place. If the circumference of the ring divided by the speed of the wave is longer than the refractory period of the medium, the wave will continue circulating around and around the ring. In a linear medium, waves can also travel along a ring. However, the amplitude of the wave will eventually diminish due to dissipation of energy, and the wave will die out. In an excitable medium, the wave may never die out.

Another geometry of waves involves propagation of spiral waves of activity (see Figure 2.12). Here the wave moves in a circuit even though there is no hole in the medium. Instead, the wave is formed into a spiral and the "hole" is a functional one created from moment to moment by areas of refractory medium. The spirals can be stable, or can meander in complex geometries, or might even break up into multiple spirals (see Figure 2.26). Such phenomena are believed to underlie pathological patterns of excitation in cardiac tissue, called **tachycardia** and **fibrillation**. In tachycardia, the heart beats much more rapidly than normal. In fibrillation, the heart does not contract in an organized way and is ineffective in pumping blood; this condition is the immediate cause of death in perhaps one in three people.

Cellular automata provide a mathematical model for excitable media. Let each node be in one of several states:

Q Quiescent but excitable. This is the state of those nodes that are not carrying a wave, but that could do so if stimulated.

E Excited. This is the state of those nodes the wave is passing through at the present instant.

R Refractory. This is the state of nodes that a wave has recently passed through, and which have not yet recovered enough to become excitable.

The rules of the automaton are simple:

- If a node is quiescent at time t, then it stays quiescent at time $t + 1$ unless one or more of its neighbors is excited at time t, in which case the node becomes excited at time $t + 1$.
- If a node is excited at time t, it becomes refractory at time $t + 1$.
- If a node is refractory at time t, it becomes quiescent at time $t + 1$. Actually, it is often desirable to have the refractory period last more than one time unit. If this is the case, then when the node first becomes refractory it is assigned a value $r = T$. If the node has value r at time t, then its value becomes $r - 1$ at time $t + 1$. When $r = 0$, the cell is quiescent. T is the refractory period.

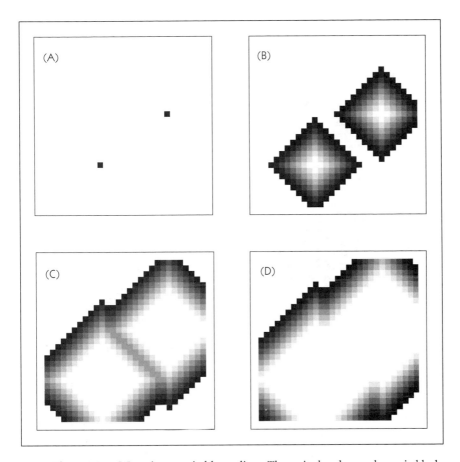

Figure 2.26 Waves in an excitable medium. The excited nodes are shown in black, the refractory nodes in shades of gray, and the quiescent nodes in white. Each node gets inputs from itself and from its four nearest neighbors. (A) Time $i = 0$. The medium is stimulated at two points to start waves. (B) Time $i = 8$. The waves spread out from each point. (C) Time $i = 14$. When the wavefronts touch, they annihilate each other. (D) Time $i = 17$. The waves will spread out until the whole medium becomes quiescent. No new wave will start until the medium is stimulated again.

These rules for cellular automata not only generate spreading waves, as seen in Figure 2.26, but also spiral waves as illustrated in Figure 2.27.

These rules can be modified to correspond to specific physical situations—for example, in heart tissue the refractory period can be made to depend on the time between excitations—but the essential rule for excitable media is simple: quiescent until excited, then refractory, then quiescent again.

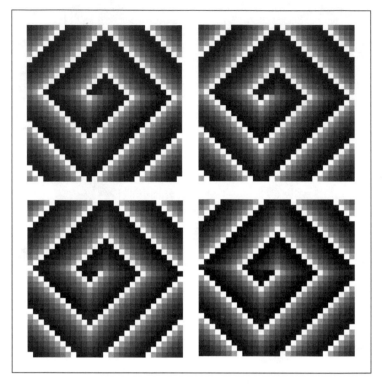

Figure 2.27 The state of the network in four successive times in a spiral wave in an excitable medium. The wave is rotating counterclockwise.

DYNAMICS IN ACTION

4 SPIRAL WAVES IN CHEMISTRY AND BIOLOGY

The study of excitable media has been one of the triumphs of applications of non-linear dynamics. For a detailed accounting, see Winfree (1987). We briefly mention two different aspects of excitable media: oscillations and waves in chemistry, and oscillations and waves in biological systems.

The earliest published report of an oscillating chemical reaction that we are aware of was published by W. C. Bray in 1921. This reaction uses very common ingredients that are easy to find. Bray's recipe is shown in the following table. Prepare a mixture at the concentrations shown. Heat to 60° C. If you follow this recipe you should be able to observe spatially homogeneous oscillations in which there is a slow buildup of a brownish color (I_2) and a rapid disappearance. It takes a bit of a time for the oscillation to set in, so be patient. We can only speculate whether periodic acid (Cotton and Wilkinson, 1980) is an intermediate in this reaction.

H_2O_2	0.19 M
KIO_3	.094 M
H_2SO_4	.073–.0961 N

The interest in oscillating chemical reactions and excitable media was stimulated in the early 1970s as news of the Belousov-Zhabotinsky reaction spread. A recipe for this reaction was given by Winfree (1972, 1980). Here is the recipe, but consult the original sources for a couple of tricks.

To 67 ml of water, add 2 ml of concentrated sulfuric acid and 5 gm of sodium bromate (total 70 ml). To 6 ml of this in a glass vessel, add 1 ml of malonic acid solution (1 g per 10 ml). Add 0.5 ml of sodium bromide solution (1 g in 10 ml) and wait for the bromine color to vanish. Add 1 ml of 25 mM phenanthroline ferrous sulfate and a drop of Triton X-100 surfactant solution (1g in 1000 ml) to facilitate spreading. Mix well, pour into a covered 90 ml Petri dish illuminated from below.

Once the reaction gets started you should see blue rings propagating from localized regions on a red background. If you give the dish a gentle shake to break up the rings, you will see spectacular geometries similar to those shown in Figure 2.25.

The observation of spiral geometries in living systems has important implications for human health. In the normal heart, a specialized region—the sinoatrial node—sets the frequency. However, in some dangerous cardiac arrhythmias, the frequency of the oscillation is set by the time it takes a wave of cardiac excitation to travel in a circuituous pathway. This type of mechanism is believed to underlie potentially fatal cardiac arrhythmias such as ventricular fibrillation. In order to record the activation of cardiac tissue in space and time, a new methodology has been developed in the past decade that promises to revolutionize the study of waves in excitable media, by using fluorescent dyes that respond to local changes in membrane potential or chemical concentrations. A dramatic demonstration of reentrant waves in cardiac tissue was given by J. M. Davidenko and coworkers (1992), who studied this type of wave in a piece of cardiac muscle in vitro (see figure on the next page). Spiral waves have been found in other biological systems, including aggregation of slime molds, where they are due to chemotactic mechanisms relying on pulsatile secretion of cyclic adenosine monophosphate (AMP). Spiral waves have also been associated with fluctuations of Ca^{2+} in amphibian oocytes.

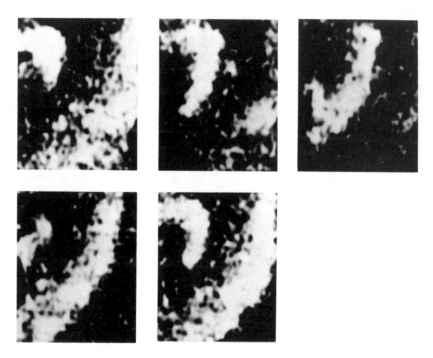

Spiral waves in cardiac tissue. From Davidenko et al. (1992). Reprinted with permission from *Nature*. Copyright 1992 Macmillan Magazines Limited.

Thus, spiral waves of activity can be observed in a wide range of different systems. These waves can be a chemical curiosity, a life-threatening condition, a vital step in the life cycle of amoeba, or of still-unknown significance (the Ca^{2+} waves). In each of these, the underlying physical and chemical mechanisms are certainly different. Yet, spiral waves emerge from the basic mechanism of wave propagation in excitable media that we have discussed and modeled in a simple way in the cellular automata. Therefore, in understanding spiral waves, it is as important to understand the mathematics of excitable media as it is to understand the specific mechanisms of halogen chemistry, the ionics of cardiac propagation, or cyclic AMP or Ca^{2+} metabolism.

2.6 ADVANCED TOPIC: EVOLUTION AND COMPUTATION

In the networks considered so far, the structure does not change in time. However, in many biological situations network structure and connectivities do change in time or **evolve**. Many unsolved problems in science involve understanding the mechanisms by which networks can change their structure.

In a biological organism, the inherited instructions are contained in the genes, and are called the **genotype**. The term **phenotype** refers to the visible properties of the organism as determined by the genotype and the environment.

Classical Darwinian evolution assumes that there is random phenotypic variation combined with selection of the fittest. Although Darwin did not know about genes, we now recognize that the phenotype is an expression of the genotype. Natural populations consist of organisms with different genotypes. The relative prevalence of a given genotype depends on the success of reproducing— the fitness—of the corresponding phenotype in preceding generations. There are two different types of mutations, point mutations and mutations in which segments of DNA recombine.

John Holland has used the term **genetic algorithm** to refer a vastly simplified computer simulation of biological evolution. Nevertheless, genetic algorithms implemented on computers preserve the following essential features of biological evolution: a population of genotypes, reproduction with mutation, and selection according to the phenotype. The presence of recombination distinguishes genetic algorithms from other types of search optimization algorithms.

In order to study the evolution of dynamical systems, investigators have studied cellular automata whose rules evolve in time. Since for a cellular automaton, the same Boolean rule is applied to every cell, we can consider the genome of a cellular automaton to be the sequence of ones and zeros in the output of the Boolean rule. A point mutation is caused when a 1 is randomly changed to a 0, and a recombination occurs when some of the ones and zeros from one rule are replaced with the ones and zeros from another. This provides all of the features for evolution, except for selection.

In nature, organisms are selected based on the ability of their phenotype to survive and reproduce in their environment. For cellular automata, we impose a selection criterion based on the performance of a computational task. One task that has been studied is the ability of a cellular automaton to perform the following computation—the determination of whether 50 percent or more of the cells in an initial condition are ON. If more than 50 percent of the cells are ON, the cellular automaton should approach a steady state in which all cells are ON. Otherwise it should approach a steady state in which all cells are OFF. If the cellular automaton has only a small local neighborhood, it is not known which cellular automaton can perform the task the best.

Norman Packard studied this problem for a cellular automaton in a class of 1-dimensional Boolean cellular automata in which the state of each element depends on itself and on its three nearest neighbors on each side—7 inputs altogether. Since there are $2^7 = 128$ different states of the inputs for each cell, there are $2^{2^7} = 2^{128}$ different cellular automata that can be constructed. This is an astronomically large number, and consequently it is impossible to study the dynamics of each member of this class. Since there is no theory that allows one to predict the dynamics of any given network without actually simulating it, it is necessary to search the space of different cellular automata.

Packard (1988) approached the problem using genetic algorithms. In the first generation a population of randomly generated cellular automata were iterated for many time steps for each of several different initial conditions. Each cellular automaton was rated based on its ability to carry out the assigned computational task. Then, in analogy to biological evolution, those cellular automata in the population that performed best were allowed to "reproduce" for the next generation. In addition, the cellular automata were allowed to interchange bits and pieces of their truth tables, and to mutate by changing entries in their truth tables. This yields a new population of cellular automata—generation 2. Once again each cellular automaton in generation 2 was tested against a set of new initial conditions. As before, the cellular automata reproduced and mutated. The process was continued for many generations.

Packard's work was preliminary and was subsequently redone and greatly extended by James Crutchfield, Raja Das, Peter Hraber, and Melanie Mitchell. Here, we present the most interesting results from the computer experiments performed by Das, Mitchell, and Crutchfield (1994). Figure 2.28 shows an illustration of the best cellular automaton that was found in generation 12. About 46 percent of the cells are OFF in the initial state and after 148 iterations, all the cells are OFF. Therefore, this cellular automaton has incorrectly classified the original distribution (though on many other initial conditions it comes up with the correct classification). This cellular automaton had a simple strategy for classifying figures. Unless there are large blocks that are all OFF cells, it will map to a state

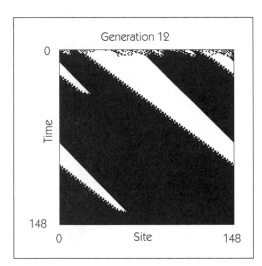

Figure 2.28
A cellular automaton that has evolved under selective pressure to perform the computational task of deciding if there are more ON or OFF cells at time zero. This one makes the wrong decision. Figure provided by James P. Crutchfield based on results in Crutchfield and Mtichell (1994) and Das, Mitchell, and Crutchfield (1994).

of all ON cells. Figure 2.29 shows the operation of the best cellular automaton in generation 18. Starting from the same initial condition, this cellular automaton correctly classifies the initial condition since all the cells converge to a OFF state. This system has developed a more sophisticated strategy for classifying the initial configuration based on transmitting information to make logical decisions about the initial condition. This is seen in the figure as the emergence over time of particles and particle interactions. The particles appear as boundaries between homogeneous regions. Their propagation and subsequent interaction implement

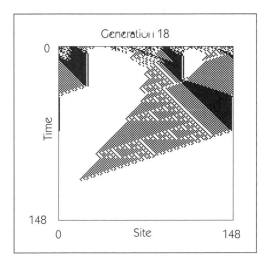

Figure 2.29
The best cellular automaton at generation 18 with the same initial condition as in Figure 2.28. This cellular automaton successfully classifies the initial condition and converges to a state in which all cells are OFF. Figure provided by James P. Crutchfield based on results in Crutchfield and Mitchell (1994) and Das, Mitchell, and Crutchfield (1994).

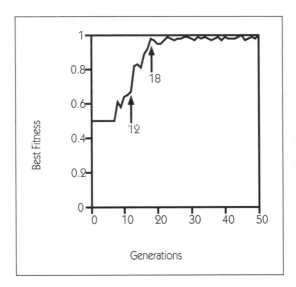

Figure 2.30 Best fitness in a population of cellular automata as a function of generation number. Generations 12 and 18 are marked with arrows. Figure provided by James P. Crutchfield based on results in Crutchfield and Mitchell (1994) and Das, Mitchell, and Crutchfield (1994).

the new computational strategy: Various logical decisions are made about large regions in which the initial condition's density was ambiguous.

What is interesting here is that over several generations, the genetic algorithm leads to an evolution in the truth tables so that the performance on this simple computational task improves over time. Figure 2.30 illustrates this evolution showing the increase of the best fitness over several generations. This is an important finding. It shows that one can simulate evolution in simple model settings. To figure out what is happening, we have to think about what strategy (computation) the cellular automata have been evolved to adopt in order to "survive"—almost as though they are alive. Thus, these sorts of simple models may provide the sorts of "data" that will help researchers formulate rules for evolution in complex systems.

SOURCES AND NOTES

To obtain an introduction to the mathematics of Boolean algebra see (Hohn, 1966).

Jacob and Monod (1961) and Monod *et al.* (1965) present early discussions of the control of cellular metabolism by gene networks. More recent texts provide introductions to genetic enzymatic regulatory mechanisms (Alberts, 1983;

Ptashne, 1986). Kauffman's (1969) original exposition of the properties of his model gene networks presents a provocative notion of how genes can be organized. The flowering of these ideas over the past quarter of a century is recounted in (Kauffman, 1993).

The analysis of excitable media is a very active area of current research with implications in physics, chemistry, and biology. Winfree (1980) gives some hints on how to get the Belousov-Zhabotinsky reaction to run (p. 301). Winfree (1987) presents a good introduction to the field with extensive references to problems in cardiac arrhythmias, aggregation of slime molds, and chemical oscillations. Gerhardt *et al.* (1990) demonstrated that many of the subtle properties of excitable media can be captured by cellular automata models and provide references to earlier studies of cellular automata models of excitable media. Experimental observation of spiral waves in cardiac tissue was carried out by Davidenko *et al.* (1992). Spiral waves of Ca^{2+} in oocytes were photographed by Lechleiter *et al.* (1991).

A discussion of logical models for lambda bacteriophage is given by Thomas, Gathoye, and Lambert (1976) and Thieffry and Thomas (1994). Thomas has been particularly interested in logical models for a variety of systems as reviewed in the monograph by Thomas and D'Ari (1990). A review of biological application of cellular automata models in diverse applications can be found in Ermentrout and Edelstein-Keshet (1993).

The study of computation and evolution has generated a significant interest among scientists and in the popular press. An important contribution was John Holland's (1975) formulation of the concept of genetic algorithms. Thinking about cellular automata from the perspective of mathematics and physics is ably reviewed by Stephen Wolfram (1983,1984), who is better known as the guiding force behind the development of Mathematica®. More recently, Packard (1988), Kauffman (1993) and others at the Santa Fe Institute in New Mexico have been pursuing the hypothesis that a simple generalization will be found that will have predictive value in explaining evolution in diverse settings. The hope is that a "law" will be found for evolution in complex adaptive systems of similar power to the second law of thermodynamics in closed chemical systems. Packard interpreted his results as indicating that on the computational task described in the text, there was evolution to the "edge of chaos". In another context, Crutchfield and Young (1989) analyzed computation at the "onset of chaos". Several recent popularizations (Waldrop, 1992; Lewin, 1992) have focused on the theme of evolution in complex systems.

In their careful studies, Mitchell, Hraber, and Crutchfield (1993) failed to reproduce the aspects of the original results of Packard that supported the argument that there was evolution to the "edge of chaos". They also gave theoretical arguments as to why Packard's results could not support the "edge of chaos" claim. Finally, they note that in finite state systems, there is no clear definition of "chaos" or the "edge of chaos".

Nevertheless, Mitchell et al. (1993) and Das et al. (1994) concluded that the conception of using genetic algorithms to evolve computation in cellular automata is an important idea, and they have made significant advances in understanding the evolution of computational strategies in cellular automata.

✐ Exercises

✐ **2.1** Explain the English-language names given to the Boolean functions of two inputs in Table 2.1. (HINT: The X in XOR stands for "exclusive." The N in NAND and NOR means "not." XNOR might make more sense if it were written NXOR, but that would be too hard to pronounce.)

✐ **2.2** Show that the network in Figure 2.31 and the following truth table are equivalent:

$(xy)_t$	$(xy)_{t+1}$	$(xy)_t$	$(xy)_{t+1}$
(00)	(10)	(10)	(11)
(01)	(00)	(11)	(01)

If the initial state at $t = 0$ is (00), then the network cycles through the states (00) → (10) → (11) → (01) → (00).... This network is frustrated, and the cycle of length 4 is the only possible activity for the network. Why?

Write down the truth table for the three-node inverting network shown in Figure 2.32, and determine all modes of behavior starting from any initial state. Is this network frustrated? What is the longest possible cycle in this network? How many possible states of the network are there? Show that there must be more than one cycle or fixed point.

✐ **2.3** Consider a single-input Boolean network with n components arranged in a loop. The nodes will be numbered $1, 2, \ldots, n$. We will write the state of

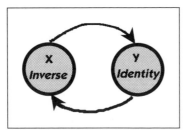

Figure 2.31

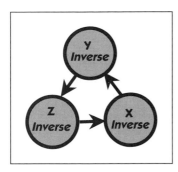

Figure 2.32

node k at time t as $x_t(k)$. The input to node 1 is node n. For all other nodes $k = 2, 3, \ldots, n$ the input comes from node $(k - 1)$. All the nodes follow the IDENTITY rule, except for node 1, which follows the INVERSE rule. This logical organization is a model for feedback inhibition, in which an end product can act to inhibit the production of an initial product. Start from an initial condition with $x_0(1)=1$ and $x_0(k) = 0$ for $k = 2, 3, \ldots, n$.

    a. What are the dynamics when $n = 2$?

    b. What are the dynamics when $n = 3$?

    c. Generalize this to all values of n.

✐   **2.4** The neural network shown in Figure 2.33 has been proposed as a model of a biological oscillator. The symbol ⊣ represents an inhibitory synapse and the symbol —< represents an excitatory synapse.

    Note that neuron 1 receives inhibitory inputs from neurons 3 and 4; neuron 2 receives excitatory inputs from neurons 1 and 3 and inhibitory input from

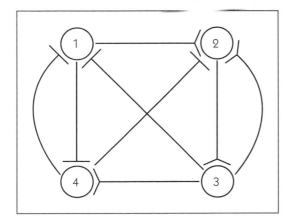

Figure 2.33

neuron 4, and so on. The truth table that relates the activity in this network at time t to the activity at time $t + 1$ is shown below.

State at time t	State at time $t + 1$	State at time t	State at time $t + 1$
(0000)	(1000)	(1000)	(1100)
(0001)	(0000)	(1001)	(0000)
(0010)	(0101)	(1010)	(0100)
(0011)	(0001)	(1011)	(0000)
(0100)	(1010)	(1100)	(1110)
(0101)	(0010)	(1101)	(0010)
(0110)	(0111)	(1110)	(0110)
(0111)	(0011)	(1111)	(0010)

    a. For each neuron, write the truth table for that neuron as a function of its inputs only.

    b. Assume that at $t = 0$ the state is (1000). Determine all future states until a steady state or cycle is reached.

    2.5 Consider a one-dimensional Boolean cellular automaton, where each cell takes input from its two neighboring cells but not from itself. The Boolean rule is

Input at time t	Output at time $t + 1$
(00)	0
(01)	1
(10)	1
(11)	0

Let there be ten cells in the network.

    a. Assume that at time $t = 0$, the state in three cells (of your choosing) is equal to 1. The rest are 0. In the chart below, follow the evolution as time proceeds for five iterations using the scheme shown below. (Remember that cell 1 is connected to cell 10, and vice versa.)

	x_1	x_2	x_3	x_4	x_5	x_6	x_7	x_8	x_9	x_{10}
$t = 0$										
$t = 1$										
$t = 2$										
$t = 3$										
$t = 4$										
$t = 5$										

Each square in your 10×6 array will have a 1 or a 0.

b. Consider the evolution of the system described above in the limit $t \to \infty$, but starting from any arbitrary initial condition at $t = 0$. Does an initial condition exist which will give rise to (i) a steady state, (ii) a cycle, (iii) or chaos (i.e., aperiodic dynamics)?

c. Give an upper limit (if one exists) for the length of a cycle in this system.

2.6 The following is a random Boolean switching network with three variables x, y, and z:

$(yx)_t$	z_{t+1}	$(yz)_t$	x_{t+1}	$(zx)_t$	y_{t+1}
(1 1)	0	(1 1)	0	(1 1)	1
(1 0)	0	(1 0)	0	(1 0)	0
(0 1)	0	(0 1)	0	(0 1)	1
(0 0)	1	(0 0)	1	(0 0)	0

a. Fill in the following table:

$(xyz)_t$	$(xyz)_{t+1}$	$(xyz)_t$	$(xyz)_{t+1}$
(111)		(011)	
(110)		(010)	
(101)		(001)	
(100)		(000)	

b. Determine the dynamics starting from all initial conditions.

c. How many steady states and cycles are there in this network?

✏ **2.7** Consider a two-dimensional 5×5 Boolean cellular automaton. The neighbors of any given cell are the four cells that share a common edge with that cell. The rule for evolution is as follows: The state of a given cell will be 1 at time $t + 1$ if the state of that cell or the state of any of its neighbors was 1 at time t. Otherwise the state of the cell will be 0 at time $t + 1$.

a. Choose three of the cells randomly and assume that the state of those cells is 1 at $t = 0$. Assume that the states of all the other cells in the network is 0 at $t = 0$. Draw a 5×5 grid and show the states of each of the twenty-five cells at $t = 0$.

b. Show the subsequent evolution of this system. At each time step, show the state of each cell (either 1 or 0) until either a steady state or a cycle is reached.

c. How many different ways could you have chosen the initial configuration in part a?

d. Find an initial condition with three cells in state 1 that gives the shortest transient until a steady state or a cycle is reached. Show this configuration, and give state the length of the transient.

✏ **2.8** A Kauffman network contains four elements w, x, y, and z where the activity of each element can be represented by a Boolean switching network.

$(yx)_t$	w_{t+1}	$(wz)_t$	x_{t+1}	$(xw)_t$	y_{t+1}	$(wy)_t$	z_{t+1}
(00)	0	(00)	1	(00)	1	(00)	1
(01)	1	(01)	0	(01)	0	(01)	1
(10)	1	(10)	0	(10)	0	(10)	0
(11)	0	(11)	1	(11)	0	(11)	1

a. Write a table that shows the state at time $t + 1$ given the state at time t for each of the sixteen possible states of the network.

b. How many fixed points and cycles are there in this network? What are they?

✏ **2.9** A Boolean switching network has three elements. The network displays the following transitions:

$$001 \rightarrow 011 \rightarrow 111 \rightarrow 110 \rightarrow 100 \rightarrow 000 \rightarrow 001 \rightarrow \cdots$$

$$010 \rightarrow 101 \rightarrow 010 \rightarrow \cdots .$$

a. Write a truth table that gives the state of the network at time $t + 1$ for each of the possible states at time t.

b. For each element of the network, indicate the inputs and the truth table that gives the output of that element as a function of the inputs.

c. Out of the 4096 different "Kauffman-type networks" with three elements and no self-input, how many will have the same dynamical behavior? Justify your answer. By "same dynamical behavior" we mean networks with two cycles, one with six states and the other with two states. In the cycle with six states, each state is different from the preceding state in one node only. The cycle of two states flips between two states that differ in all three nodes. HINT: This requires some thought. There are a couple of ways to get the answer. You might wish to think about different ways of generating frustrated networks with three elements.

✐ **2.10** What does it mean to pick a "random" Boolean function? A Boolean function of k inputs gives the output for any given combination of ones and zeros. For example, one of the Boolean functions of two inputs, AND, is $(00) \rightarrow 0$, $(01) \rightarrow 1$, $(10) \rightarrow 0$, and $(11) \rightarrow 0$. We know that for two inputs there are four possible input states (00), (01), (10), (11). If we adopt the convention that the input states will always be written in increasing order (in base 2), we can make a shorthand notation for this Boolean function of (0001), which reflects the output of the function for each of the four possible input states. Thus, the sixteen possible Boolean functions of two inputs can be written as

$$0000, 0001, 0010, 0011, \ldots, 1110, 1111.$$

If we read this in base 2, then these sixteen Boolean functions are just $0, 1, 2, 3, \ldots, 14, 15$. So, each possible Boolean function of two inputs has a unique identifying number.

Consider Boolean functions of k inputs, and describe how to generate the unique identifying number for them.

In studying random Boolean networks, we may not want to use the Boolean functions CONTRADICTION and TAUTOLOGY. Show that for Boolean functions of k inputs, these two functions have the identifying numbers 0 and $2^{2^k} - 1$, respectively.

COMPUTER PROJECTS

Project 1 Write a program to generate random Boolean switching networks where each element receives 2 inputs. Restrict yourself to networks in which there is no self input. Starting from an initial condition iterate the network until a steady state or cycle is reached. Your program should allow you to change the number of elements in the network.

Project 2 Generate 100 different random networks with 10 elements. For each network count the number of different cycles that you find starting from different initial conditions. It is necessary to test a large number of different initial conditions to guarantee that you have found all possible attractors. Find the mean number and standard deviation of the number of attractors per network.

Project 3 Now consider the influence of changing the number of elements of the network. As the number of elements increases, it is possible that the cycle can get astronomically long (but this does not happen too often). You will want to increase the number of elements in your network in a rather gradual manner, and figure out what to do if you never find a cycle. You might wish to consider the possibility of looking for cycles in a clever way. For example, suppose you just keep track of which elements change their states at each time step. What would happen if there is a periodic cycle? When Kauffman (1969) carried out this computation computers were rather primitive. You might wish to test your computing skills and your computers abilities to see how far up you can push the number of elements. Test to see if the cycle length and the number of cycles per network increase as the square root of the number of elements as was found by Kauffman.

Project 4 Generate random Boolean networks in which the number of inputs per element is different from 2. What happens to the cycle length and the number of cycles per network as a function of the size of the network?

Project 5 The game of "Life" and extensions provide students and recreational mathematicians with an interesting exercise: write a program to simulate the game of life. In doing this you should assume a geometry with cyclic boundary conditions. Generate random initial conditions and see what happens under subsequent iterations. How many different patterns can you find that represent repeating cycles?

Project 6 The following project is a difficult one, but would be a challenge to someone with interests in finite mathematics. Consider cellular automata that follow rule 90 with cyclic boundary conditions. Write a program to determine the number of different steady states and periodic orbits that are found for networks of different size as $t \rightarrow \infty$. In doing this you should try to take account of the cyclic symmetry so that two periodic cycles that only differ by their location on the ring are counted the same. Explore the way the number of attractors changes as the number of cells changes.

Project 7 Write a computer program to simulate wave propagation in excitable media. Vary the size of the neighborhood that can excite a given cell, the number of inputs that have to be active in the neighborhood of a cell to excite the cell, and the duration of time each element is excited or refractory. Assign different colors to excited states, excitable states and refractory states. Try to find an initial condition that will evolve to spiral waves. One way to do this is to start from an initial condition in which a wave of excitation covers a some of the space, but a free end is left dangling into the rest of the media. How close can you come to simulating spiral waves such as are observed in the Belousov-Zhabotinsky reaction?

CHAPTER 3

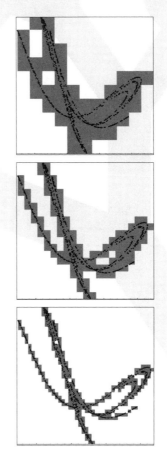

Self-Similarity and Fractal Geometry

If you cut a limb off a tree, the resulting object will resemble—in miniature—the tree itself. If you cut a branch off this limb, the shape of the resulting object will be similar to the limb and to the entire tree. If you cut a twig off this branch, it too will resemble the entire tree. The term **self-similar** describes the geometry of objects in which a small part when expanded looks like the whole.

Many objects encountered in nature and biology are self-similar. Examples include the geometry of the vascular system, the branching system of bronchi in the lungs; and the network of creeks, streams, and rivulets that flow into rivers. All these objects have treelike shapes.

But self-similarity is not limited to objects with treelike geometry. Some types of clouds are self-similar. Mountains often have small outcroppings that resemble the mountain as a whole. The shore of a lake or ocean often has inlets or bays, which often contain inlets or bays of smaller size themselves, and so on.

Of course, not everything is self-similar. If you remove a part from an automobile, the part will not look like a smaller version of the car. A single house in a neighborhood does not look like the neighborhood itself. An arm or a leg does not look like an entire body.

In this chapter we will discuss the geometry of self-similar objects, called **fractal geometry**. We will introduce the concept of **dimension** to describe the scaling of self-similar objects, and we will describe the relationship between fractal geometry and dynamics.

3.1   DESCRIBING A TREE

Suppose you were asked to develop a method for describing the shapes of trees. The reason for doing this might be to help in creating a theory that would link the shapes of trees to their environment—the stresses on branches from wind and snow, the availability of sunlight.

One way to describe the shape of a tree is to consider sections of branches as cylinders and to write down the length, diameter, and orientation of each cylinder. This might provide an accurate description, but not only would it require you to keep a long list of many cylinders, it would also be difficult to compare two trees to see if they are similar.

Another method for describing the shape of a tree is to look at the shape of the volume of space that contains the tree. For example, many types of fir trees resemble cones, while some deciduous trees roughly resemble spheres. Although this type of description is not very detailed, it makes it easy to compare the overall shapes of different trees.

Another possible type of description makes use of the self-similar structure of many trees. Since the structure of each limb or branch looks like the tree as a whole, but in miniature, you might quantify the self-similarity by use of a **scale factor**. For example, at the end of each branch many trees have two smaller branches separated by a certain angle. To describe the local geometry of the tree, you would need to use only two numbers: the angle between the two smaller branches, and the scale factor that tells how large the smaller branches are compared to the larger branch from which they stem. (To determine the scale factor, we take the ratio of the **lengths** of the parent and child branches, not their volumes or areas.) For three-dimensional trees, it makes sense to measure a second angle, which represents how the plane containing the two smaller branches intersects the plane containing the parent branch and its twin. To describe the whole tree, two additional numbers would be needed: the size of the main trunk and the size of the smallest twig. Given just these five numbers—two angles, a scaling factor, and the largest and smallest sizes—it is possible to write a computer program that draws realistic-looking trees.

How is this done? Assume for a moment that you have already written a program to draw a self-similar tree in two dimensions, and that it has the following name:

```
simpleTree(x, y, angle, length)
```

(The notation here is described in Appendix B.) This program will draw a tree with the base of its trunk at position (x, y), whose main branch (i.e., the trunk) goes at direction `angle`, and which has a height `length`. Let's also assume that the type of tree this program draws has a high degree of self-similarity: It looks like a trunk of length `length` and two copies of the whole tree, shrunk by a scale factor of $\frac{1}{2}$, growing out of the trunk's end, each at angle `theta` to the original. This suggests writing `simpleTree` as three parts:

1. Draw the branch.

2. Draw a copy of the whole tree coming out the top of the branch at the current angle plus θ.

3. Draw another copy of the whole tree coming out the top of the branch at the current angle minus θ.

As a computer program, this might be written as follows:

```
simpleTree(x, y, angle, length)
 double x, y, angle, length;
{  double topx, topy;
    topx = x + length*cos(angle);
    topy = y + length*sin(angle);
    drawLine(x, y, topx, topy);
    simpleTree(topx, topy, angle+theta, length/2);
    simpleTree(topx, topy, angle-theta, length/2);
}
```

A computer program of this sort is **recursive**, which means that the program is defined in terms of itself. Recursive programs are, therefore, self-similar. A very simple example of a recursive program is given in Appendix B.

You may be thinking that we still haven't adequately defined `simpleTree`, and you are right, but we are very close. An important point to keep in mind about real trees is that they are only self-similar up to a point. Small twigs don't have even-smaller twigs growing from them; they have leaves. We can finish our definition of `simpleTree` by specifying that if `length` is smaller than some predefined twig size, then instead of drawing the two small copies of the whole tree, we should draw a leaf. We can do this just by putting a dot at the position (x, y). The whole program now looks as follows:

```
simpleTree(x, y, angle, length)
 double x, y, angle, length;
{  double topx, topy;
```

```
if (length < twigSize)
    drawDot(x,y);
else{
    topx = x + length*cos(angle);
    topy = y + length*sin(angle);
    drawLine(x, y, topx, topy);
    simpleTree(topx, topy, angle + theta, length/2);
    simpleTree(topx, topy, angle-theta, length/2);
}
}
```

Now we have a complete definition of `simpleTree`, and we can set the computer to work. Figure 3.1 shows some results.

It would be silly to claim that the tree in Figure 3.1 is realistic; it is obviously extremely stylized. There are several reasons for this: Real trees are three-dimensional and are not perfectly self-similar; the branches of real trees are not line segments but have some amount of thickness, which decreases as one gets closer to the leaf; and the approximate self-similarity of real trees appears to require more than the three parameters used here (angle, relative length of each child branch).

Making the program only slightly more complicated allows us to draw a variety of much more realistic trees. The complication mostly involves specifying the angles of the branches in three-dimensional space. In addition, the branches are drawn with a thickness that depends on their length. Figure 3.2 depicts three-dimensional drawings of trees.

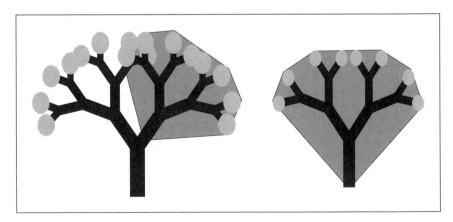

Figure 3.1 The simple two-dimensional tree shown here is self-similar. Each of the branches of the whole tree is a small copy of the whole tree.

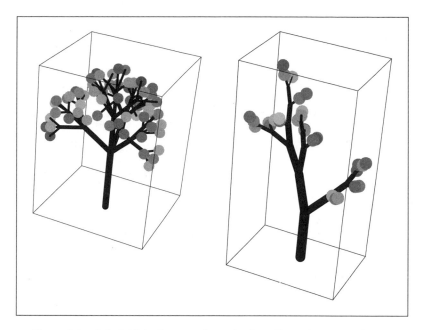

Figure 3.2 *Left*: Self-similar trees drawn in three dimensions. At each generation, four copies of the entire tree are drawn. One is vertical and the other three are tipped toward the base of the parent branch. *Right*: At each generation, two copies of the entire tree are drawn. The larger copy continues almost straight from the parent branch, while the smaller copy is tipped more towards the base of the parent branch.

This type of self-similar description of a tree is in many ways superior to a description based on cylinders, cones, or spheres. It is capable of representing realistic details of the structure of trees but at the same time requires only a few numbers, enabling ready comparisons between different trees. There is also an appealing possibility that the self-similar description is close to the biological mechanisms that generate the shape of a tree, since presumably the global structure of trees (e.g., spheres, cones) is a result of a purely local branching mechanism.

3.2 FRACTALS

Although the `simpleTree` program was recursive, it was not completely self-similar. At each step, in addition to drawing two smaller copies of the tree, we also drew a trunk.

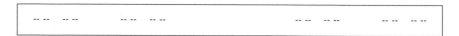

Figure 3.3   The Cantor set.

There are objects that are completely self-similar: They consist exclusively of smaller copies of themselves. One of the simplest of these self-similar shapes is called the **Cantor set**. The Cantor set consists of two copies of itself, and the length of each copy is one third the length of the whole set, separated by an empty region whose length is also one third that of the whole set (see Figure 3.3). We can write this as a recursive computer program.

We will introduce a new variable, t, that keeps track of how many times we allow the computer to make the recursive copies of the set. In an ideal mathematical sense, the true Cantor set puts no limit on t. For our computer representation of the set, because we have a limited amount of time and memory, we use t to limit the **depth of the recursion**.

We will start with t $= n$, and at each generation where we make recursive copies of the set, we will decrease the value of t by 1. When t == 0 we will stop the recursion and draw a line from x to x + length. The computer program for this follows:

```
drawCantorSet(x, length, t)
  double x, length, t;
{
    if (t == 0)
```

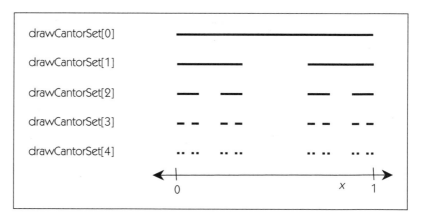

Figure 3.4   Computer approximations to the Cantor set, showing the sets produced by a recursive generation of the Cantor set with recursion depth set as indicated in brackets. Note that drawCantorSet[1] consists of two copies of drawCantorSet[0], and that drawCantorSet[2] consists of two copies of drawCantorSet[1] and so on. The true Cantor set is $\lim_{n\to\infty}$ drawCantorSet[n].

```
      drawLine(x, 0, x+length, 0);
  else {
      drawCantorSet(x              , length/3, t-1);
      drawCantorSet(x + 2*length/3, length/3, t-1);
  }
}
```

The output produced by this program for various values of t is shown in Figure 3.4.

It's easy to imagine how to construct self-similar shapes where more than two copies are made at each generation.

Interesting self-similar shapes can be drawn in two dimensions. The "Sierpiński gasket" is a shape that consists of three copies of itself, each of which is half the size of the whole set. Each of the three copies is placed at the vertex of an equilateral triangle. The program to generate this is:

```
drawGasket(x, y, length, t)
  double x, y, length, t;
{   double newx, newy;
   if (t == 0)
      drawTriangle(x, y, length);
   else {
      drawGasket(x,          y,                    length/2, t-1);
      drawGasket(x+length/2, y,                    length/2, t-1);
      drawGasket(x+length/4, y + 0.433012*length, length/2, t-1);
   }
}
```

The only complicated part of this program is the calculation of where to put the various copies of the set. The variables x and y hold the position. The particular values used (e.g., 0.433012) can be found by trigonometry. To limit the depth of the recursion, we will draw a triangle of the appropriate size when t reaches 0. See Figure 3.5 for sample output.

As another example, the "Koch snowflake" is a self-similar shape that consists of four copies of itself, each of which is one third the size of the whole set. Figure 3.6 shows an emerging approximation to the ideal set.

3.3 DIMENSION

In Euclidean geometry, a *point* is zero-dimensional, a *line* is one-dimensional, a *plane* is two-dimensional, and so on. What is the dimension of the various self-similar sets shown in Section 3.2? The traditional view of the meaning of "the dimension of an object" is that it gives the number of values needed

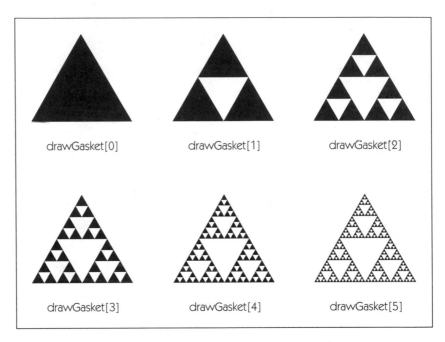

Figure 3.5 Computer approximations to the Sierpiński gasket set. drawGasket[1] consists of three copies of drawGasket[0] and so on. Although in this figure draw-Gasket[0] is drawn as a triangle, any shape of the appropriate size could be used.

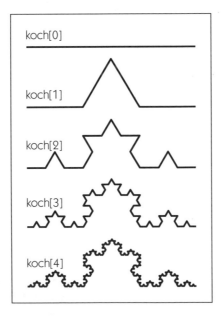

Figure 3.6
Computer approximations to the Koch snowflake. koch[t] gives a recursive generation of the set to recursion depth t. Note that koch[1] is made of four smaller copies of koch[0], koch[2] is four smaller copies of koch[1], and so on.

to specify the position of a point on the object. For instance, one value needs to be given to specify the position of a point on a line, two values (the "x" and "y" coordinates) need to be given to specify the position of a point on a plane, and so on.

Here, we will explore another meaning of "dimension," which is based on the idea of self-similarity, but which reduces to the traditional meaning when applied to familiar Euclidean objects such as lines and planes. To make a connection between self-similarity and the concept of dimension, consider how to give a self-similar description of a one-dimensional object: a line segment. One way to do this is to say that a line segment of length l consists of two copies of itself, each of length $\frac{l}{2}$:

```
lineSegment(x, length, t)
 double x, length, t;
{
    lineSegment(x,              length/2, t-1);
    lineSegment(x + length/2, length/2, t-1);
}
```

The progression of line segments drawn this way all look the same.

Now, imagine how to draw a familiar two-dimensional object: a filled-in square. We can give a self-similar description as four copies of itself, each of length $\frac{l}{2}$:

```
filledSquare(x, y, length, t)
 double x, y, length, t;
{
    filledSquare(x,              y,              length/2, t-1);
    filledSquare(x+length/2, y,              length/2, t-1);
    filledSquare(x,              y+length/2, length/2, t-1);
    filledSquare(x+length/2, y+length/2, length/2, t-1);
}
```

Two quantities characterize each of the self-similar shapes we have studied:

- the number of self-similar copies: N
- the edge length of the original relative to each copy: ϵ.

The following formula can be used to define a dimension D for an object:

$$D \equiv \frac{\log N}{\log \epsilon}. \tag{3.1}$$

Applying this definition to the various self-similar objects we have studied here, we can make the following table of values for N, ϵ, and D:

Object	N	ϵ	D
Line segment	2	2	1
Filled square	4	2	2
Cantor set	2	3	0.631
Gasket	3	2	1.585
Snowflake	4	3	1.262

For the line segment and the filled square, the definition of dimension in Eq. 3.1 gives the same value as the familiar concept of dimension. For the Cantor set, the gasket, and the snowflake, the dimension is a fraction. For this reason, these objects are called **fractals**. Obviously, it's hard to interpret a fraction as "the number of variables needed to specify a position on the object." The definition of dimension in Eq. 3.1 provides an extension of the concept of dimension from the familar Euclidean objects of lines and planes to the world of self-similar objects.

Where does the definition of dimension in Eq. 3.1 come from? Recall that the area of a square of edge-length l is l^2, and that the volume of a cube of edge-length l is l^3, and that the length of a line of length l is, obviously, just l. Let's use the word **bulk** to refer to an abstract concept of which length, area, and volume are examples. For Euclidean objects of dimension D, the bulk of an object with an edge-length l is proportional to l^D:

$$\text{``bulk''} \quad \text{is proportional to} \quad l^D.$$

(The constant of proportionality depends on the particular shape of the object. For example, the area of a circle of diameter l is $\frac{\pi}{4} l^2$ and the volume of a sphere of diameter l is $\frac{\pi}{6} l^3$.) For self-similar objects, one way to measure the "bulk" is to count the number of self-similar copies. If there are N copies each with a characteristic edge length ϵ, then we expect that the total bulk is related to the dimension of the object:

$$N \quad \text{is proportional to} \quad \epsilon^D.$$

Taking the log of both sides leads to Eq. 3.1, which concludes the explanation of how that equation was derived.

DYNAMICS IN ACTION

5 THE BOX-COUNTING DIMENSION

Equation 3.1 gives a formula for calculating the dimension of a fractal object if we know the number of self-similar copies, N and the size of the original relative to each copy, ϵ. But suppose we have only an object, such as a lung with its treelike branches, or a river, or a snowflake. How do we estimate the dimension of an object?

One simple technique for calculating the dimension of an object is directly motivated by the definition of dimension given in Eq. 3.1. The procedure is as follows:

1. "Cover" all the points in the object with boxes of edge-length ϵ_0. If the object is a photograph or a map, then the boxes will be squares. If the object lives in the three-dimensional world, then the boxes will be cubes. Count how many such boxes there are, calling the result $N(\epsilon_0)$.

2. Repeat step (1), using boxes that have edge-length $\epsilon_1 = \frac{\epsilon_0}{2}$. Then repeat again using $\epsilon_2 = \frac{\epsilon_1}{2}$, and again with $\epsilon_3 = \frac{\epsilon_2}{2}$, and so on. By doing this, we construct a function $N(\epsilon)$ sampled at the values $\epsilon = \epsilon_0, \epsilon_1, \ldots$.

3. In theory, the dimension D is the number such that

$$\lim_{\epsilon \to 0} N(\epsilon) = A\epsilon^{-D},$$

where A is a constant. In practice, D can be estimated as

$$D = \frac{\log N(\epsilon_{i+1})/N(\epsilon_i)}{\log \epsilon_i/\epsilon_{i+1}}. \tag{3.2}$$

The difficult part is selecting an appropriate value for i. In general, one chooses i to be as large as possible in order to approximate the limit $\epsilon \to 0$. But keep in mind that for physical objects, it may not make sense to make the boxes infinitely small. For example, in studying the fractal shapes produced in growth (see the *Dynamics in Action* 8 box, later in this chapter), it is inappropriate to make the boxes smaller than a single cell or particle.

The example in the figures shows a calculation of the box-counting dimension for a fractal object, the chaotic attractor of the Ikeda map. The Ikeda Map is described in Chapter 6. For now, it simply serves as a convenient way of generating a fractal object whose self-similarity is not obvious to the eye.

$$x_{i+1} = 1 + 0.7(x_i \cos t_i - y_i \sin t_i) \tag{3.3}$$

$$y_{i+1} = 0.7(x_i \sin t_i + y_i \cos t_i) \tag{3.4}$$

where $t_i = 0.4 - \frac{6}{(1+x_i^2+y_i^2)}$. Using numerical iteration, the program generated 1000 points and plotted them out as pairs (x_{i+1}, x_i).

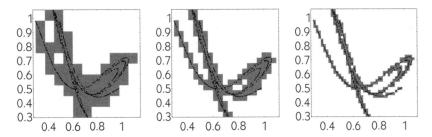

Left: The attractor of the Ikeda map, covered with boxes of edge-length $\epsilon_0 = 0.08$. Forty-three boxes are needed. *Middle*: One hundred ten boxes of edge-length $\epsilon_1 = 0.04$ are needed. *Right*: Two hundred fifty boxes of edge-length $\epsilon_2 = 0.02$ are needed.

By covering the Ikeda attractor as shown in the figures, we find that for $\epsilon_1 = 0.04$ there are 110 boxes used to cover the object, and that for $\epsilon_2 = 0.02$ there are 250 boxes used. Substituting these values into Eq. 3.2, we find that the dimension is $D \approx 1.2$. Note that in this case, it does not make sense to set the dimension of the boxes much smaller than $\epsilon_2 = 0.02$, because at some point only one of the 1000 points will be in each box, and making the boxes smaller will not increase the number of boxes needed to cover the points.

3.4 STATISTICAL SELF-SIMILARITY

In geometry the word "similar" means "not differing in shape but only in size or position." The fractals we have studied in the previous section are self-similar in this geometric sense.

In everyday language, "similar" means "alike" and does not have as narrow a meaning as in geometry—two things can be alike even if they are slightly different. The self-similarity of real trees makes use of this common meaning of "similar."

We do not expect that all branches of a tree will look the same, just that they will look somewhat like the tree as a whole.

It is often worthwhile to consider self-similarity in a statistical sense, and say that an object is self-similar if its parts, on average, are similar to the whole. For example, the coastline of a continent contains gulfs and bays, and the gulfs and bays themselves contain smaller bays and inlets, which themselves contain coves and other small structures.

DYNAMICS IN ACTION

6 SELF-SIMILARITY IN TIME

Imagine a whale, a human, and a bat listening to the same sound. Will all three hear the same thing? The auditory systems of all three mammals are roughly the same, but owing partly to the extreme differences in size, they hear different frequency ranges. Whales are tuned to very low frequencies that propagate well for long distances through the ocean; bats are highly developed to hear the very high frequency sounds that are used in echolocation; and humans hear best in the familiar 20–20,000 cycles-per-second (hertz) frequency range that we call the "audio range." So, if the whale, human, and bat were listening to, say, Mozart's "Clarinet Concerto in A," the human would hear the music, while the whale and the bat might hear something that sounds very different. Since there are other frequencies in music besides the audio ranges, whales and bats would also hear sound but it would probably not sound much like Mozart as we know it.

Let us think about the music in a more general way. The music is a *signal*, that is, a quantity that varies in time. There are lots of different frequencies in the music. It is common to analyze signals by considering how "loud" different frequency bands are. A more precise meaning for "loud" is the energy of a signal in a given frequency range. For example, in many concerts and recording studios the energy in specific frequency ranges can be amplified separately (this is what goes on in those complex sound equalizers that you see people fiddling with in concerts). Of course, the amount of energy in each frequency band is a very crude measure of the signal generated. Therefore, from this perspective the music of Mozart would likely be very similar to that of Guns 'n' Roses.

We have already seen how spatial structures, such as the Cantor set, can be self-similar in space. It is also possible for temporal signals to be **self-similar in time** in a statistical sense, but here the meaning is a bit different. We say that a temporal signal is self-similar when it has, for example, the same energy in the 20–200 Hz range as it has in the 200–2000 Hz range, and in the 2–20 Hz range and any other range from kHz to 10 kHz. This self-similarity is often termed **1/f noise**.

Mozart and Guns 'n' Roses are not self-similar when the audio range is considered. However, very low frequency fluctuations in their loudness are indeed self-similar. Voss and Clarke (1975) looked at the loudness of different types of music in the frequency range from 0.001 Hz to 0.1 Hz and found that it was $1/f$.

Signals that display $1/f$ noise are surprisingly common and are observed in all sorts of different situations such as the arrival times of telephone calls, the intrinsic noise in semiconductors, the density of urban automobile traffic, the level of the Nile river, and the rate of the human heartbeat. In all these cases the mechanisms responsible for $1/f$ noise are still being investigated.

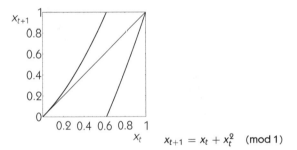

$$x_{t+1} = x_t + x_t^2 \quad (\text{mod } 1)$$

The name "$1/f$ noise" suggests that the signal is generated by a random process. Indeed, it is impossible to imagine that clustering characteristics of telephone calls made by independent individuals arise from a deterministic process. It seems unlikely that only one mechanism will be universally applicable to such diverse situations. Indeed, a number of different deterministic and random processes have been shown to produce $1/f$ noise. To give some idea about the various ways of producing $1/f$ noise, we illustrate one deterministic model and one random model that generate $1/f$ noise.

A simple, deterministic, one-dimensional finite-difference equation, proposed by I. Procaccia and H. G. Schuster (1983), generates $1/f$ noise. Procaccia and Schuster

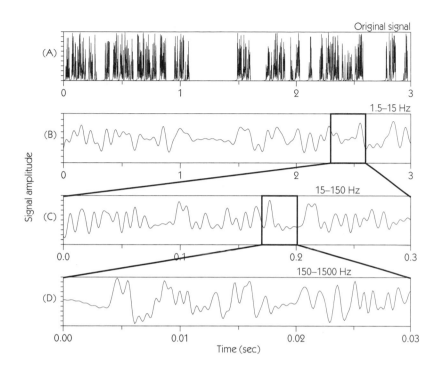

(A) A signal generated by Eq. 3.5. (B) The signal in (A) filtered to include only the range 1.5–15 Hz. (C) The signal in (A) filtered to include only the range 15–150 Hz. Note that the time scale is 10 times larger than in (B). (D) The signal in (A) filtered to include only the range 150–1500 Hz. Note that the time scale is 100 times larger than in (B).

considered the equation

$$x_{t+1} = x_t + x_t^2 \bmod 1, \tag{3.5}$$

the graph of which is shown on the previous page. If x_0 is near zero, then x_t grows very slowly at first, then faster, and then shows a kind of "bursting" behavior where x_t oscillates very rapidly until it is "reinjected" back near zero. Then, the phase of slow growth starts again, and the cycle repeats. However, the duration of the slow-growth phase depends sensitively on how close to zero the reinjected value of x is. This results in slow-growth phases of varying lengths, as seen in Figure A above.

We can take the signal shown in Figure A and filter it to include only those components in a given frequency range. If we take the range from 1.5 to 15 Hz (where we have assumed that one iteration of Eq. 3.5 takes 0.0001 sec), then the signal shown in Figure B results. Figures C and D show the results of filtering using higher frequency ranges. Note that all three filtered signals look similar, even though they are plotted on very different time scales.

Self-similar signals can also be generated by random processes. A simple example involves computer random-number generators. We take a set of random-number generators and arrange the first so that it makes a new random number every time step, arrange the second so it makes a new random number every second time step, the third so that it changes every *fourth* step, the next so it changes every *eighth* step, and so on. At each time step, the output of all of the random numbers is totaled.

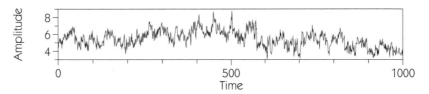

A self-similar signal generated using random numbers.

Let us now consider a physiological signal—the heartbeat. Since the heartbeat can easily be recorded by placing electrodes on the surface of the body, it is possible to record heartbeats continuously over one or more days. Of course, although it is easy to record the heartbeats, it is not so easy to interpret the signals. Since heart disease is a deadly problem, computer calculations are cheap, and doctors' fees are high, there is a great deal of interest in determining computer algorithms that can aid diagnosis based on the timing of heartbeats. The figure on the next page shows a recording of one of the authors' heart rates.

There is a practical limit to the ranges over which signals can be self-similar. For instance, the human heart rate is self-similar for frequency ranges as low as one cycle per day (and maybe lower—the long measurements needed to find out are rare) and as high as one cycle every sixty seconds. For the frequency ranges where self-similarity appears, it may offer an important clue to the dynamics of the systems that generate the signal.

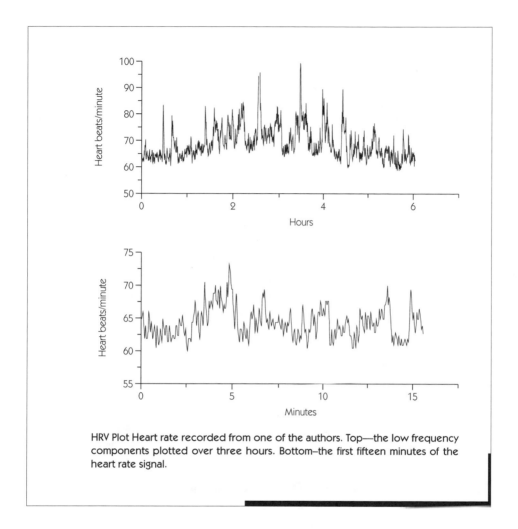

HRV Plot Heart rate recorded from one of the authors. Top—the low frequency components plotted over three hours. Bottom–the first fifteen minutes of the heart rate signal.

3.5 FRACTALS AND DYNAMICS

As we have seen, the term **fractal** refers to the geometry of objects that are self-similar. The term **dynamics** refers to how things change in time. Fractals and nonlinear dynamical systems are related in quite subtle and fascinating ways. In this section, we will give some examples of the relationship.

THE "FRACTAL GAME"

Consider a simple game introduced by M. F. Barnsley: Draw an equilateral triangle on a piece of paper and label the vertices A, B, and C. Make a mark anywhere inside the triangle. Now toss a die. If it comes up 1 or 2, place a new mark halfway between the old mark and A; if the die comes up 3 or 4, place the new mark halfway between the old one and B; if the die comes up 5 or 6, place the new mark halfway between the old one and C. Repeat this many times, always using the latest mark as the reference point for placing the next mark. After many tosses of the die, the resulting picture will look like the Serpinski gasket in Figure 3.5. Figures 3.7 and 3.8 depict the results after 3, 100, 1000, and 5000 rolls of the die, respectively.

How can this simple game produce a structure with as much detail as the Serpinski gasket? Since a random die is involved, why is the result of the game always almost exactly the same whenever it is played?

The "Fractal game" is a discrete-time dynamical system similar in many respects to the finite-difference equations studied in Chapter 1.* As shown in Figure 3.9, the initial position is somewhere in the ABC triangle. If the first toss of the die gives A, then regardless of where the initial position was in ABC, the new mark must be made in the top triangle. If the first toss of the die gives B, the new mark must be in the lower left triangle, and if the toss gives C, the new mark must be in the lower right triangle. Thus we know for certain that independent of the outcome of the first die toss, the new mark will be somewhere in the set `drawGasket[1]`.

The same logic applies to the second toss of the die—but this time we already know that the previous mark was `drawGasket[1]`. Exactly where the mark will be placed depends both on the initial position and on whether the first two tosses of the die were AA, AB, AC, BA, BB, BC, CA, CB, or CC. But after the second toss, the mark will be somewhere in `drawGasket[2]`. Similarly, after three tosses of the die, the mark will be somewhere in `drawGasket[3]`, and so on. This means that

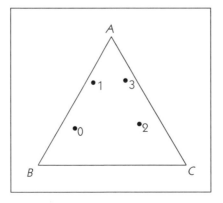

Figure 3.7
The initial condition and first three moves of the "Fractal Game."

---

* The game is also different in many respects from the systems studied in Chapter 1. Those systems were deterministic, meaning that given the state at time t, the state at time $t + 1$ could be calculated. In the Fractal Game, there is a random or stochastic element, and so the dynamics are not deterministic.

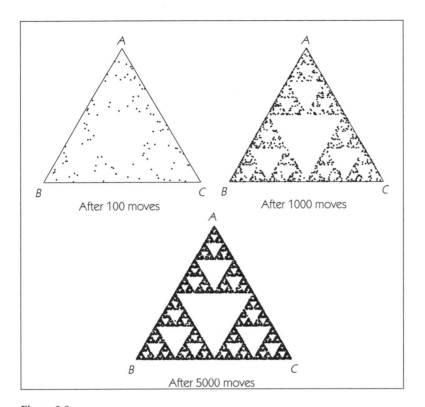

Figure 3.8

drawGasket [n] is an attractor that we are guaranteed to reach after *n* steps of the game.

So we know that after *n* steps the mark (and all future marks) will be somewhere on drawGasket [n]. Why aren't the points that we draw concentrated in some small region of drawGasket [n]? This is where the random nature of the die comes in. After each die toss, the new mark is placed in the part of drawGasket [1] identified with the letter that came from that toss. As long as the die tosses include at least one A, B, or C, then at least one mark will be made in each of the three triangles. After each *pair* of die tosses, the new mark is placed in the one of the nine triangles of drawGasket [2] that corresponds to the appropriate pair of letters (see Figure 3.9). As long as the series of die tosses includes at least one of each of the nine possible pairs AA, AB, AC, BA, BB, BC, CA, CB, and CC, then each of the nine triangles in drawGasket [2] will have a mark placed in it. If we have many more than nine die tosses, then we're virtually certain to represent all the triangles. Similarly, triplets of die tosses correspond to the twenty-seven triangles of drawGasket [3], and so on.

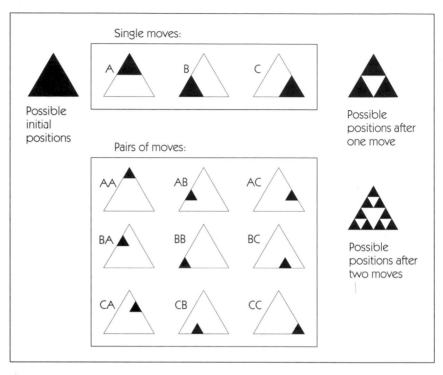

Figure 3.9   The initial position in the fractal game can be anywhere in the triangle. After the first toss of the die, the new mark must be in one of the three smaller triangles. After two tosses, the new mark must be in one of the nine very small triangles.

CELLULAR AUTOMATA

The three-input Boolean cellular automaton with rule 90 (see Section 2.5) generates self-similar patterns. The process starts with a single ON-site, and then two ON-sites appear after the first iteration. Already we see the seeds of self-similarity: One parent has led to two children. These two children go on produce two children, but with sufficient space between them that their offspring can have the same configuration as the original ON-site. The two children produced by the fourth iteration are spaced exactly the right distance apart to reproduce the whole configuration, eventually producing two points that again reproduce the whole configuration, and so on (see Figures 3.10 and 3.11).

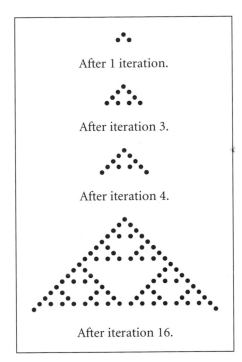

After 1 iteration.

After iteration 3.

After iteration 4.

After iteration 16.

Figure 3.10
Dynamics of the three-input Boolean cellular automaton with rule 90, with a single ON-site as an initial condition.

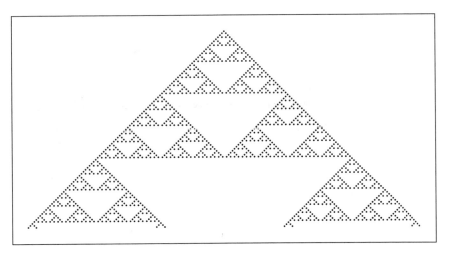

Figure 3.11   The cellular automaton generates an approximation to the Sierpiński gasket that improves as the number of iterations increases.

DYNAMICS IN ACTION

7 RANDOM WALKS AND LÉVY WALKS

If we put a crystal of colored soluble salt in a clear liquid solution, ions spread out in the liquid, leading to a slow coloration of the liquid. This process is an example of **diffusion**. Diffusion plays an important role in many processes in biology, for example the exchange of oxygen and carbon dioxide in the lungs, the absorption of some liquids and nutrients in the gut, and the transport of drugs from the blood to target organs. Diffusion occurs on a molecular scale. This is different from other processes such as bulk fluid flow in which there is motion of macroscopic volumes of fluid associated with an expenditure of energy. Diffusion requires no expenditure of energy and will continue until all differences in concentration are eliminated.

Although we now understand that the physical mechanism underlying diffusion is random displacements due to collisions occurring on a molecular scale, the original observations of the random motions that underly diffusion were not at all understood and make for a fascinating story in the history of science. In his botanical studies in 1827, Robert Brown used a microscope to observe pollen grains in water. He saw them moving about in an erratic fashion. Since the pollen grains were derived from a plant, the first guess was that the movement of the pollen reflected a "vital force" and that the pollen grains were "alive". To test this hypothesis, Brown first looked at particles derived from organic sources. In recounting his findings he wrote, "Reflecting on all the facts with which I had now become acquainted, I was disposed to believe that the minute spherical particles or Molecules of apparently uniform size, . . . were in reality the supposed constituent or elementary molecules of organic bodies, first so considered by Buffon and Needham . . . " However, a control experiment was needed. Brown continues, "Rocks of all ages, including those in which organic remain have never been found, yielded the molecules in abundance. Their existence was ascertained in each of the constitutent minerals of granite, a fragment of the Sphinx being one of the specimens observed." The open-minded Brown rejected his original hypothesis.

Brown was a botanist and did not realize that the motions he saw were associated with collisions between the particles and liquid. It took another 75 years before Albert Einstein recognized the connections between the random motions observed by Brown and the physical process of diffusion. Nevertheless, Brown's careful observations immortalized his name. We now call random motions similar to those observed by Brown **Brownian motion** or a **random walk**.

The mathematics of Brownian motion is often studied using simple models. The simplest is called the drunk random walker. The drunk random walker takes steps of equal size in any direction. Before each step he chooses a new random direction and takes a step. Imagine a large number of drunk random walkers all starting out from the same place at the same time (with deference to Einstein, we might call this a *gedrunken* experiment.) As time proceeds the initial high concentration of random walkers spreads out, invading regions of lower concentration. There are two important questions concerning this process: What is the distribution of random walkers as a function of time? and What is the average distance that a single walker is expected to go in a given time?

The spatial distribution of random walkers is well described by a bell-shaped, Gaussian distribution. This type of distribution arises in many fields and we will discuss it in more detail in Chapter 6 and Appendix A. For the moment we only consider the walkers' displacement from the start to the end of their walks. Although the walkers are assumed to be moving at a constant velocity, their path takes so many twists and turns that the total displacement is, on average, proportional to $\sqrt{t}$.

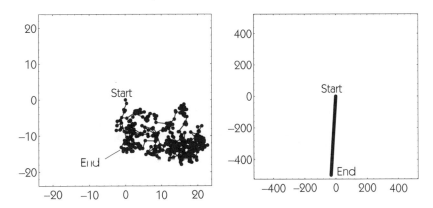

Left: A random walker starts from $(0, 0)$ and takes steps in a random direction. The steps tend to cancel each other out, and the walker does not get very far. On average, if the walk lasts for t time units, the distance between the start and the end is proportional to $\sqrt{t}$. 500 steps are shown. *Right*: A purposeful walker starts from $(0, 0)$ and takes steps in a single direction. The distance between start and end is proportional to t. 500 steps are shown.

For purposeful movement, the start-to-end displacement increases at a rate proportional to t. The drunk random walker therefore does not get very far compared to his sober friends walking at a constant velocity.

The result found for a drunk random walker—that when walking for duration t, the average start-to-end displacement is proportional to $\sqrt{t}$—does not depend on all steps being the same size. For example, suppose that the step size itself varies randomly from step to step, with each step size being drawn from a Gaussian distribution. In this case, we obtain the same results as above (but the constant of proportionality different is different).

Since the total walk has a gaussian probability distribution, and each step has a gaussian probability distribution, the whole is similar to each of the parts. In this sense, a gaussian random walk is self-similar. Likewise, a purposeful walk is self-similar—each step looks like a miniature copy of the whole walk.

There are other situations in which a random walk is self-similar. For example, suppose that the distribution of step sizes, $p(R)$, is proportional to $(R^{3-\alpha})$, where $p(R)$ is the probability that the step size will be between R and $R + dR$. This is a **power law** distribution of steps, and for $2 < \alpha < 3$, the start-to-end displacement is proportional to $t^{\frac{4-\alpha}{2}}$. The random walk with a power-law distribution of steps is in between the purposeful walking case (corresponding to $\alpha = 2$) and the drunken random walker (corresponding to $\alpha = 3$).

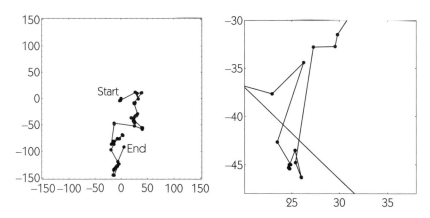

Left: A walker takes steps in random directions, with the length of each step chosen from a self-similar power-law distribution $p(R) = R^{3-\alpha}$. Here, $\alpha = 2.03$. 500 steps are shown. *Right*: A magnification of a small part of the random walk shown in Figure .

The above figure shows a power-law random walk with $\alpha = 2.03$. There are 500 steps shown in the walk, although it appears that there are many fewer steps. Most of the steps are very small, and the dots appear to overlap. If we zoom in on a small section of the walk, we can see the smaller steps in more detail, and that even on short segments of the walk there is additional detail that is similar to the walk as a whole. These self-similar walks were originally discussed by the mathematician Paul Lévy. Random walks with self-similar dynamics and power-law scaling are now called **Lévy walks**.

One difficulty in studying power-law walks is that there is no typical step size— steps of all sizes occur. For instance, the mean step size for a power-law walk is infinite. This can make it difficult to compare power-law walks with other types of walks. In the figures shown here, it has been assumed that the walker's velocity is constant on each step, so that large steps take longer than short steps. Thus, if the path traced out by each of the walkers were straightened out, each path would be the same length.

The recognition that some physical processes are best described by Lévy walks has important implications in the observation of time series. Very large jumps are possible. Even though very large jumps may be very rare, they nevertheless inevitably occur and contribute quite substantially to the start-to-end displacement. As a consequence of the large steps, the estimate of the average displacement found for small times can be considerably different from the estimate of the average displacement found for large times.

ESCAPE!

In Chapter 1, we studied the finite-difference equation

$$x_{t+1} = Rx_t(1 - x_t).$$

Because we interpreted x_t to be the population density of flies at time t, we imposed the restriction $0 < R \leq 4$. As long as $0 < R \leq 4$, any value of x_t in the range $0 \leq x_t \leq 1$ would produce a value of x_{t+1} in that same range. By iteration, we can see that if x_t is in that range, all future values will also be in that range.

Consider the case where $R > 4$. This makes it possible for x_{t+2} to become negative even when $0 \leq x_t \leq 1$. (Of course, this doesn't make physical sense if we interpret x as the population density of flies, but there are other situations where it might make physical sense.) For example, examine the case where $x_0 = \frac{1}{2}$. This produces $x_1 = R/4$, which is greater than 1 if $R > 4$. Iterating once again, we see that $x_2 = \frac{4R^2 - R^3}{16} < 0$. Since $x_2 < 0$, all future values will be less than zero and will asymptotically approach $-\infty$.

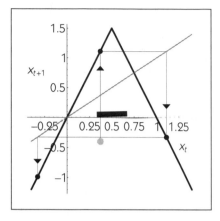

Figure 3.12
The tent map with $b = 3$. Initial conditions in the darkened interval will escape to $-\infty$.

The quadratic map is not the only map that has escapes to $-\infty$. Consider the **tent map** (see Figure 3.12):

$$x_{t+1} = \begin{cases} bx_t & \text{if } x_t \leq 1/2 \\ -bx_t + b & \text{if } x_t > 1/2. \end{cases} \tag{3.6}$$

The iterates of the tent map can escape to $-\infty$ for $b > 2$. For this example, we will set $b = 3$.

We can use the cobweb method of iteration to demonstrate that if the initial condition is anywhere in the darkened interval $[\frac{1}{3}, \frac{2}{3}]$, the iterates will escape to

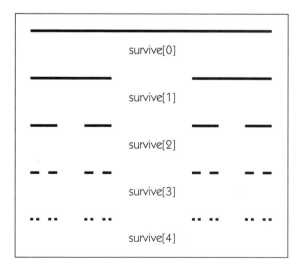

Figure 3.13   Initial conditions that do not escape from $[0, 1]$ after the indicated number of iterations.

$-\infty$. Are there any other points in the interval from 0 to 1 that will also escape? The answer is yes. Any initial condition that gets mapped into the darkened interval will eventually escape to $-\infty$.

Are the points that escape to $-\infty$ rare or common? To answer this question, consider all the points that do not escape the interval $[0, 1]$ after one iteration. Call these points survive[1], because they survive for *at least* one iteration in the interval $[0, 1]$. It's easy to see that survive[1] consists of all points in $[0, 1]$ that are not in $[\frac{1}{3}, \frac{2}{3}]$. (survive[0] is the whole interval $[0, 1]$.)

What does the set survive[2] look like? Look at Figure 3.14, which shows that it is the set of points that get mapped into survive[1] by a single iteration. The points in survive[2] are called the **preimages** of the points in survive[1]. If we draw survive[1] on the vertical axis, then we can see what points get mapped into survive[1] by tracing backward to the map and then down. Because the tent map consists of two segments (one sloping up, and the other sloping down), survive[2] consists of two copies of survive[1].

A similar argument allows us to derive survive[3] from survive[2], and, generally, survive[n] from survive[n-1], see Figure 3.13 for the results. The process is exactly like drawing the Cantor set. The set of points that survive forever is $\lim_{n \to \infty}$ survive[n], which is the ideal Cantor set.

We know that the Cantor set has a dimension $D = \frac{\log 2}{\log 3} \approx 0.631$. You might think this means that the probability of a randomly chosen initial condition having iterates that never escape is 63.1 percent. This is wrong. In fact, the probability that a randomly selected initial condition will survive for n iterations is given by the total length of the line segments that comprise survive[n]. There are 2^n segments, each of which has a length $(\frac{1}{3})^n$, giving a total length of $(\frac{2}{3})^n$. As $n \to \infty$, this total length approaches zero. For example, the probability that a randomly selected initial condition in $[0, 1]$ will survive for 20 iterations is $(\frac{2}{3})^{20} = 0.0003$. Points that survive the dynamics of the tent map for many iterations are very rare. The fact that the dimension of $\lim_{n \to \infty}$ survive[n] is 0.631 means that between any two points of $\lim_{n \to \infty}$ survive[n] there is an interval of points that do escape.

❏ **EXAMPLE 3.1**

For $b = 3$, calculate the dimension of the set of points that *do* escape to ∞ in the tent map, as well as the dimension of the set of points that do *not* escape.

Solution: To find the dimension of the set of points that escape, start by noticing that you need one segment of length $\frac{1}{3}$ to cover the set of points that escape $[0, 1]$ in one iteration, and five segments of length $\frac{1}{9}$ to cover the set of points that escape in two or fewer iterations. At any iteration t, let N_t be the number of segments needed to cover the set of points that escape, and let

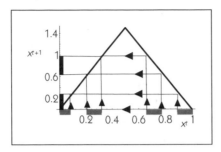

Figure 3.14   The tent map transforms the points in survive[2] (shown in gray) into the points in survive[1] (shown in black). By drawing survive[1] on the vertical axis and using the cobweb method in reverse, we can derive the intervals that are in survive[2]. survive[2] consists of two smaller copies of survive[1]; one arises from the left side of the map and the other arises from the right side of the map.

each segment be smaller by a factor of $\epsilon = 3$ than the segments in the previous iteration. By inspecting Figure 3.13 carefully, we can conclude that $N_{t+1} = 3N_t + 2^t$. This situation is different from the cases we have studied so far, where $\frac{N_{t+1}}{N_t}$ is a constant. Here, there is no single fractal dimension for finite t, but if we consider $\lim_{t \to \infty}$, we find that the dimension is

$$\frac{\log \left(\lim_{t \to \infty} \frac{N_{t+1}}{N_t} \right)}{\log 3} = \frac{\log(3 + \lim_{t \to \infty} 2^t/N_t)}{\log 3} = \frac{\log 3}{\log 3} = 1.$$

To see that the term $\lim_{t \to \infty} 2^t/N_t = 0$, we note that since $N_t > 3^{t-1}$, then

$$0 \geq \frac{2^t}{N_t} < \frac{2^t}{3^{t-1}} = 2 \left(\frac{2}{3} \right)^{t-1}.$$

The rightmost term $\to 0$ as $t \to \infty$, therefore $0 \geq \frac{2^t}{N_t} < 0$ as $t \to \infty$.

We have already seen that the points that do not escape are a Cantor set, which has dimension 0.631. It may seem paradoxical that the line segment between 0 and 1, a one-dimensional object, can be divided into two sets, one with dimension 1 and the other with dimension 0.631, but keep in mind that the set of points that do not escape form a "disconnected dust."

FRACTAL BASIN BOUNDARIES

Many of the dynamical systems we have studied can have more than one eventual outcome, depending on the starting condition. Sometimes the initial conditions that lead to different asymptotic states are neatly distinct; sometimes, as in the dynamics of escape in the quadratic map, the different basins of attraction are interleaved in a complicated way. In the case of the logistic map, there is only a "dust" of initial conditions that eventually leads exactly to the unstable fixed point at the origin or at $(R-1)/R$. Similarly, a "dust" of points lies on unstable periodic cycles (see Figures 1.26 to 1.29) or leads exactly to such points. All other initial conditions result in escape to $-\infty$. For other maps, though, two or more basins of attraction may be interleaved in a fractal way, without one of the basins being a "dust."

As an example we consider a one-dimensional, nonlinear, finite-difference equation such as we studied in Chapter 1. The equation

$$x_{t+1} = x_t + a + b\sin 2\pi x_t \qquad \text{(mod 1)} \qquad (3.7)$$

is often used as a theoretical model for the interaction of two oscillators. Here, a and b are real constants, and (mod 1) means that we consider only the fractional part of the expression. (For example, 1.27 mod 1 is 0.27.) Therefore, starting from any initial condition x_0, we generate a sequence of numbers that lie between

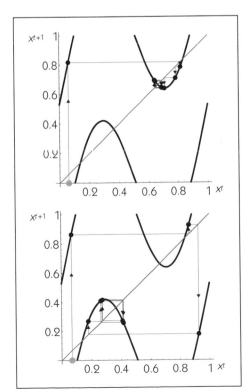

Figure 3.15
Dynamics of Eq. 3.7 for two nearby initial conditions:
Top—$x_0 = 0.06$ leads to a cycle of period 2.
Bottom—$x_0 = 0.07$ leads to a cycle of period 4. Any initial condition $0 \le x_o \le 1$ will lead to one of these two cycles.

0 and 1. The study of the dynamics of this equation as a function of a and b is a difficult problem that is still not completely understood. Here we look at a small aspect of this problem by considering the dynamics starting from different initial conditions and seeing what happens asymptotically in the limit $t \to \infty$. Consider the case for which $a = 0.53$ and $b = 0.62$. The graph of the equation is shown in Figure 3.15. There are two different stable periodic cycles in this map: a cycle of period 2 ($x_t \approx 0.667$, $x_{t+1} \approx 0.651$) and a cycle of period 4 ($x_t \approx 0.399$, $x_{t+1} \approx 0.298$, $x_{t+2} \approx 0.420$, $x_{t+3} \approx 0.248$). Starting from any initial condition such that $0 \leq x_0 \leq 1$, the dynamics will approach one of the two different stable behaviors: There is multistability. For example, when $x_0 = 0.06$ we approach the cycle of period 2, and when $x_0 = 0.07$ we approach the cycle of period 4.

Now we consider what happens when starting from all initial conditions. Figure 3.16 shows which initial conditions lead to the cycles of period 2 and to those of period 4; initial conditions that approach the period-2 cycle are shaded black, and all initial conditions that approach the period-4 cycle are shaded white. Clearly there are large regions where it appears that two nearby initial conditions lead to the same eventual result. If we zoom in on a small region of the set of initial conditions, we can see that there are often gaps in the regions that appear continuous. As we try to define more precisely the boundary between black and white, we see an increasingly fractured boundary. One cannot draw a single line

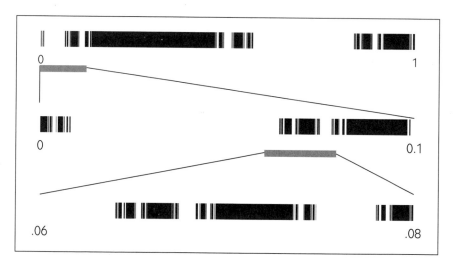

Figure 3.16 The initial conditions $0 \leq x_0 \leq 1$ of Eq. 3.7 that eventually lead to the cycle of period 2 are marked in black, while conditions that lead to the cycle of period 4 are white. Zooming in on a small section (for example, $0 \leq x_0 \leq 0.1$) reveals additional structure and shows that the seemingly continuous black zones are in fact broken into smaller zones interrupted by white. A further zooming-in to initial conditions shows still further structure. This example is based on Martinez-Mekler et al. (1986).

as the boundary, no matter how finely we search. The basins of attraction for both the period-4 and period-2 cycles are fractal—and are a type of Cantor set.

THE MANDELBROT SET

The dynamics of Eq. 3.7 produce a complicated interweaving of attractor basins in one dimension. Even more complicated and beautiful patterns can be produced in two dimensions. Consider the map

$$z_{t+1} = z_t^2 + c. \tag{3.8}$$

Since we haven't specified the value of c, we actually have a family of maps, parameterized by c.

Using the tools we developed in Chapter 1, we can easily find the fixed points of this family of maps and their stability. We find the fixed points, z^* by solving $z_{t+1} = z_t^2 + c$ to get

$$z^* = \frac{1 \pm \sqrt{1 - 4c}}{2}. \tag{3.9}$$

The stability is given by the value of

$$\frac{dz_{t+1}}{dz_t} = 2z_t$$

at the fixed points. Any fixed point that has a value $|z^*| < \frac{1}{2}$ will be stable because $\left| dz_{t+1}/dz_t \right|_{z^*} \right| < 1$. With a little algebra, we can show that a fixed point of Eq. 3.8 is stable for $-\frac{3}{4} < c < \frac{1}{4}$. For values of $c < -2$ or $c > \frac{1}{4}$, the iterates of Eq. 3.8 escape to ∞.

Notice that there are some values of c for which the values of the fixed points in Eq. 3.9 are **complex**. For example, for $c = 0.26$, the fixed points are at $z^* = 0.5 \pm 0.1i$, where $i \equiv \sqrt{-1}$. If we take z_0 to be purely real, then there is no way to reach these complex fixed points, because all future values of z_t will be real. However, if we allow z_0 to be complex, then future values of z_t can also be complex. Alternatively, if we allow c to be complex, then the complex fixed points of Eq. 3.8 are relevant to the dynamics.

One way to explore the dynamics of Eq. 3.8 for complex numbers is to iterate Eq. 3.8 starting at the initial condition $z_0 = 0$ for many different values of c, and look to see whether the iterates escape to ∞. Since each value of c is a point in the complex plane, we can draw a picture, placing a black dot at that point if the iterates escape to ∞ and a white dot if the iterates do not escape. The pictures drawn in this way show a complicated structure, with increasing detail becoming evident when looking at smaller and smaller regions of c. The set of values of c for which the iterates of Eq. 3.8 do not escape to ∞ is called the **Mandelbrot set**. (For a precise description of the manner in which the Mandelbrot set can be drawn, see the Computer Project 3.)

Benoit Mandelbrot is the mathematician who coined the word "fractal." He has had a tremendous influence on the development of the mathematics of fractals and the realization of the importance of fractals in describing the geometry of natural objects. His brilliant manifesto, *The Fractal Geometry of Nature* (1982), has become a classic and can be read with enjoyment and interest by both the mathematically naïve and the mathematically sophisticated.

The Mandelbrot set has quite a subtle relationship to the finite-difference equation, Eq. 1.6. For any purely real value of c, Eq. 3.8 is equivalent to Eq. 1.6.

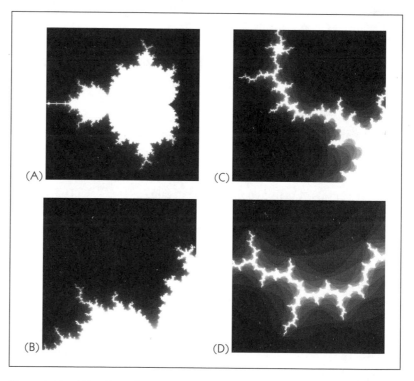

Figure 3.17 (A) Values of c in Eq. 3.8 for which $x_0 = 0$ eventually escapes to ∞ are marked in black. (Well, almost. See Computer Project 3.) Corner is $c = -1.8 - 1.3i$ and the upper right corner is $c = 0.8 + 1.3i$. (B) Zooming in to the rectangle $c = 0 - 1.5i$ to $c = 1 - 0.5i$ shows further detail. (C) Zooming in to $c = 0.25 - 1.3i$ to $c = .4 - 1.15i$ shows more detail still. (D) Zooming in to $c = 0.345 - 1.29i$ to $c = 0.36 - 1.275i$ shows further detail.

For any single map (corresponding to a specified value of the parameter c), one can ask which initial conditions eventually escape to ∞. It may be, as in Section 3.5, that the set of initial conditions that do not escape is a disconnected dust. For any one map, either this set of points is a dust or it is not. The Mandelbrot set describes for what values of c (i.e., which specific maps in the family of maps given by Eq. 3.8) the set of initial conditions that do not escape is a disconnected dust.

DYNAMICS IN ACTION

8 FRACTAL GROWTH

The next time you take a hike in the mountains, look carefully at the lichens, the trees, the rocks, the clouds, the rivers. The shapes of these objects are much more complicated than the shapes you studied in elementary Euclidean geometry courses. In the natural world fractal geometries abound. Yet, it is not clear how the objects have grown and evolved to the fantastic shapes you will observe. As a step toward understanding the generation of fractal geometries, we consider two simple schemes for growing objects. Although each scheme is easy to state and readily implemented on a computer, mathematical analysis of the geometries of each scheme are difficult problems treated only using advanced mathematical techniques.

The first steps in an Eden growth model.

The **Eden model** for growth assumes that one starts with a single cell and that this divides into two cells, the daughter cells divide, and so forth (Eden, 1961). To simulate the process, Murray Eden programmed 1960s-vintage computers. He assumed that there is a square lattice. Initially, at $t = 0$, there is one cell in the lattice. At $t = 1$, a single cell is added randomly to one of the four positions adjacent to the initial filled square, giving rise to a configuration in which two cells are filled. At $t = 2$, a third cell is randomly added to one of the six squares that are adjacent to the two cells filled at $t = 1$. The process continues in similar fashion, always adding a cell in a randomly chosen location adjacent to cells already filled, as shown in the figure on the previous page. Although this process is extremely simple, the resulting geometries have fractal boundaries! Is this simple model at all relevant to any growth process observed in nature?

Eden growth after 500 steps.

Vicsek et al. (1990) believe that it is. They carried out experiments with the bacteria *E. coli*. They started out with a line of cells inoculated in a nutrient-rich agar solution. After four days the *E. coli* colony displayed the geometry outlined in the figure on page 140. This can be contrasted with the geometry obtained from numerical simulation of the Eden model, which also starts from a line of initial cells. Statistical analysis of the two geometries reveals that there are some differences, reflecting differences in the growth processes between the model system and the bacterial colony. For example, in the bacterial colony growth can occur in the vertical direction (i.e., out of the two-dimensional grid), so that the samples consist of many layers leading to a smoother surface in the two-dimensional projection.

In the above situation, the medium is nutrient-rich. However, in similar experiments, dramatic changes were noticed depending on the growth occurring in nutrient-rich or nutrient-poor solutions. Matsuura and Miyazima (1993) carried out experiments in which the fungus *Aspergillus oryzae* was grown under a variety of conditions

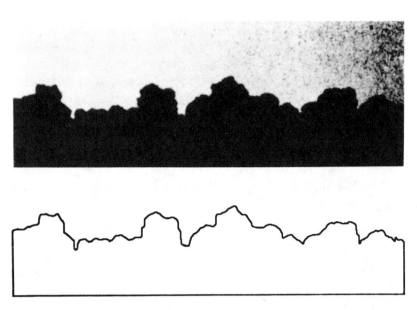

Growth in an *E. coli* colony. From Viscek et al. (1990).

of nutrient, temperature, and medium stiffness. When the nutrient was rich, top panel, they observed similar geometries to those found earlier for the growth of bacteria. However, when the nutrient was poor, the geometry displayed elaborate branching patterns. It is easy to understand one reason why there should be differences. In a nutrient-rich case, all points on the boundary have adequate nutrition and an equal probability of growing—this gives rise to "Eden" growth. In a nutrient-poor medium, points on the boundary that grow out will have a growth advantage over neighboring points, because they will deplete their immediate surrounding region of nutrient. New nutrient will diffuse in and will not be available elsewhere. Consequently, once the initial outgrowths get started, they will thrive in comparison to neighboring regions, giving rise to exotic efflorescence. Of course, this does not provide a complete picture since the resulting geometry depends in subtle ways on rates of growth as a function of nutrient, medium stiffness, and temperature.

A detailed theoretical model for growth in fungi has not yet been developed. However, a simple theoretical model for growth closely related to the Eden model reproduces geometries similar to the fungal growth. As before, we assume that there is initially a single seed. Particles are added and randomly diffuse until they are adjacent to the seed. If they are adjacent to the seed, then they will stick. This process, called **diffusion limited aggregation** (DLA) (Witten and Sander, 1981), differs from the Eden model because the new growth will preferentially occur on the outgrowths since the probability that a diffusing particle will reach a point adjacent to an outgrowth is higher than the probability that a diffusing particle will reach a point shielded by the outgrowth (see the figure on the next page). With a bit of imagination, we can see why the geometries generated by DLA might be found in a wide range of different structures from riverbeds, to blood vessels, to nerve cells.

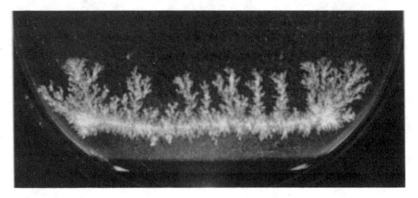

Growth in an *A. oryzae* colony in a nutrient-poor medium. From Matsuura and Miyazima (1993).

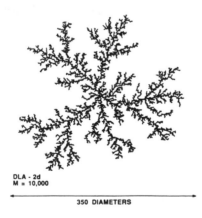

DLA - 2d
M = 10,000

350 DIAMETERS

The result of a computer simulation of diffusion limited aggregation. From Meakin (1988).

These simple models show that fractal structures of extraordinarily rich geometry can be generated by very simple growth rules. Since fractal growth seems to be a general outcome of these simple rules, simply noticing fractals does not pin down the exact mechanism of growth. In pursuing applications, people are carrying out detailed studies to try to determine the growth rules more precisely, and to correlate the growth rules with the actual geometries that are observed in the physical and biological systems.

SOURCES AND NOTES

The coining of the word "fractal" by Benoit Mandelbrot in the 1970s, helped to focus a large body of mathematical work that had been developing over the preceding century, and to draw attention of natural scientists to the possibility for a mathematics of the often bizarre and complex shapes that are found in such diverse areas as the geometry of river beds, neurons, or snow flakes. Mandelbrot's original presentation (1977) has been updated and expanded (Mandelbrot, 1982). Both books are written in Mandelbrot's inimitable style and contain many important insights as well as fascinating historical references. Anyone wishing to study the original precursors to the modern era, will benefit from consulting the collection (Edgar, 1993). The artistic possiblities of fractals has been developed by many. An art exhibit that circulated widely during the 1980s brought fractals to the attention of many in the general public; several pictures from that exhibit along with a description of the underlying mathematics are contained in Peitgen and Richter (1986).

Because of profound mathematics that underlie fractal geometry, the far-reaching scientific implications of fractals, and the beautiful graphics that can be generated, the number of books on this topic is increasing rapidly. Peitgen, Jürgens and Saupe (1992) provide a good elementary introduction. Barnsley's text (1992) is more advanced, but provides a rigorous and brilliant foundation to the mathematics of fractal sets. Applications of fractals to biology and medicine can be found in Bassingthwaighte, Liebovitch, and West (1994).

Simulations of growth models that yield fractals date back to Eden (1961). More recently, this work has been developed in a variety of directions, with particular success in the study of diffusion limited aggregation (Witten and Sander, 1981). Useful collections of related papers are Family and Vicsek (1991), and Stanley and Ostrowsky (1988).

The analysis of $1/f$ noise has been a topic of interest for a century. Mandelbrot (1977, 1982) offers many insights into the history of this concept and recalls early studies. Voss and Clarke (1975) demonstrate $1/f$ noise in music. A deterministic model that gives $1/f$ noise is in Procaccia and Schuster (1983), while a summary of mechanisms in physical systems is in Wolf (1978).

Our recounting of the observations of Robert Brown is based on (Nelson, 1967), which should be consulted for further historical discussion of our understanding of the physics and mathematics of random walks. For a recent review of Lévy walks with references to the original papers see Shlesinger, Zaslavsky, and Klafter (1993). An experimental observation of Lévy walks in a hydrodynamic experiment is in Solomon, Weeks, and Swinney (1993).

✐ EXERCISES

✐   **3.1** A fractal game that will sketch out a Cantor set is this: Mark two points, A and B. From an initial condition on the line between the two points, move two-thirds of the way towards A or B, depending on whether a coin comes up heads or tails, and place a mark there. Iterate, using the previously drawn mark as the initial condition.

You can use Figure 3.18 to play this game. Put a mark on the gray line, and move two-thirds of the way towards the A-end or the B-end of the line. Above the gray line is drawn a fattened approximation to a Cantor set, so you can see how close you are to the set.

1. If you take your initial condition at point x, then the initial condition is not on the Cantor set. How many iterations do you need to play the game before you are on the set? How much closer do you move to the set after each iteration? How long does it take before you are closer to the set than the size of the dots you mark?

2. Take your initial condition at point y, which we will assume is on the Cantor set. Will you move off of the set in future iterations?

3. Suppose you picked an initial condition at random. What is the probability that this initial condition would be exactly on the ideal Cantor set?

✐   **3.2** On a piece of paper, draw some fractal objects of dimension 1. Can you draw fractal objects of dimension 2 on a piece of paper?

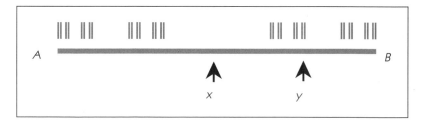

Figure 3.18

3.3 Calculate the dimension of the objects shown in Figure 3.19. Design a fractal game to draw these objects.

COMPUTER PROJECTS

Project 1 Write a computer program to play the fractal game. The program should read in a list of the x and y coordinates of target points, e.g., (A_x, A_y), (B_x, B_y), (C_x, C_y), ... The program should also read in a fraction ϵ between zero and one.

Start at an initial position, whose coordinates are given by (x_0, y_0), and draw a dot on the computer screen at this position. Iterate the following procedure:

1. Randomly pick one of the target points.

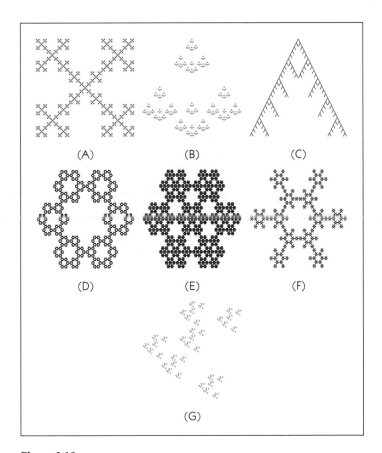

(A) (B) (C)

(D) (E) (F)

(G)

Figure 3.19

2. Calculate the next position (x_{t+1}, y_{t+1}) by moving towards the selected target point by the fraction ϵ. For instance, if the target point is (A_x, A_y), then

$$x_{t+1} = x_t + \epsilon(A_x - x_t)$$

$$y_{t+1} = y_t + \epsilon(A_y - y_t).$$

3. Draw a dot on the computer screen at (x_{t+1}, y_{t+1}).

Experiment with different sets of target points and different values for ϵ. You may also want to make ϵ different for the different target points. If you have a color display, you might make the color of each dot depend on the value of the *previous* target point.

Project 2 Write a computer program that draws fractals deterministically. As in Computer Project 1, the program can read in a set of target points. Let's assume that you have N target points. Start with an initial position (x_0, y_0). Now, make N new points, which are found by moving the initial position towards each of the target points. Repeat this process, for all N new points. This will produce N^2 points. Iterating again will produce N^3 points, and so on.

When you have a satisfactory number of points, draw a dot at each of them, using only the points in the last iteration.

More attractive results can be had if, instead of drawing a dot at each point, you draw a small shape that reflects the overall shape of the fractal (for example, a triangle for the Serpinski gasket). One way to do this is to make a list of the outer corners of the polygon described by the target points, and at each iteration, replicate this polygon by moving each of the points towards each target point in turn.

Project 3 Write a computer program to draw a picture of the Mandelbrot set. It is useful to remember the following facts about arithmetic with complex numbers:

addition $a + ib$ added to $x + iy$ gives $(a + x) + i(b + y)$.

multiplication $a + ib$ multiplied by $x + iy$ gives $(ax - by) + i(bx + ay)$. (Remember, $i \cdot i = -1$.)

real part   The real part of $a + ib$ is a.

imaginary part   The imaginary part of $a + ib$ is b.

absolute value $|a + ib| = \sqrt{a^2 + b^2}$.

To draw the set, you will want to loop over possible values of the complex variable c. Most computer languages do not have complex arithmetic built-in, so you will have to keep track of the real and imaginary parts separately. Thus, if we write z_j as $x_j + iy_j$ and c as $a + ib$, we have the set of equations

$$x_{j+1} = x_j^2 - y_j^2 + a \tag{3.10}$$

$$y_{j+1} = 2x_j y_j + b \tag{3.11}$$

which can easily be programmed on a computer.

Obviously, it is impractical to follow the iterates of $z_0 = 0$ until they actually reach ∞. Instead, you should iterate the map corresponding to each c a certain number of times, n and look to see whether at the end of the iterations the value of z_n suggests that future iterates will tend to ∞. As it happens, if $|z_n| > 2$ then it is certainly the case that future iterates will escape to ∞.

Each value of c corresponds to a pair of numbers (a, b), so the "position" of each value of c corresponds to a point in a plane, called the "complex plane." If the value of c is such that the iterates are escaping to ∞, then color the point at $c = (a, b)$ black. Otherwise, color this point white.

Computer displays can display only a fixed number of points (typically, roughly 500 pixels by 500 pixels) and so it is only possible to display a fixed number of values of c at one time ($500 \times 500 = 25000$). If you want look at the set in greater detail, you will have to zoom in on a small section of it. Note that as you zoom in, you will have to increase the value of n that you use to decide whether the map is causing $z_0 = 0$ to escape to ∞.

You can refine the pictures of the Mandelbrot set in the following way. Rather than iterating each map a fixed number of times n, stop at the first iteration for which $|z_j| > 2$ (but don't go further than n iterations, since some maps will never have $|z_j| > 2$). Then, you can color each point according to the number j at which it first reached $|z_j| > 2$.

CHAPTER 4

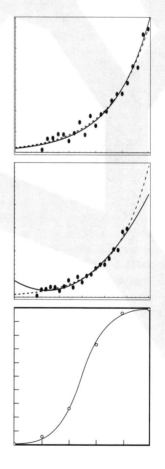

One-Dimensional Differential Equations

A molecular biology student is conducting experiments using radioactive adenosine triphosphate (ATP). The radioactive isotope is P^{32}, which has a half-life of fourteen days. He has been told to complete his experiments within four weeks, before the isotope decays away. Ordinarily, the ATP is stored in a freezer at $-20°$ C. The student believes—incorrectly—that the radioisotope will last longer if the ATP is frozen at $-70°$ C. To test this hypothesis, he takes 1 μl of the ATP, containing about 10 μcuries of the P^{32}, and puts it in the $-70°$ freezer. He keeps the remaining 24 μl of the lab's supply (containing roughly 240 μcuries) in the $-20°$ C freezer. He takes daily readings of the radioactivity by counting the number of radioactive decays from each sample for one minute. After four weeks, his measurements clearly show that the $-20°$ sample has many more counts than the $-70°$ sample (see Figure 4.1). Since each count represents the decay of one atom of P^{32}, the $-20°$ sample is decaying faster than the $-70°$ sample.

The student approaches his advisor with this evidence that storage in colder temperatures slows radioactive decay. The advisor looks at the graphs with interest for a minute, then says that the graphs show that the half-life of the radioisotope does not depend on the temperature. "Remember," the advisor says,

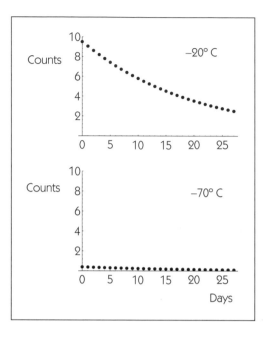

Figure 4.1
Daily measurements of the number of radioactive counts ($\times 10^5$) in one minute.

"the radioactive decay rate is proportional to the amount of P^{32} in the samples." The reason there is a greater decay rate in the warmer sample is because that sample is bigger.

Mathematically, this statement can be written as an equation:

$$\frac{dx}{dt} = -bx, \tag{4.1}$$

where x is the amount of P^{32} at any instant. Since this amount changes with time t, we will sometimes explicitly write x as a function of time, $x(t)$. The rate of change in the amount of $x(t)$ is the derivative $\frac{dx}{dt}$; since this is positive when x is increasing, the "decay rate" is $-\frac{dx}{dt}$. Equation 4.1 says that the decay rate is proportional to x. The constant of proportionality is b.

4.1   BASIC DEFINITIONS

Equation 4.1 is an example of a **differential equation**. A differential equation is an equation in which the derivative of a variable appears. There are many types of differential equations. The type we shall study in this chapter are "first-order, ordinary differential equations of a single variable." The term **first-order** means that the derivative that appears in the equation is a first-order derivative, like $\frac{dx}{dt}$, and not a higher-order derivative like $\frac{d^2x}{dt^2}$. (In Chapter 5 we will study some second-order differential equations and equations that involve multiple variables.) The term **ordinary** refers to the type of derivative involved in the equation. In **partial** differential equations, there are partial derivatives included. Partial differential equations are used to describe phenomena such as diffusion, fluid flow, and wave propagation.

In this chapter, we will take two complementary approaches to studying first-order, ordinary differential equations. The first is to find the algebraic solution to an equation—this means finding a function $x(t)$ that satisfies the equation. This approach is straightforward for equations such as Eq. 4.1. The second approach is a geometrical one where the information one seeks is not the detailed solutions $x(t)$ but rather information about what fixed points there are, and whether they are stable.

4.2 GROWTH AND DECAY

Differential equations of the form of Eq. 4.1 are often used as models of growth or decay. Consider some quantity $x(t)$, which might be, for example, the number of bacteria in a test tube at time t, the amount of money in a bank account, or the amount of a radioactive isotope. If $\frac{dx}{dt} > 0$, then x is growing. If $\frac{dx}{dt} < 0$, then x is decaying. If $\frac{dx}{dt} = 0$, then x remains constant: Such a value for x is called a **fixed point**. Recall that in Chapter 1, a fixed point of the finite-difference equation $x_{t+1} = f(x_t)$ was a point that satisfied $x_t = f(x_t)$. For both finite-difference and differential equations, a fixed point is where the state variable x remains constant and corresponds to steady-state behavior.

CONSTANT GROWTH OR DECAY

Suppose there is a swimming pool that is being emptied by a pump that removes w liters of water per minute. If $x(t)$ is the amount of water in the pool, then an appropriate differential equation is

$$\frac{dx}{dt} = -w, \tag{4.2}$$

where x is measured in liters and t is measured in minutes.

The solution to Eq. 4.2 can be easily found using the tools of calculus. Write Eq. 4.2 as $dx = -w\,dt$ and integrate both sides of the equation using the limits 0 to t:

$$\int_0^t dx = \int_0^t -w\,dt \implies x(t) - x(0) = -wt,$$

giving

$$x(t) = x(0) - wt.$$

This equation says simply that starting from an initial condition $x(0)$ at time t, the volume of water decreases proportional to the elapsed time (see Figure 4.2). Obviously, Eq. 4.2 can be right only as long as there is water in the pool, that is, as long as $x > 0$, although in other situations it might make sense physically to allow x to become negative.

The equation for linear growth is very similar:

$$\frac{dx}{dt} = w,$$

which gives a solution of

$$x(t) = x(0) + wt.$$

Figure 4.3 shows a graph of linear growth.

It is important to appreciate that the basic method to solve differential equations is to **integrate** them, just as integrating a function is the inverse of differentiation.

EXPONENTIAL GROWTH AND DECAY

In the description of radioactive decay in Eq. 4.1, the number of radioactive counts per unit time is proportional to the amount of the radioactive substance. So, rather than having a constant rate of decay, the rate of decay changes, decreasing as the surviving amount of the radioactive substance decreases.

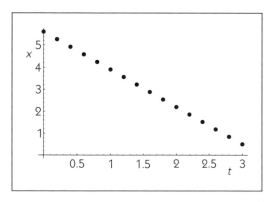

Figure 4.2   Linear decay $\frac{dx}{dt} = -1.7$.

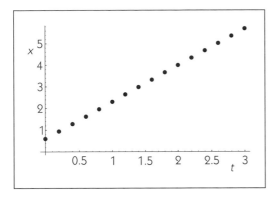

Figure 4.3 Linear growth $\frac{dx}{dt} = 1.7$.

Similarly, in many models of growth, the rate of growth is proportional to the amount of the substance. For example, the increase of funds in a bank account is proportional to the amount of money in the account—the constant of proportionality a is related to the interest rate. Another example is given by bacterial reproduction. Bacteria divide at a constant rate, and the change in the number of bacteria is proportional to the number of bacteria—the constant of proportionality a is related to the rate of cell division.

The differential equation

$$\frac{dx}{dt} = ax \tag{4.3}$$

describes a situation in which the rate of growth of x is proportional to the amount of x. This is a linear equation.

Both Eqs. 4.3 and 4.1 can be solved algebraically in the same manner. In order to solve Eq. 4.3 analytically, we multiply both sides of this equation by $\frac{dt}{x}$ to obtain

$$\frac{dx}{x} = a\,dt.$$

Integrating this equation, using as the limits of integration 0 and t, we have

$$\int_0^t \frac{dx}{x} = a \int_0^t dt.$$

Since, $\int \frac{dx}{x} = \ln x$, the "natural logarithm" of x, we can find

$$\ln x(t) - \ln x(0) = at. \tag{4.4}$$

Raising both sides of the above expression to the power e, we obtain the solution of the equation for exponential growth and decay:

$$x(t) = x(0)e^{at}, \tag{4.5}$$

where $x(0)$ represents the value of x at the initial time, $t = 0$, and a is a constant, which is positive if there is exponential growth and negative if there is exponential decay.

FITTING DATA TO EXPONENTIAL GROWTH AND DECAY

In practical situations one may be presented with data and asked to fit the data to an appropriate mathematical expression. For the case of the exponential function, this entails finding an appropriate value of the constant a that gives good agreement with the data. An example is the pharmacokinetics of how a drug is eliminated from the body. One would often wish to determine the value of a that best describes the kinetics of a given drug. This information would be important in order to decide how frequently a drug should be administered.

The constant of proportionality a in Eq. 4.3 describes the rate of growth or decay. $\frac{1}{a}$ is called the **time constant**. Another description of this rate is called the **half-life** in the case of decay, and the **doubling time** in the case of growth. The half-life gives the length of time needed for x to decay from its initial value to one half its initial value. A remarkable feature of exponential decay is that the half-life is independent of the initial value. Call $t_{\frac{1}{2}}$ the half-life. Since $x(t_{\frac{1}{2}}) = 0.5x(0)$, we obtain

$$0.5x(0) = x(0)e^{at_{1/2}},$$

or

$$t_{\frac{1}{2}} = \frac{-\ln 2}{a}.$$

Similarly, the doubling time is the time required for x to increase to twice its initial value. The doubling time is also independent of the initial value of x.

There are two ways that are most commonly used to determine a. The first involves fitting the data to a straight line. Let us assume that we have measured the values of x as a function of time. From Eq. 4.4 we know that the graph of $\ln x(t)$ versus time is a straight line with slope a and x-intercept $\ln x(0)$. To find the values of a and $\ln x(0)$, we choose the straight line that represents the "best" fit of the straight line to the data (see Figures 4.4 and 4.5). Here "best" has a definite meaning and refers to the straight line for which the sum of the squares of the deviations of the individual values is minimized. When we carry out this

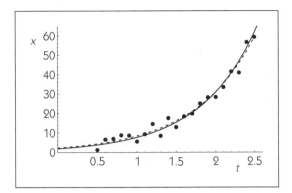

Figure 4.4   Data generated from the system $\frac{dx}{dt} = 1.3x$. To simulate a real measurement process, a small random number has been added to each measurement. The solid line shows the best fit to the measured data, $\frac{dx}{dt} = 1.39x$. The dashed line shows the theoretical solution to $\frac{dx}{dt} = 1.3x$ and almost coincides with the fitted curve.

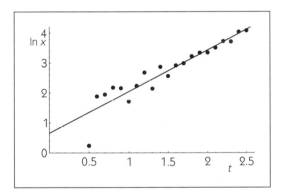

Figure 4.5   The above data plotted as ln x versus t. The line shows the best linear fit to the data and has slope 1.39.

computation, small discrepancies of individual points from the theoretical curve do not lead to large errors in the determination of a, since all experimentally measured points contribute to the final determination.

❏ **EXAMPLE 4.1**

The amount of a radioactive isotope that survives to time t is described by the function

$$x(t) = x(0)e^{-\alpha t},$$

where α is a positive constant. The half-life for U^{235} is 7.04×10^8 years. What is the value of α?

Solution: Since $t_{\frac{1}{2}} = \frac{\ln 2}{\alpha}$, we have $\alpha = \frac{\ln 2}{t_{\frac{1}{2}}} = 9.85 \times 10^{-10}$ years^{-1}.   ☐

❑ EXAMPLE 4.2

If the doubling time t_{DT} of a tumor is 60 days, how long does it take for a tumor's volume to increase to 2.5 times its initial volume?

Solution: Using the same argument for the half-life used in Example 4.1, we find that $a = \frac{\ln 2}{t_{DT}}$. Therefore, $a = 1.15 \times 10^{-2}$ days^{-1}. For this problem we have

$$2.5x(0) = x(0)e^{at},$$

where t is the time needed for the volume to multiply by 2.5 times its initial value. Therefore, we find that $t = \frac{\ln 2.5}{a} = 79.8$ days.   ☐

❑ EXAMPLE 4.3

Chemists use the notation $A \underset{k_{-1}}{\overset{k_1}{\rightleftharpoons}} B$ to indicate that compound A is transformed into compound B, and vice versa. k_1 is called the rate constant in the "forward" direction, and k_{-1} is the rate constant in the "reverse" direction.$[A]$ denotes the concentration of compound A in the reaction vessel, and similarly $[B]$ denotes the concentration of B. The total concentration of A and B together is constant, $[A] + [B] = M$. In this situation, we can write a differential equation for $[A]$:

$$\frac{d[A]}{dt} = -k_1[A] + k_{-1}[B].$$

Substituting $[B] = M - [A]$, we have

$$\frac{d[A]}{dt} = -(k_1 + k_{-1})[A] + k_{-1}M.$$

If we define two new variables $\alpha = k_1 + k_{-1}$ and $\beta = k_{-1}M$, and rename $[A]$ as x, the equation takes on a quite simple form,

$$\frac{dx}{dt} = \beta - \alpha x. \tag{4.6}$$

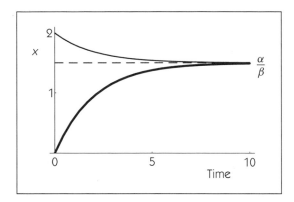

Figure 4.6   Solutions to $\frac{dx}{dt} = 3 - 2x$ for two initial conditions, $x(0) = 0$ (heavy line) and $x(0) = 2$ (thin line). The dashed line is drawn at $x = \frac{\beta}{\alpha} = \frac{3}{2}$.

Assume that at the beginning of an experiment, the reaction vessel contains only compound B. This means that $x(0) = [A(0)] = 0$. Starting from this initial condition that $x(0) = 0$ at time $t = 0$, determine the dynamics for all future times.

Solution: Equation 4.6 is an important equation, and there are a few different methods that can be used to solve it. One simple method involves transforming the equation by defining a new variable,

$$y(t) = x(t) - \frac{\beta}{\alpha}.$$

Since $\frac{dy}{dt} = \frac{dx}{dt}$, we derive the differential equation

$$\frac{dy}{dt} = -\alpha y.$$

We already know that the solution of this equation is $y(t) = y(0)e^{-\alpha t}$. Now substituting back to express the solution in terms of $x(t)$, we find

$$x(t) = \frac{\beta}{\alpha} + \left(x(0) - \frac{\beta}{\alpha} \right) e^{-\alpha t}.$$

Note that this solution is the same sort of exponential decay that we saw as the solution to Eq. 4.5, but here the decay is not to zero but to $\frac{\beta}{\alpha}$. See Figure 4.6.

For another interpretation of the equation $\frac{dx}{dt} = \beta - \alpha x$, see Section 4.7.

$\square$

DYNAMICS IN ACTION

9   TRAFFIC ON THE INTERNET

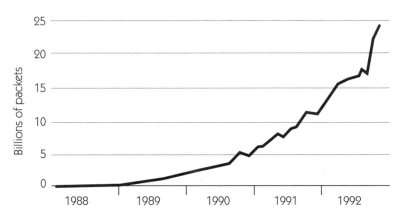

The number of message packets transmitted on the Internet. Adapted from *The Montreal Gazette.*)

An example of exponential growth is provided by the Internet, a very large network of computers. The amount of traffic on the network is measured in "packets," each of which contains a message or part of a message. The figure here shows that the number of packets is increasing rapidly. Although the source of the data did not give the important information about whether the units are in billions of packets per day, month, year, or second, from the shape of the graph it can be seen that the doubling time is roughly one year. If this rate were continued until the year 2000, the amount of traffic on the network would be roughly 6000 billion packets. However, if we assume that future growth will be linear rather than exponential, a reasonable estimate for the traffic on the network in the year 2000 would be 125 billion packets. Obviously, the form of growth that is assumed has a tremendous impact on the projected traffic.

The half-life or doubling time of data provides a quick-and-dirty method of estimating the rate of decay or growth. It is usually easy to "eyeball" a value of $t_{\frac{1}{2}}$ or t_{DT} from a graph of data. Although this is very useful for "back-of-the-envelope calculations," the problem with this method for determining the rate of decay or growth is that it does not make maximal use of our knowledge of the data. For example, an error in the measurement of the initial value $x(0)$ would be

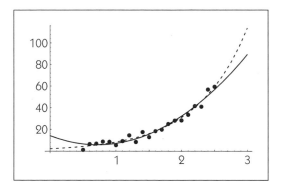

Figure 4.7 Data from a system with exponential growth fitted to an exponential curve (dashed line) and a parabola (solid line). Although both curves fit the data well, outside of the range of measured data the parabolic fit deviates substantially from exponential growth.

reflected directly in the determination of $t_{\frac{1}{2}}$ or t_{DT}. The method of estimating a by fitting a line to the logarithm of the measurements makes use of all the data, and so is not unduly influenced by an error in any of them.

Fitting experimental data to exponential curves is a ubiquitous practice in diverse fields such as neurophysiology, microbiology, pharmacology, and physiology. Sometimes, even advanced students and researchers do not have a clear conception of why one chooses to fit functions to an exponential curve rather than some other curve that might have a similar geometrical form (such as the parabola for growth or the hyperbola for decay); see Figure 4.7. One reason is that exponential functions represent the solution of a linear one-dimensional differential equation and as such arise in a variety of circumstances in which the rate of change of a variable is proportional to the value of the variable. Even though a hyperbola or a parabola may fit the measured data as well as an exponential curve, if the physical mechanism that generates the data is not related to the type of curve used, then extrapolation of the curve is likely to be in error.

The equation for exponential growth and decay is probably the most important dynamical model in biology. Even though it is mathematically simple, it is relevant in a wide range of circumstances. Yet, careful examination of the data shows that exponential functions frequently are only approximations to the data. Specification sheets for drugs usually give the half-life of the drugs but will rarely mention how well the kinetics are described by an exponential curve. Since many drugs may be eliminated by a variety of pathways, exponential functions provide only an approximation for the kinetics of drug elimination.

DYNAMICS IN ACTION

10 OPEN TIME HISTOGRAMS IN PATCH CLAMP EXPERIMENTS

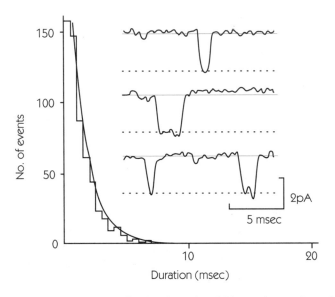

Potassium ion currents flowing through a single membrane channel. The three small insets show the channel current recorded during three events; the current is zero most of the time, but changes to −2.4 picoamps (the dotted line) when the channel opens. The open-time histogram is constructed from many such events and shows how likely the channel is to stay open for the given duration. It is well described by exponential decay. Adapted from Sakmann et al. (1983). Reprinted with permission from *Nature*. Copyright 1983 by Macmillan Magazines, Limited.

The equations for exponential growth find application even in the study of single molecules, where there is no reproduction or decay. In nerves, muscles, and other excitable tissues, the cell membrane is perforated by proteins that serve as channels for ionic currents. These channels open and shut, regulating the amount of ionic current that flows through the membrane. By placing a micro-electrode directly on the cell surface and applying gentle suction, it is possible to obtain a high-resistance electrical seal. This method is called the **patch clamp** technique; it allows the current flowing through a single channel to be measured, as shown in the figure. The sharp changes in current show the opening and closing of a single channel in the membrane. By measuring the time that the channel stays open during each such event, one can construct a histogram that shows the probability that the channel will open for a given amount of time. In the figure it can be seen that the majority of open times are short, under 2 msec. In the example shown in the figure, the histogram can be well fit by an exponential function,

$$N(t) \propto e^{-t/\tau}.$$

τ is called the time constant.

There are many possible mechanisms that could give rise to an exponential histogram. The simplest assumption is that once a channel opens, the probability that it will close during any time interval is a constant (i.e., the probability does *not* depend on how long the channel had been open). This is directly analogous to the decay of radioactive molecules—the probability that any given molecule will decay in a unit of time is always constant. The difference is that in radioactive decay the radioactivity is eventually depleted, while membrane channels can open and close repeatedly. To characterize the dynamics of membrane channels more completely, one would study the distribution of closed times, which are also often well described by exponential functions.

❏ **EXAMPLE 4.4**

Estimate the time constant for the open time histogram of the potassium channels shown in the figure in *Dynamics in Action* 10.

Solution: The length of time for $N(t)$ to decrease by 50 percent is approximately 1.2 msec. Therefore we have

$$\frac{1}{2} = e^{-1.2/\tau}.$$

Taking the logarithm of both sides, we find that $\tau = -\frac{1.2}{\ln 2}$ msec, or $\tau = 1.73$ msec.

❏

LIMITS TO EXPONENTIAL GROWTH

Although one can imagine physical and biological processes in which exponential decay can occur for long times, exponential growth must always be of limited duration. The reason for this is simple: The doubling of population sizes in fixed times eventually leads to astronomically large numbers. A good rule of thumb is that in 10 generations (i.e., 10 times the doubling time) a population will multiply by 1000; in 20 generations by 1,000,000; and in 30 generations by 1,000,000,000. (The precise values are $2^{10} = 1024$; $2^{20} = 1,048,576$; $2^{30} = 1,073,741,824$, but this precision is warranted only when the doubling time is known with great precision.)

Thus, assuming a doubling time of a cancer tumor of 60 days, it takes 60 months, or 5 years, for a tumor to increase its volume by one billion times its original volume. Even starting with a single cell, this represents a significant mass after 5 years. If the tumor kept growing in the same way for another 5 years, it would be significantly larger than the person carrying it—obviously this is not possible.

❏ Example 4.5

The bacterium *E. coli* divides approximately every 20 minutes under optimal conditions. Starting with one bacterium, how many bacteria would there be after 48 hours?

Solution: The doubling time for *E. coli* is $t_{DT} = 20$ minutes, so that in 48 hours there are 3×48, or 144, doublings. Therefore,

$$N(48) = 2^{144} = 2.23 \times 10^{43}.$$

To give some appreciation for the magnitude of this number, consider that the diameter of *E. coli* is roughly 10^{-6} m, so that 2.23×10^{43} *E. coli* would take up a volume of 1.17×10^{25} m^3. The volume of the earth is roughly 1×10^{21} m^3. ❏

It is not surprising that natural growth processes do not show exponential growth for extended periods of time. Rather, though many growth processes are initially exponential, after a time duration that may be relatively small, they slow down and may sometimes reach a steady state, or even decrease. In this section we discuss two simple theoretical models that account for this slowing of growth.

Verhulst growth or **logistic growth** is described by

$$\frac{dx}{dt} = kx - \alpha x^2, \tag{4.7}$$

where k and α are positive constants. This equation captures the same idea that we encountered in Chapter 1 when describing crowding effects in finite-difference equations modeling population dynamics. For high population levels, the growth rate must slow down due to such factors as crowding or limited resources. However, in the current case we have a differential equation, rather than a finite-difference equation, and surprisingly the dynamics in Eq. 4.7 are much simpler than the dynamics in Eq. 1.6.

The solution of Eq. 4.7 is as follows:

$$x(t) = \frac{kx(0)}{(k - \alpha x(0))e^{-kt} + \alpha x(0)}.$$ (4.8)

This solution can be obtained by direct integration of Eq. 4.7.

Figure 4.8 is a classic graph from early in this century in which the growth of a bacterial culture was fit to the logistic curve. Note that for short times this curve is similar to the exponential function (this is often called the **log phase** of the growth), whereas for long times the value of the population reaches a fixed level, which from Eq. 4.8 is $\frac{k}{\alpha}$. Note that if $x(0) > \frac{k}{\alpha}$, Eq. 4.7 will lead to *decay* to $\frac{k}{\alpha}$ rather than growth.

You should appreciate the differences between the dynamics in the Verhulst differential equation here and its cousin, the logistic finite-difference in Eq. 1.6 which we encountered in Chapter 1. In the differential equation, values of the variables change continuously in time. If the initial value is less than $\frac{k}{\alpha}$ there will be a monotonic increase up to the value $\frac{k}{\alpha}$, and if the initial value is greater than

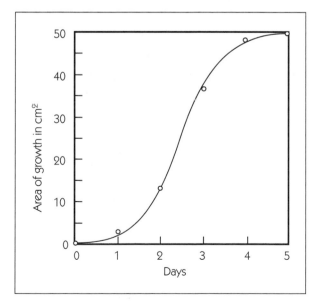

Figure 4.8 Bacterial growth. Adapted from Lotka (1956).

$\frac{k}{\alpha}$ the population will decay to the value $\frac{k}{\alpha}$. There is no way that this equation can show oscillation or chaotic dynamics, in striking contrast to Eq. 1.6. This subject is discussed in more detail in Section 4.6.

□ **Example 4.6**

Figure 4.8 gives experimental data concerning the area of growth of a bacterial colony. The data points have been fit to the logistic function,

$$y(t) = \frac{a}{b + e^{-\gamma t}},$$

where a, b, and γ are positive constants.

a. In terms of a, b, and γ, what is the value of $y(t)$ when $t = 0$ and $t = \infty$?

b. Show that the expression for $y(t)$ given above is a solution of the one-dimensional, nonlinear, ordinary differential equation

$$\frac{dy}{dt} = k_1 y - k_2 y^2,$$

where $k_1 = \gamma$ and $k_2 = \frac{b\gamma}{a}$.

c. In Figure 4.8 $a = 0.25$ cm^2, $b = 0.005$, and $\gamma = 2.1$ day^{-1}. Find the numerical values of k_1 and k_2.

d. According to the differential equation in part b, what would be the area of growth as $t \to \infty$ starting from an initial area of 100 cm^2?

Solution:

a. By direct substitution, we compute the limiting values of $y(t)$: $y(0) = \frac{a}{b+1}$, and $y(\infty) = \frac{a}{b}$.

b. Direct substitution of $y(t)$ into the differential equation yields

$$\frac{-a(-\gamma)e^{-\gamma t}}{(b + e^{-\gamma t})^2} = \frac{k_1 a}{b + e^{-\gamma t}} - \frac{k_2 a^2}{(b + e^{-\gamma t})^2}.$$

Simplifying terms, we find that

$$\frac{a\gamma e^{-\gamma t}}{(b + e^{-\gamma t})^2} = \frac{k_1 ab + k_1 ae^{-\gamma t} - k_2 a^2}{(b + e^{-\gamma t})^2}.$$

In order for the left-hand side to equal the right-hand side, the coefficients of the exponential terms in the numerators must be equal.

This will only be the case if $a\gamma = k_1 a$ or $k_1 = \gamma$. Further, in order for the right-hand side to equal the left-hand side, it is necessary that $k_1 ab - k_2 a^2 = 0$. This is only the case if $k_2 = \frac{b\gamma}{a}$.

c. Substituting for the values above, we find $k_1 = 2.1$ day^{-1} and $k_2 = 4.2 \times 10^{-2}$ cm^{-2} day^{-1}.

d. Starting from any initial condition, the size in the limit $t \to \infty$ is 50 cm^2.

❏

The **Gompertz equation** is another theoretical model for self-limiting growth, but it uses a different mathematical idea. Gompertz growth can be summarized as follows: The growth rate is proportional to the current value, but the proportionality factor decreases exponentially in time so that

$$\frac{dx}{dt} = ke^{-\alpha t}x, \tag{4.9}$$

where k and α are positive constants. The Gompertz equation can be solved to yield

$$x(t) = x(0) \exp[\frac{k}{\alpha}(1 - e^{-\alpha t})]. \tag{4.10}$$

For Gompertz growth, x approaches $x(0)e^{\frac{k}{\alpha}}$ as $t \to \infty$. Thus, the asymptotic value depends on, and is always greater than, the initial value. (In contrast, the asymptotic value for Verhulst growth is always $\frac{k}{\alpha}$, independent of the initial condition.)

DYNAMICS IN ACTION

11 GOMPERTZ GROWTH OF TUMORS

Gompertz growth has been used as a theoretical model for the growth of animals and the growth of tumors (A. Laird (1964)). The figure shown here gives experimental data on the growth of an Ehrlich ascites tumor in tissue culture. The logarithm of the number of cells is plotted as a function of time. If the tumor were growing exponentially, the graph would be a straight line and the slope of the line would give the rate of growth (see Figure 4.5). This is clearly not the case. Rather, there appears to be a steady decrease in the growth rate—the graph gets flatter as time proceeds. The experimental points are well fitted by the theoretical expression for Gompertz growth.

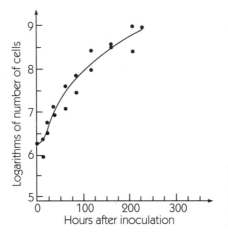

Growth of Ehrlich ascites tumor. Log of the number of tumor cells plotted against time. Adapted from Laird (1964) based on Klein and Révész (1953).

4.3 MULTIPLE FIXED POINTS

In a 1977 article on the applications of nonlinear ordinary differential equations to ecology, Robert May asks, "Is the human story largely a deterministic tale of civilisations marching to Toynbee's tune, three and a half beats to disintegration, or did the hinge of history turn on the length of Cleopatra's nose?"

May thus introduced the notion that in dynamical systems, the dynamics as $t \rightarrow \infty$ may depend on the initial condition. For example, imagine a single cow in a field of modest size. If the cow were introduced to the field after the field had lain fallow for a time, there would be ample vegetation. The cow could eat a bit here and a bit there, but there would be adequate vegetation so that the cow would be well nourished and the vegetation would continue to grow. Suppose, however, that the same cow was placed in the same field after a herd of cows had grazed for several weeks. There would be little vegetation when the cow was introduced to the field, and the grazing cow might eat new grass blades as they appeared. Neither the cow nor the field would flourish. This shows how the initial condition, in this case the state of the field when the cow is introduced, might affect the final outcome.

May developed a theoretical model for the dynamics in this system. He assumed that the growth of the vegetation is a result of the balance between two terms: A growth term for the vegetation that is modeled by the Verhulst equation, and a grazing term in which the vegetation that is consumed is described by an increasing sigmoidal function (see Appendix A). Thus, May was led to an equation to describe the dynamics of the amount of vegetation V:

$$\frac{dV}{dt} = G(V) - Hc(V), \tag{4.11}$$

where $G(V)$ describes the growth of vegetation, $c(V)$ is the consumption of vegetation per cow, and H is the number of cows in the herd. The vegetation growth function is

$$G(V) = rV(1 - \frac{V}{K}),$$

where r and K are positive constants, and the consumption function has a sigmoidal shape

$$c(V) = \frac{\beta V^2}{V_0^2 + V^2},$$

where β and V_0 are constants. Even though the resulting equation is quite complicated, a theoretical analysis of the qualitative properties of the equation can be easily carried out.

The system will be at a steady state whenever the amount of vegetation V is such that consumption $Hc(V)$ equals the production $G(V)$, so that the derivative in Eq. 4.11 is zero. In Figure 4.9 we show the functions $G(V)$ and $Hc(V)$

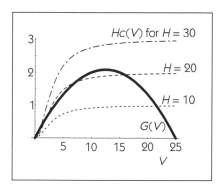

Figure 4.9
Growth $G(V)$ (heavy line) and consumption $Hc(V)$ (broken lines) for different herd sizes for the parameters $r = \frac{1}{3}$, $K = 25$, $\beta = 0.1$, and $V_0 = 3$.

superimposed for low, moderate, and high values of H. A careful examination of the graph shows that when $H = 10$, there are two possible steady states, one at $V = 0$ (no vegetation, starving cows) and one near $V = 22$ (well-fed cows who wouldn't eat much more even if it were available—we know this because the consumption curve is almost flat). When $H = 30$, the steady states are at $V = 0$ and $V = 1$. (You have to look very closely to see this on the graph, but you can verify it algebraically.) At the $V = 1$ fixed point, the cows are hungry: The fact that the sigmoidal consumption curve has a positive slope at $V = 1$ means that the cows would eat more if it were available. When $H = 20$, there are four fixed points, at $V = 0$, $V \approx 2$, $V \approx 7.5$, and $V \approx 16$. At $V \approx 7.5$ or $V \approx 16$ the cows are well fed. At $V \approx 2$ they are hungry.

It is perhaps surprising that the same cows in the same field might be starving or well fed depending on which steady state they happen to reach—the two outcomes are both possible. For a land resources manager (or a cow), it would be important to know what the outcome will be. The cow's fate can easily be found using geometric analysis, as shown in the next section. We will see that the outcome depends entirely on the amount of vegetation present when the cows are first placed in the field.

4.4 GEOMETRICAL ANALYSIS OF ONE-DIMENSIONAL NONLINEAR ORDINARY DIFFERENTIAL EQUATIONS

We now consider the geometrical analysis of one-dimensional nonlinear ordinary differential equations. The style of analysis parallels exactly the analysis of the fixed points and stability in the one-dimensional finite-difference equations in Chapter 1. However, although the approach is similar, the dynamics in the nonlinear differential equations are so simple that we can give a complete analysis of all possible behaviors.

We consider the equation

$$\frac{dx}{dt} = f(x), \tag{4.12}$$

where $f(x)$ is a single-valued continuous function of x. ("Single-valued" means that, for any given x, the function $f(x)$ has a single, unique value. This value can be different for different x.) For example, $f(x)$ may appear as the complex landscape in Figure 4.10. Notice that if $f(a) > 0$, then starting at point $x = a$, x will increase. (This follows immediately from the differential equation; a positive derivative indicates that x is increasing.) On the other hand, if $f(a) < 0$, then starting at $x = a$, x will decrease. The increase or decrease will continue until a fixed point is reached. A **fixed point** x_0 is any value for which $f(x_0) = 0$. In

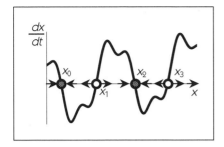

Figure 4.10 Geometrical picture of the nonlinear differential equation $\frac{dx}{dt} = f(x)$. If $f(x) > 0$ then x increases and if $f(x) < 0$, then x decreases. Thus, from the graph of $f(x)$, we can determine all the fixed points and their stability. Open symbols represent unstable fixed points and closed symbols represent stable fixed points.

Figure 4.10 we label the fixed points as x_0, x_1, x_2, $\cdots$. Since more than one fixed point can be stable, we can have multistability.

Returning to the cows, Figure 4.11 shows the graph of the right-hand side of Eq. 4.11 for three different herd sizes. From the graph of $\frac{dV}{dt}$ as a function

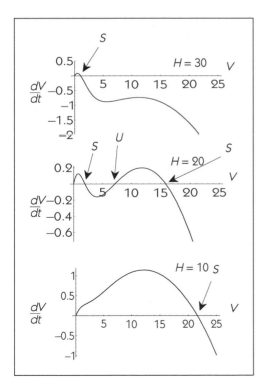

Figure 4.11
$\frac{dV}{dt} = G(V) - Hc(V)$
for different herd sizes.
The stable fixed points are
marked with **S**, and the
unstable fixed point with **U**.

of V, it is straightforward to figure out what the dynamics will be. If $\frac{dV}{dt} > 0$, V will increase; if $\frac{dV}{dt} < 0$, V will decrease; and if $\frac{dV}{dt} = 0$, V will remain unchanged (i.e. it is a fixed point). When the herd size H is high, there will always be a movement to very low values of V. Conversely, when H is low, the stable steady state for V is high. For intermediate values of H there are two possible stable behaviors. When the initial condition of V is above the unstable fixed point (marked with a **U**), V will approach a moderate value. Other initial conditions will lead to an evolution to very low values of V. Thus, in this case, the dynamics depend on the initial state, and very different outcomes result from the different initial conditions.

The beauty of this geometrical approach is that we can determine many important features of the nonlinear differential equation, Eq. 4.11, without actually integrating the equation (numerically or analytically). Just as in the cobweb method for one-dimensional finite-difference equations, the geometry underlying the dynamics is easy to grasp.

4.5   ALGEBRAIC ANALYSIS OF FIXED POINTS

The position and stability of fixed points of one-dimensional ordinary differential equations can also be found using algebraic techniques. The method is completely analogous to that used in Section 1.5 to study the existence and stability of fixed points in one-dimensional finite-difference equations.

In a differential equation, a fixed point occurs when

$$\frac{dx}{dt} = 0.$$

So, given a differential equation $\frac{dx}{dt} = f(x)$, one can find the fixed points by solving $f(x) = 0$ for x. We will denote such values of x by $x^\star$. There may be more than one value of $x^\star$ that satisfies $f(x^\star) = 0$.

For each fixed point $x^\star$ we can carry out a Taylor series expansion of $f(x)$ in the neighborhood of the fixed point $x^\star$:

$$f(x) = f(x^\star) + \left.\frac{df}{dx}\right|_{x=x^\star} (x - x^\star) + \frac{1}{2} \left.\frac{d^2 f}{dx^2}\right|_{x=x^\star} (x - x^\star)^2 + \cdots .$$

At a fixed point, $f(x^\star) = 0$. Very close to $x^\star$, the term $(x - x^\star)^2$ and all of the higher-order terms are much smaller than $(x - x^\star)$, so $f(x)$ can be approximated as

$$f(x) = m(x - x^\star),$$

where $m = \frac{df}{dx}\big|_{x=x^*}$. Defining a new variable $y = x - x^*$ makes the differential equation become

$$\frac{dy}{dt} = my. \tag{4.13}$$

Equation 4.13 should be familiar since it is the linear equation for exponential growth or decay. Therefore, we already know the behavior of this equation. If $m > 0$, there is a monotonic exponential departure from the fixed point x_0; if $m < 0$, there is a monotonic exponential approach to the fixed point. Consequently, the fixed point is stable if $m < 0$ and is unstable if $m > 0$.

❑ EXAMPLE 4.7

Consider the differential equation

$$\frac{dx}{dt} = \exp(-ax) \sin(2\pi x), \qquad 0 \le x, \quad 0 < a.$$

a. Sketch the function on the right-hand side of this equation.

b. Based on this sketch, determine the fixed points.

c. What is the stability of these fixed points?

d. Start at an initial condition of $x(0) = 1.1$. In the limit $t \to \infty$, what is the value of $x(t)$?

Solution:

a. The right-hand side is the product of an exponential function that is greater than 0 for x finite, and a sinusoidal function that oscillates, with zeroes at $x = 0, \frac{1}{2}, 1, \frac{3}{2}, \cdots$. Therefore, the graph is a decaying oscillatory function as shown in Figure 4.12.

b. The fixed points occur where the function is 0, or at $x = 0, \frac{1}{2}, 1, \frac{3}{2}, \cdots$.

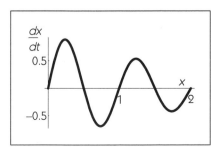

Figure 4.12
$f(x) = \exp(-\alpha x) \sin(2\pi x)$.

c. The graph shows that the slope of the right-hand side is positive when x is an integer, so that all the fixed points where x is an integer are unstable. In contrast, when $x = \frac{n}{2}$, where n is an integer, the slope of the right-hand side is negative so that these fixed points are stable.

d. Starting at $x = 1.1$, x will increase and asymptotically approach the value $x = 1.5$.

❑ EXAMPLE 4.8

In a mathematical model for the control of ovulation, Lacker (1981) proposes the equation

$$\frac{dx}{dt} = f(x) = x + \alpha x^3.$$

In this equation x represents the amount of hormone and α is a constant that can be either positive or negative.

a. Sketch $\frac{dx}{dt}$ as a function of x.

b. Analytically compute the location of all fixed points.

c. Algebraically determine the stability of these fixed points.

d. From an initial condition of $x = 1$, describe the dynamics as $t \to \infty$.

Solution:

a. For $\alpha > 0$, $f'(x) > 0$ for all x, so there are no extremal points and the function always has a positive slope (see figure 4.13).

For $\alpha < 0$, we can set $f'(x) = 0$, and we find that there are extremal points at $x = \pm\sqrt{\frac{-1}{3\alpha}}$ for $\alpha < 0$. To decide if these extrema are maxima, minima, or inflection points, we look at the second derivative,

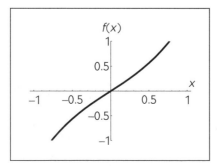

Figure 4.13
$f(x) = x + 0.5x^3$.

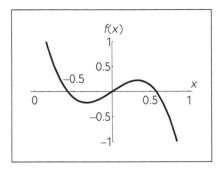

Figure 4.14
$f(x) = x - 3x^3$.

$f''(x) = 6\alpha x$. It is negative for $x = \sqrt{\frac{-1}{3\alpha}}$, so this point is a maximum. Similarly, the second derivative is positive at $x = -\sqrt{\frac{-1}{3\alpha}}$, so this point is a minimum. The second derivative is zero at the origin, which is an inflection point. A graph is shown in Figure 4.14.

b. The fixed points are found by setting $f(x) = 0$. This yields the cubic equation

$$x + \alpha x^3 = 0.$$

There are three solutions: $x = 0$, and $x = \pm\sqrt{\frac{-1}{\alpha}}$. Therefore, for $\alpha \geq 0$ there is only one fixed point at the origin, and for $\alpha < 0$ there are three fixed points.

c. The stability is determined by

$$\frac{df}{dx} = f'(x) = 1 + 3\alpha x^2$$

evaluated at the fixed points. At $x = 0$, $f'(x) = 1$, so the fixed point at the origin is unstable. For $\alpha < 0$ the slope at the other two fixed points is

$$f'(x) = 1 + 3\alpha \left(\frac{-1}{\alpha} \right) = -2,$$

and so the other two fixed points are stable fixed points.

d. For any positive initial condition, $x(t) \to \infty$ for $\alpha > 0$, and $x(t) \to \sqrt{\frac{-1}{\alpha}}$ for $\alpha < 0$.

4.6 DIFFERENTIAL EQUATIONS VERSUS FINITE-DIFFERENCE EQUATIONS

In Chapter 1 we saw that the finite-difference equations

$$x_{t+1} = f(x_t) = Rx_t - bx_t^2$$

can generate many sorts of behavior: fixed points and unlimited growth to $\pm\infty$, periodic cycles, and chaos. Yet, in differential equations of the form

$$\frac{dx}{dt} = f(x) \tag{4.14}$$

we see only fixed points and growth to $\pm\infty$. One-dimensional, ordinary differential equations of this form cannot generate periodic cycles or chaos. Why not?

A differential equation can be approximated by a finite-difference equation. This fact allows us to compare the dynamics of differential equations and finite-difference equations. The key step is to define a discrete-time variable $x_t \equiv x(t)$ for $t = 0, \Delta, 2\Delta, \ldots$, and write

$$\frac{dx}{dt} = \lim_{\Delta \to 0} \frac{x_{t+1} - x_t}{\Delta}$$

Although the mathematical definition involves a limit $\Delta \to 0$, as an approximation we can take Δ as small but finite. We have not yet said what "small" means, but this will turn out to be the crux of the matter.

The differential equation in Eq. 4.14 can be approximated as

$$\frac{x_{t+1} - x_t}{\Delta} = f(x_t),$$

giving

$$x_{t+1} = f(x_t)\Delta + x_t. \tag{4.15}$$

If Δ is small enough, the dynamics of Eq. 4.15 will be just like the dynamics of Eq. 4.14. Here, "small enough" means that $\Delta \to 0$. Note that writing "$\Delta \to 0$" is different from writing "$\Delta = 0$." If $\Delta = 0$, then Eq. 4.15 becomes $x_{t+1} = x_t$, which is not a good approximation to Eq. 4.14. Figure 4.15 shows the differential equation for Verhulst growth. Figure 4.16 shows a finite-difference approximation.

Analyzing Eq. 4.15 using the techniques studied in Section 1.5 reveals the following:

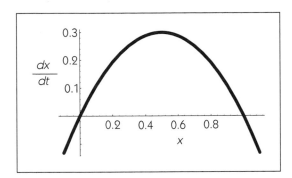

Figure 4.15 The graph of the differential equation $\frac{dx}{dt} = 1.2(x - x^2)$.

- Fixed points in the finite-difference equation occur when $f(x_t) = 0$. This is the same criterion as for fixed points in the original differential equation. Let the location of the fixed points be denoted by x^*.

- The stability of a fixed point at x^* depends on

$$\frac{dx_{t+1}}{dx_t}\bigg|_{x^*} = \Delta \frac{df}{dx}\bigg|_{x^*} + 1.$$

Whatever the value of $\frac{df}{dx}\big|_{x^*}$, by making Δ small enough, we can make $\frac{dx_{t+1}}{dx_t}$ very close to 1. This means that for Δ small, Eq. 4.15 shows a monotonic approach to or departure from the fixed point, and never the alternating approach or departure as seen in Figures 1.21 or 1.22 for cases where $\frac{dx_{t+1}}{dx_t}\big|_{x^*} < 0$. (When Δ is not small, the finite-difference equation may not represent the dynamics well. See Exercise 4.27.)

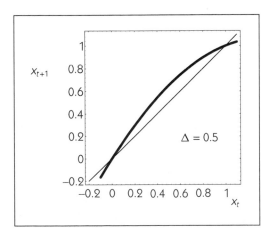

Figure 4.16
The finite-difference approximation to the differential equation sketched in Figure 4.16 for $\Delta = 0.5$.

- A fixed point at $x^\star$ is stable when $\frac{df}{dx}\big|_{x^\star} < 0$, and unstable when $\frac{df}{dx}\big|_{x^\star} > 0$, reflecting whether $\frac{dx_{t+1}}{dx_t}\big|_{x^\star}$ is greater than or less than zero. This criterion for the stability of fixed points in the finite-difference approximation is the same as in the original differential equation. See the graph in Figure 4.16.

- Cycles of period 2 are found by looking for cases were $x_{t+2} = x_t$ and $x_{t+1} \neq x_t$. But,

$$x_{t+2} = \Delta f(x_{t+1}) + x_{t+1} = \Delta f(x_{t+1}) + \Delta f(x_t) + x_t.$$

Again, as $\Delta \to 0$ the only points that satisfy $x_{t+2} = x_t$ also satisfy $x_{t+1} = x_t$. So, there are no cycles of period 2 in the dynamics, only fixed points. The same is true for any cycle of period $n > 1$.

We see that the somewhat limited types of dynamical behavior of single-variable ordinary differential equations arise from the restriction that $\Delta \to 0$. One way to understand this is with the concept of **state**. The state of the system $\frac{dx}{dt} = f(x)$ at time t is simply $x(t)$. A differential equation like Eq. 4.15 says that the change of state $\frac{dx}{dt}$ is a function of the state. One can imagine the state as a bead on a wire. The wire represents all the possible states (the real numbers) and $\frac{dx}{dt}$ tells the speed and direction of the state's movement. The position of the bead indicates the current state. Since $\frac{dx}{dt}$ is a function of position on the wire, at any point on the wire $\frac{dx}{dt}$ has a single, fixed value. The requirement that $\Delta \to 0$ says that the bead has to move continuously on the wire; it cannot jump from one spot to another, faraway spot. On the other hand, since $\frac{dx}{dt}$ has a single, fixed value at any point on the wire, the bead can never back up; if the bead could back up, then $\frac{dx}{dt}$ would have one value the first time the bead passed and another value of the opposite sign when the bead passes in the other direction. So, the only possible motion for the bead is to move steadily in one direction, either heading to $\pm\infty$ or ending up at a fixed point.

4.7   DIFFERENTIAL EQUATIONS WITH INPUTS

Most of the differential equations we have studied so far have the form $\frac{dx}{dt} = f(x)$. The derivative $\frac{dx}{dt}$ is a function only of x. In particular, the function $f(x)$ does not change in time—although obviously x itself may change in time and with it the value of the function at any instant. The only equation we have seen where the function itself changes in time is Eq. 4.9, where the function $f(x) = ke^{-\alpha t}x$. Differential equations where the function changes in time are very common in science and technology. Of particular importance are cases where the function contains some factor that can be interpreted as an "input." As a simple example, consider a patient who has been told to take a pill "once every four hours." Assume that after the drug is taken, it is eliminated from the bloodstream at a rate proportional to its concentration. A differential equation describing this situation is

$$\frac{dx}{dt} = \alpha x + I(t), \tag{4.16}$$

where $I(t)$ is the input and $\alpha < 0$ is the elimination rate for the drug once it enters the bloodstream (see Figure 4.17). In this case, the input is zero most of the time but has a spike every four hours. The area under this spike corresponds to the amount of drug in a single pill, and the width of the spike corresponds to the time it takes for the drug to enter the bloodstream after the pill is ingested (see Exercise 4.19).

LINEAR SYSTEMS AND SUPERPOSITION OF INPUTS

A general form for a one-dimensional, ordinary differential equation with an input is

$$\frac{dx}{dt} = f(x, I(t)).$$

If f is nonlinear, this type of equation can often be solved only using numerical methods on a computer.

However, when f is linear, there are elegant mathematical techniques that not only provide a solution, but also give powerful insight into how the solution is related to the input. For a one-dimensional system, there is only one form for f that is linear, as given in Eq. 4.16. This produces exponential growth ($\alpha > 0$) or decay ($\alpha < 0$).

The principle used to solve Eq. 4.16 is **linear superposition of solutions.** The idea is this: Write the input $I(t)$ as a summation of N different input

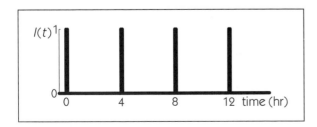

Figure 4.17 The input function $I(t)$ for drug concentration for a patient taking a pill every four hours.

functions,

$$I(t) = \sum_{i=1}^{N} I_i(t).$$

For example, the input function for the preceding drug example might be written as a sum of four inputs each consisting of a single spike (see Figure 4.18).

Suppose that we know how to solve the differential equation for each of the $I_i(t)$ individually. This means that we have a function $x_i(t)$ that satisfies the equation $\frac{dx_i}{dt} = \alpha x_i + I_i(t)$. Making use of the fact that

$$\frac{d\sum x_i}{dt} = \sum \frac{dx_i}{dt},$$

we can see that the sum of the individual solutions $\sum x_i$ is also a solution. That is,

$$\frac{d\sum x_i}{dt} = \alpha \sum x_i + \sum I_i(t).$$

So, if we can find a way to break down $I(t)$ into a sum of simple functions, and if we can solve Eq. 4.16 for each of these simple functions, then we can easily find the solution for the sum of the inputs.

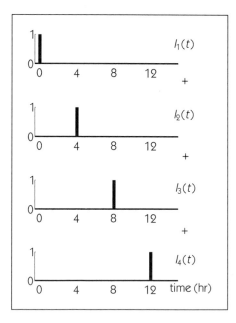

Figure 4.18
The input function in Figure 4.17 written as the sum of four simpler input functions.

TRANSIENT RESPONSE

No matter how we choose to decompose the input $I(t)$ into simple functions, there is always one simple function that must always be included. This is

$$I_0(t) = 0.$$

Although this function does not add anything to the input, it is very important for bookkeeping purposes because it covers the **transient response** of the differential equation from its initial condition in the absence of any input. As we have already seen, the solution to Eq. 4.16 in the absence of input is

$$x(t) = x(0)e^{\alpha t}, \qquad (4.17)$$

where $x(0)$ is the initial condition. By including this transient response in the summation that leads to the solution of the Eq. 4.16, we account for the complete role that the initial condition $x(0)$ plays in the solution.

THE IMPULSE RESPONSE FUNCTION

One of the most powerful ways of decomposing an input function $I(t)$ is to use components that have the form of a spike or **impulse**. The easiest case is when the impulse occurs at time $t = 0$. In this case the solution can be written in two parts:

$$x(t) = \begin{cases} 0 & \text{for } t < 0 \\ A_{\text{imp}}(0)e^{\alpha t} & \text{for } t \geq 0. \end{cases} \qquad (4.18)$$

As we will show, $A_{\text{imp}}(0)$ is the area under the impulse $I(0)$. The graph of this solution is shown in Figure 4.19.

If you differentiate each part of this solution, you will see that each part separately satisfies the equation $\frac{dx}{dt} = \alpha x$ when $t \neq 0$. But what is the derivative at time $t = 0$? We can write the derivative as

$$\frac{dx}{dt}\bigg|_{t=0} = \lim_{h \to 0} \frac{x(t + h/2) - x(t - h/2)}{h}\bigg|_{t=0} \qquad (4.19)$$

$$= \lim_{h \to 0} \frac{A_{\text{imp}}(0)e^{\alpha h/2}}{h} = \lim_{h \to 0} \frac{A_{\text{imp}}(0)}{h}. \qquad (4.20)$$

Since $\lim_{h \to 0} \frac{1}{h}$ is infinite, Eq. 4.19 implies that $\frac{dx}{dt}\big|_{t=0} \to \infty$. This is consistent with the very rapid rise shown in Fig. 4.19, but it can be a little hard to interpret

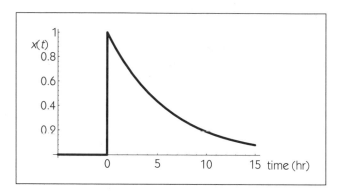

Figure 4.19 The reponse to a spike input as given by Eq. 4.18. The area of the input impulse is 1, and the half-life of the dynamics is six hours.

physically. As long as h is finite (corresponding, in the above example, to the fact that it takes a finite amount of time for the drug from the ingested pill to enter the bloodstream) there is no problem mathematically. What is the relationship between $A_{\mathrm{amp}}(0)$ and the spike input $I(0)$? If the spike has a rectangular shape and lasts for duration h, then the area under the spike is $hI(0)$. If we set $A_{\mathrm{imp}}(0)$ to be $hI(0)$—the area under the spike—then

$$\lim_{h \to 0} \frac{A_{\mathrm{imp}}(0)}{h} = \lim_{h \to 0} I(0) = I(0).$$

Using Eq. 4.19, and $A_{\mathrm{imp}} = hI(0)$, we see $\frac{dx}{dt}\big|_{t=0} = I(0)$. This is consistent with the original differential equation (Eq. 4.16) given that our solution at time $t = 0$ is $x(0) = 0$.

To find the solution to Eq. 4.16 when the input is an impulse of area $A_{\mathrm{imp}}(s)$ at time $t = s$, we simply translate the solution that we obtained for the impulse at time $t = 0$, getting

$$x(t) = \begin{cases} 0 & \text{if } t \le s; \\ A_{\mathrm{imp}}(s)e^{\alpha(t-s)} & \text{otherwise.} \end{cases} \tag{4.21}$$

CONVOLUTION

When the input $I(t)$ can be decomposed into a finite number of impulses, the solution to Eq. 4.16 is easy—simply add together the solutions for each of the individual impulses as given by Eq. 4.21. For example, if impulses occur at times s_i with areas A_i for $i = 1, \dots, N$ (N impulses altogether), then the solution of

Eq. 4.16 is

$$x(t) = x(0)e^{\alpha t} + \sum_{s_i \le t} A_i e^{\alpha(t-s_i)}. \tag{4.22}$$

When we write $\sum_{s_i \le t}$ we mean that the sum should be performed only for those impulses that occurred at or before time t. The impulses that occur later than time t do not contribute to the summation. The term $x(0)e^{\alpha t}$ is the transient response to the initial condition at time $t = 0$.

In the example of the patient taking a pill every four hours, the exponential decay of the drug from each pill ingested goes on independently of the other pills. However, the response from each pill is added to the decaying response from the pills consumed earlier (see Figure 4.20).

Surprisingly, perhaps, any form of input $I(t)$, even one that is smooth, can be written as a sum of impulses, although there may be an infinite number of them. In this case, the finite sum in Eq. 4.22 is replaced with an integral, giving

$$x(t) = x(0)e^{\alpha t} + \int_0^t I(s)e^{\alpha(t-s)}ds. \tag{4.23}$$

This integral is called a **convolution integral**. Note that the variable s is a "dummy variable," and that the time t appears in the upper limit of integration. The term $e^{\alpha(t-s)}$ is called the **convolution kernel** or **impulse response**—note that the kernel is the same as the response to an impulse at time s. This particular form for the term is only valid for the differential equation in Eq. 4.16. A general technique in solving linear differential equations with inputs is to find the impulse response, and then find the complete solution using the convolution integral.

RESPONSE TO SINE WAVE INPUT

It is often convenient to regard an experimental or field system as a **black box**, whose inner dynamics are unknown but which provides an output for any

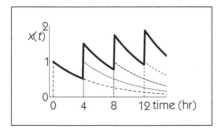

Figure 4.20
Buildup of a drug administered at times 0, 4, 8, and 12. The dark line shows the total concentration, which is a linear summation of the decaying exponentials (dashed lines) from each of the drug administrations.

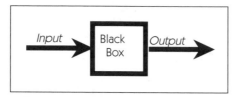

Figure 4.21

given input. One way to understand such black box systems is to provide a variety of functions as inputs and to study the output provided by each type of input.

An important special case is when the input is a sinusoidal function of time,

$$I(s) = A \sin \omega s,$$

where A and ω are positive constants (see the graph in Figure 4.20). When the sinusoidal input is substituted in Eq. 4.23, the right-hand side can be integrated to obtain

$$x(t) = x(0)e^{\alpha t} + \frac{Ae^{\alpha t}}{\alpha^2 + \omega^2} \left[e^{-\alpha s}(-\alpha \sin \omega s - \omega \cos \omega s) \right]\Big|_0^t,$$

which can be rewritten as

$$x(t) = \left(x(0) + \frac{\omega A}{\alpha^2 + \omega^2} \right) e^{\alpha t} + \frac{A}{\alpha^2 + \omega^2} (-\alpha \sin \omega t - \omega \cos \omega t). \quad (4.24)$$

This solution is often rewritten in a slightly different format using the trigonometric identity

$$\sin(\omega t - \phi) = \sin \omega t \cos \phi - \cos \omega t \sin \phi.$$

Let us now try to find ϕ such that

$$\cos \phi = \frac{\alpha}{C}, \qquad \sin \phi = \frac{\omega}{C}.$$

The above expression is solved to give

$$\phi = \tan^{-1} \frac{\omega}{\alpha}, \qquad C = \sqrt{\alpha^2 + \omega^2}.$$

Using the above substitutions, Eq. 4.24 can be evaluated to yield

$$x(t) = \left(x(0) + \frac{\omega A}{\alpha^2 + \omega^2} \right) e^{\alpha t} + \frac{A}{\sqrt{\alpha^2 + \omega^2}} \sin(\omega t - \phi). \quad (4.25)$$

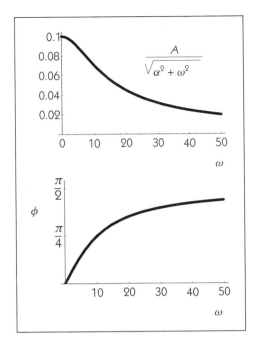

Figure 4.22
The amplitude and phase of the sine wave solution to $\frac{dx}{dt} = -10x + \sin \omega t$.

The above result says that when the input for a linear differential equation system such as Eq. 4.16, is a sine wave, the output will also be a sine wave of the same frequency, but perhaps of a different amplitude and phase. (Also, a transient response will be in the output, but for $\alpha < 0$ it approaches zero for sufficiently large t.) Further, both the amplitude of the solution, $\frac{A}{\alpha^2+\omega^2}$, and the phase shift ϕ depend on the driving frequency ω. Figure 4.22 shows these functions.

The preceding discussion suggests general methods to characterize linear systems. These methods are referred to under the general name of **system identification**. The idea is to provide a sinusoidal input to the system and measure the output. If the output is a sine wave with the same frequency as the input, then the system can be characterized by linear differential equations. In the current case, there is only one parameter α, and a measurement of the response as a function of frequency can be used to determine α. In doing this procedure, you should realize that to carry out this type of experiment you need not have any detailed understanding of the system being studied. You are treating it as a black box.

DYNAMICS IN ACTION

12 HEART RATE RESPONSE TO SINUSOID INPUTS

An interesting example of the application of system identification techniques is the control of the heart rate by the vagus nerve. Activity in the vagus nerve leads to release of the neurotransmitter acetylcholine and slows the heart rate. To study vagal control of heart rate in cats, G.F. Chess and F.R. Caleresu (1971) cut the vagus nerve and stimulated the part of the nerve still connected to the heart. They measured the heart rate in response to sinusoidally modulated stimulation at different frequencies (see the figure on the next page). In response to the stimulus, the heart rate is also sinusoidally modulated with the same period as the stimulus input, but the amplitude and phase angle of the heart rate output depend on the frequency of the input. The amplitude and phase angle of the output can be plotted as a function of the input frequency.

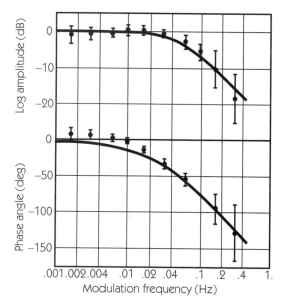

Phase angle of the heart rate response to sinusoidally modulated stimulation of the vagus nerve. Adapted from Chess and Caleresu (1971).

The solid line in the figure on this page shows the best fit to the data based on Eq. 4.25. Further analysis shows that this data corresponds to an exponentially decaying impulse response, with a time constant of 3.15 sec. The response is

sumably reflect the nerve synapse processes involved in the release, transmission, and destruction of acetylcholine.

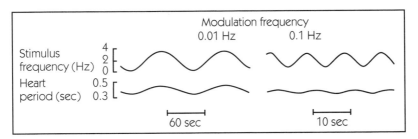

Stimulus (input) and heart rate (output) at two different stimulus frequencies. Adapted from Chess and Caleresu (1971).

4.8 ADVANCED TOPIC: TIME DELAYS AND CHAOS

In the one-dimensional ordinary differential equations we have been studying, the rate of change of a quantity depends on its present value. However, in some circumstances it is reasonable to assume that the rate of change of a quantity depends not only on its value at the present time, but also on its value at some time in the past. For example, let us assume there is a variable x that decays at a rate proportional to its own concentration (just as in exponential decay) but is produced at a rate that is a function of its value τ time units in the past. This gives a **delay differential equation**

$$\frac{dx}{dt} = P(x(t - \tau)) - \alpha x(t), \qquad (4.26)$$

where P is the function that controls the production of x and α is a decay constant. This equation was used by M. C. Mackey and L. Glass in 1977 as a theoretical model for physiological control.

As an example, let $x(t)$ be the number of mature blood cells in circulation at time t. Blood cells have a certain half-life, but new replacements are always being made. Since it takes roughly four days for a new blood cell to mature, there is a delay in the dynamics governing the number of mature blood cells.

The goal of many control systems is to maintain a quantity at a constant level. Assume that the goal of the system described by Eq. 4.26 is to produce blood

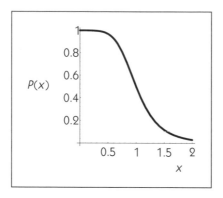

Figure 4.23
A monotonically decreasing sigmoidal function.

cells so that the total level x maintains a constant value θ. If $x(t - \tau) < \theta$, the control system might be designed to produce large quantities of new blood cells in order to bring x up to the value θ. Thus, P would be at a high value. On the other hand, if $x(t - \tau) > \theta$, we would want P to be at a low value.

To think about this, imagine a furnace heating a house in winter. When the furnace is on, the house is getting warmer. When the furnace is off, the house cools down. Furnaces are controlled by thermostats that set the desired temperature—the thermostat turns on the furnace when the inside temperature is too low, and turns off the furnace when the temperature is too high. Real furnaces (especially old ones) take a significant amount of time to turn on and to turn off. This correponds to the delay τ. By the time the furnace actually turns on, the temperature has fallen below the value set by the thermostat. When the furnace is on, the temperature will have risen above the set value before the furnace actually turns off. The result is an oscillation around the set value.

A furnace is either on or off, but biological systems can have intermediate values. It is reasonable to suppose that P is a monotonically decreasing sigmoidal function (see Figure 4.23). When a monotonically decreasing function is substituted in Eq. 4.26, one of two different behaviors has been observed: either an

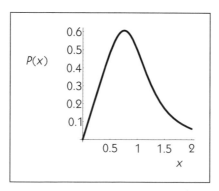

Figure 4.24
A single-humped function.

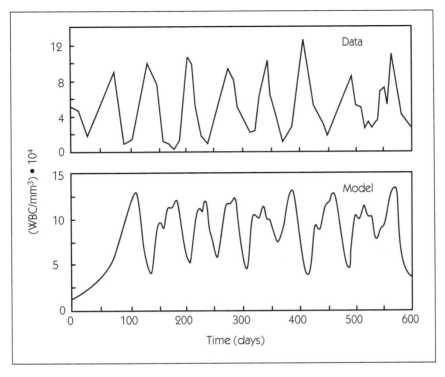

Figure 4.25 *Top*: Count of circulating white blood cells versus time in a 12-year-old girl with diagnosed chronic granulocytic leukemia. *Bottom*: Numerical solutions of $\frac{dx}{dt} = \frac{0.2x(t-20)}{1+x(t-20)^{10}} - 0.1x(t)$. Adapted from Mackey and Glass (1977). Original figure copyright 1977 by the AAAS.

approach to a fixed point or a stable periodic oscillation. One obtains the oscillatory solution if a product of the time delay and the slope of the control function exceeds a critical value. The mathematical analysis of the stability is in the same style that we carried out for the ordinary differential equation, by considering stability of a linear equation, but the analysis is more difficult as a consequence of the time delay.

In some cases, a monotonic decrease of the control function P might not be realistic. Then if x is too low, the individual might be very sick and consequently unable to produce new cells at a high rate. At intermediate values of x, the individual is healthy enough to produce new blood cells, and at large values of x there is no need to produce blood cells. Therefore, an appropriate form for the function P is a single-hump (see Figure 4.24). Mackey and Glass found that when a single-humped production function was substituted in Eq. 4.26, the dynamics could be much more complex, potentially including fixed points, cycles, period-doubling bifurcations, and chaotic dynamics (see Figure 4.25). In fact, there are striking similarities between the dynamics in this system and those in the finite-difference equation that we studied in Chapter 1.

This range of behaviors is possible in delay-differential equations, but not in one-dimensional differential equations without delays, as discussed in Section 4.6. The reason for this involves the state of a delay-differential equation. Whereas the state at time t_0 of a nondelay, one-dimensional differential equation is a single number $x(t_0)$, the state of a delay-differential equation at time t_0 is given by a function $x(t_0 - s)$ for s in the range 0 to τ. Thus, the state of a delay-differential equation is infinite-dimensional.

DYNAMICS IN ACTION

13 NICHOLSON'S BLOWFLIES

The Australian scientist A. J. Nicholson carried out a set of experiments in the 1950s to study the dynamics of fly populations. Nicholson grew cultures of the sheep blowfly *Lucilia cuprina*, carefully feeding them regularly and counting the number of adults and larvae over extended periods of time. Despite the fact that the environment was maintained constant, Nicholson observed large fluctuations in the numbers of blowflies, as shown in the figure. This type of laboratory experiment, in which population levels can be accurately measured and experimental conditions can be carefully controlled and manipulated, can offer great insight into population dynamics, although it lacks the romance of field studies in exotic locales.

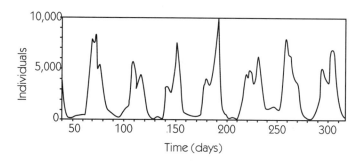

Observed number of flies in one of Nicholson's experiments. Adapted from Gurney et al. (1980). Based on Nicholson (1954). Reprinted with permission from *Nature*. Copyright 1980 by Macmillan Magazines, Limited.

In order to interpret Nicholson's experimental observations, Gurney et al. (1980) assumed that:

1. Adults die off at a rate proportional to the current adult population;

2. The number of eggs laid depends only on the current size of the adult population;

3. All eggs that develop into sexually mature adults take exactly the same length of time τ to do so;

4. The probability of a given egg maturing into a viable adult depends on the number of competitors of the same age: The larger the number of eggs, the smaller is the probability that a given egg will mature to adulthood.

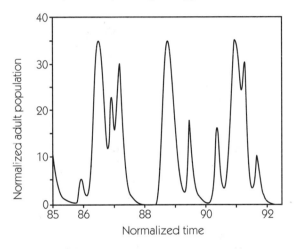

Size of the model fly population. Adapted from Gurney et al. (1980).

Very few adults means there will be few eggs laid, and even though a large fraction of the eggs will mature, there will be only a small number of new adults τ time units in the future. Very many adults means there will be many eggs, but few future adults will be produced because each egg has only a small probability of maturing. For an intermediate number of adults, the largest number of eggs mature to adulthood. Thus, the number of adults produced at any time is a single-humped function of the number of adults τ time units previously. We will write this function as $P(x(t - \tau))$.

Adding together the change in adult population due to maturing eggs ($P(x(t - \tau))$) and due to death ($-\alpha x(t)$), we arrive at

$$\frac{dx(t)}{dt} = P(x(t - \tau)) - \alpha x(t),$$

which is the same as Eq. 4.26. Gurney and colleagues were able to solve the equation to demonstrate that dynamics in the theoretical model were qualitatively similar to the dynamics in the laboratory experiments. Thus, it can be seen that plausible assumptions about reproduction, maturation, and death can lead to population fluctuations even when environmental conditions are constant.

Experiments such as Nicholson's, where a population is maintained in a laboratory environment, are rare. More commonly, scientists try to study populations in their native environment. However, difficulties in measuring populations accurately, as well as uncontrollable environmental fluctuations, make understanding ecological dynamics extremely difficult.

SOURCES AND NOTES

Mathematical models of growth have been studied throughout this century. Lotka's 1924 book contains many basic notions about limited growth, and contains references to studies by Lotka's contemporaries (Lotka, 1956). One area in which this type of analysis has practical significance is in the analysis of tumor growth. Early studies of the dynamics of tumor growth were carried out by Laird (1964). For a clinical perspective on the utility of mathematical models of growth to lung cancer see Chahinian and Israel (1976).

The qualitatitive theory of one-dimensional ordinary differential equations is very elementary and hence is often not discussed at length in mathematics books. However, the analysis of this problem provides the conceptual foundation for the more difficult problem of qualitative theory of differential equations in higher dimensions, and as such is an important topic. One application of the theory to analyze multistability in ecological systems was given by May (1977).

Systems analysis techniques are often used in physics and engineering. In the 1960s there was significant development of applications of systems analysis to the biological sciences (Grodins, 1963; Milhorn, 1966). Textbook introductions to systems analysis from an engineering perspective are contained in Chen (1984) and Franklin, Powell, and Emami-Naeni (1994). Classical systems analysis methods are suitable for many applications, for example see the applications to the analysis of control of heart rate in Chess and Caleresu (1971) and Berger, Saul, and Cohen (1989). However, since complex systems usually have nonlinearities, methods of nonlinear dynamics are frequently essential for understanding complex rhythms.

✏ **EXERCISES**

✏ **4.1** Show algebraically that linear differential equations can have only one fixed point.

✏ **4.2** Are the following data better described by linear growth or exponential growth? Write down the differential equation, complete with numerical values for the parameters, that describes this data.

t	x	t	x
0.5	1.27	1.6	18.45
0.6	6.58	1.7	19.85
0.7	7.00	1.8	25.03
0.8	8.83	1.9	28.14
0.9	8.66	2.0	28.31
1.0	5.53	2.1	33.41
1.1	9.33	2.2	41.43
1.2	14.57	2.3	40.87
1.3	8.51	2.4	56.71
1.4	17.61	2.5	59.32
1.5	12.94		

✏ **4.3** Bacteria are inoculated in a petri dish at a density of 10/ml. The bacterial density doubles in twenty hours. Assume that this situation is described by the differential equation

$$\frac{dx}{dt} = Cx,$$

where x is the bacterial density and C is a constant.

a. Integrate this equation giving x as a function of time.

b. Find the value of C.

c. How long does it take for the density to increase to eight times its original value? To ten times?

✐ **4.4** This question deals with radiocarbon dating, which archeologists use for estimating the age of once-living artifacts such as wood or bone. The radioisotope C^{14} decays to C^{12} with a half-life of 5720 years. Assume that in the atmosphere the ratio of $\frac{C^{14}}{C^{12}}$ is 1.6×10^{-12} and that this ratio has remained constant. As long as an organism is living, the $\frac{C^{14}}{C^{12}}$ ratio in the organism is the same as in the atmosphere. Once the organism dies, no new C^{14} is incorporated into the body and the existing C^{14} decays exponentially to C^{12}, which is not radioactive. Thus, the $\frac{C^{14}}{C^{12}}$ ratio can be used to estimate when the organism died.

A preserved sample of organic material is obtained in which the ratio $\frac{C^{14}}{C^{12}}$ is 0.4×10^{-12}.

    a. Give the equation for the radioactive decay of C^{14}. Determine the value of all constants in this equation.

    b. How long ago was the material in the sample formed from the atmospheric carbon.

✐ **4.5** This question is based on the closing of single ion channels (Cooper and Shrier, 1985). Suppose N channels are open at time $t = 0$ and that all of the channels will eventually close. The number that will close in a time interval between t and $t + \delta t$ is $N p \delta t$, where p is the solution of the differential equation,

$$\frac{dp}{dt} = \frac{-p}{\tau},$$

where τ is a constant to be determined.

    a. Integrate this equation to find $p(t)$.

    b. Find $p(0)$ in terms of τ. HINT: $\int_0^\infty p(t)dt = 1$ since all channels will close by $t = \infty$.

    c. The histogram in Figure 4.26 shows the number of events recorded having open time durations given on the abscissa and the graph in Figure 4.27 shows the percentage of channels that open at $t = 0$ and that

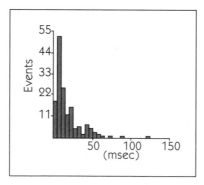

Figure 4.26
Adapted from Cooper and Shrier (1985).

close by the time shown on the abscissa. Using the expression found in part a, derive a theoretical expression for the percentage shown in the graph.

d. Using any technique you wish, estimate τ in this data.

4.6 This question deals with a mathematical model for ionic currents found during action potentials in cardiac muscle; it was developed by Noble and Tsien (1969). They hypothesized that the membrane current during the plateau phase of the action potential can be separated into two components $x_1(t)$ and $x_2(t)$ described by the differential equations

$$\frac{dx_1}{dt} = \alpha_{x_1}(1 - x_1) - \beta_{x_1} x_1, \tag{1}$$

$$\frac{dx_2}{dt} = \alpha_{x_2}(1 - x_2) - \beta_{x_2} x_2, \tag{2}$$

and where α_{x_1}, α_{x_2}, β_{x_1}, and β_{x_2} are constants set from experimental data.

a. Show by direct substitution into Eq. (1), that solution of its (1) can be written as

$$x_1(t) = A_\infty \left[1 - \exp\left(\frac{-t}{\tau_1} \right) \right],$$

where A_∞ and τ_1 are constants that depend on α_{x_1} and β_{x_1}. Express A_∞ and τ_1 as a function of α_{x_1} and β_{x_1} (see Figure 4.28).

b. Consider the graph that gives $\ln\left(\frac{A_\infty - x_1(t)}{A_\infty} \right)$ as a function of t. Write the equation for, and sketch, this graph.

c. Call $t_{\frac{1}{2}}$ the time that is necessary for $x_1(t)$ to increase from its initial value to a value halfway between the initial value and the final value. Find $t_{\frac{1}{2}}$ in terms of A_∞, τ_1.

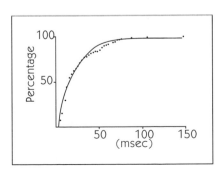

Figure 4.27
Adapted from Cooper and Shrier (1985).

d. The solution to Eq. (2) is

$$x_2(t) = B_\infty \left[1 - \exp\left(\frac{-t}{\tau_2} \right) \right],$$

where B_∞ and τ_2 are constants. Figure 4.28 is reproduced from the Noble and Tsien article. The filled circles represent experimental measurements of $x_1(t) + x_2(t)$; the solid line that overlaps the solid circles at the end of the record is a theoretical estimate of $A_\infty + x_2(t)$; and the filled triangles represent an estimate of $B_\infty + x_1(t)$. Estimate τ_1 and τ_2 (a very rough estimate within 20 percent of their value is fine). HINT: There are many ways to do this, but it is easiest to use the result in part c of this problem.

4.7 The Hodgkin–Huxley equations (Hodgkin and Huxley, 1952) describe the electrical potential across the cell membrane in a nerve cell axon. They represent an outstanding example of the application of nonlinear ordinary differential equations to biology.

The axon membrane—as are all excitable cells—is perforated by proteins that conduct specific ions. The ability of the proteins to conduct the ions depends on the voltage across the membrane. The voltage, in turn, depends on the levels of the various conductances applicable to each species of ion. In this problem, we will deal with only part of the Hodgkin–Huxley system of equations relating to the conductance of potassium ions through the membrane. The units for measuring conductance are *mho*. In order to account for the size of the axon, it is convenient to present conductance in $m.mho/cm^2$.

The potassium conductance, g_k, is given by

$$g_k = \overline{g}_k n^4, \tag{4.27}$$

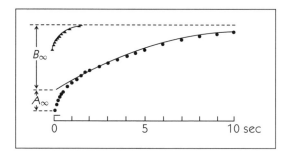

Figure 4.28   Adapted from Noble and Tsien (1969).

where

$$\frac{dn}{dt} = \alpha_n(1 - n) - \beta_n n. \tag{4.28}$$

Here $\bar{g}_k$ is a constant and α_n and β_n are constants that depend on voltage.

a. Assume that β_n is a function of the form

$$\beta_n = C_1 \exp\left(\frac{V}{C_2}\right).$$

Find C_1 and C_2 from the following table reproduced from the original article. The original article reported $C_1 = 0.125$ msec^{-1} and $C_2 = 80$ mv. If you do this correctly, your results will differ somewhat from the reported values. You might enjoy checking the original article and tracking down the origin of the discrepancy.

	V (mV)	β_n (msec^{-1})
A	-109	0.037
B	-100	0.043
C	-88	0.052
D	-76	0.057
E	-63	0.064
F	-51	0.069
G	-38	0.075
H	-32	0.071
I	-26	0.072
J	-19	0.072
K	-10	0.096
L	-6	0.105

b. Solve Eq. 4.28 and express the result as a function of the initial value n_0.

c. Using the solution of Equations 4.27 and 4.28, show that g_k can be given by

$$g_k = \left\{ (g_{k_\infty})^{\frac{1}{4}} - \left[(g_{k_\infty})^{\frac{1}{4}} - (g_{k_0})^{\frac{1}{4}} \right] e^{\frac{-t}{\tau_n}} \right\}^4. \qquad (4.29)$$

Give the values of g_{k_∞}, g_{k_0}, and τ_n in terms of $\overline{g}_k$, α_n, β_n, and n_0.

d. Plot Eq. 4.29 for $g_{k_0} = 0.09$ m.mho/cm^2, $g_{k_\infty} = 7.06$ m.mho/cm^2, and $\tau_n = 0.75$ msec.

✏ **4.8** The diffusion equation can be written as

$$\frac{\partial C}{\partial t} = D \frac{\partial^2 C}{\partial x^2},$$

where D is a diffusion coefficient and C is the concentration of a chemical compound. For a particular initial condition, a solution of this equation for a tube of length L, $0 \le x \le L$, is

$$C(x, t) = C_0 \left[1 - \frac{2}{\pi} \cos\left(\frac{\pi x}{L}\right) e^{\frac{-\pi^2 D t}{L^2}} \right].$$

a. Show that $C(x, t)$ above is a solution of the diffusion equation.

b. What is the concentration at $t = 0$? At $t \rightarrow \infty$?

c. Show that the flux across the boundary (equal to $D \frac{\partial C}{\partial x}$) is zero at $x = 0$ and $x = L$.

d. At all points in the tube (except $x = \frac{\pi}{2}$) the evolution from the initial concentration to the asymptotic concentration as $t \rightarrow \infty$ follows an exponential curve. Determine the time needed to go one-half way from the initial to the final concentration at each point (except $x = \frac{\pi}{2}$) for $D = 10^{-5}$ cm^2/sec for a tube with $L = 10$ cm.

✏ **4.9** The graph in Figure 4.29 gives experimental data concerning the growth of the yeast *Schizosaccharomyces kephir*. The data points have been fit to the logistic function

$$N(t) = \frac{a}{1 + be^{-\gamma t}},$$

where a, b, and γ are positive constants.

a. Determine the values of k_1 and k_2, in terms of a, b, and γ, such that the above expression is a solution of the nonlinear differential equation

$$\frac{dN}{dt} = k_1 N - k_2 N^2.$$

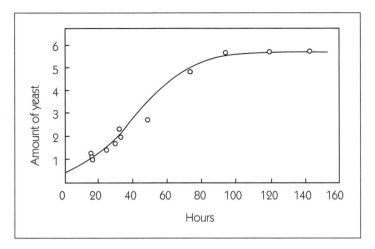

Figure 4.29   Adapted from Gause (1932). (Company of Biologists, Limited)

b. Define $t_{\frac{1}{2}}$ as the value of t for which

$$N(t) = N(0) + 0.5(N(\infty) - N(0)).$$

Analytically calculate the value of $t_{\frac{1}{2}}$ in terms of a, b, and γ.

c. Estimate numerical values for a, b, and γ.

4.10 The following equation has been proposed to describe growth of a bacterial population in culture:

$$\frac{dx}{dt} = Ktxe^{-\alpha^2 t^2},$$

where x is the density of bacteria, K and α are positive constants chosen to agree with experimental data, and t is the time. The solution of this equation is

$$x(t) = x(0) \exp\left[\frac{K}{2\alpha^2}(1 - e^{-\alpha^2 t^2})\right],$$

where $x(0)$ is the density at $t = 0$.

a. Show by direct substitution of the solution into the left- and right-hand sides of the differential equation that this is a solution of the original equation.

b. Suppose that a graph is constructed in which $\ln x(t)$ is plotted as a function of time, $0 \le t$. Sketch this graph. Be sure to show the values at $t = 0, t = \infty$, and at the inflection point.

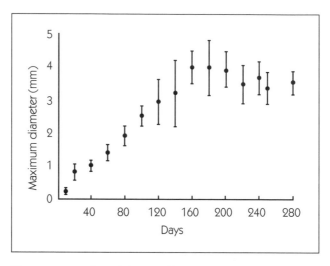

Figure 4.30 Adapted from Folkman and Hochberg (1973). Reproduced from *The Journal of Experimental Medicine* by copyright permission of The Rockefeller University Press.

4.11 Figure 4.30, from Folkman and Hochberg (1973), shows data on the growth of spherical tumor nodules grown in tissue culture.

a. Try to find a set of parameters for Gompertz growth which can be used to fit the data. Plot the theoretical Gompertz curve in the same fashion as the experimental data.

b. Carry out the same steps as in part a but with Verhulst growth.

4.12 A spherical tumor grows at a rate proportional to its volume.

a. Write down and solve the differential equation for the tumor growth.

b. Assume that the doubling time for the tumor volume is 138 days. Derive the equation that gives the radius as a function of time.

c. For the parameters above, when the natural logarithm of the radius of the tumor is plotted against time (in days), the result is a straight line. What are the slope and y-intercept of this line?

4.13 The yearly total of new cases of AIDS reported per year from 1979 to 1988 is shown in Figure 4.31. Assume that the total number of new cases of AIDS is growing exponentially.

a. Using the data provided derive a theoretical expression for the total number of new AIDS cases that will be reported yearly starting from 1989 onward.

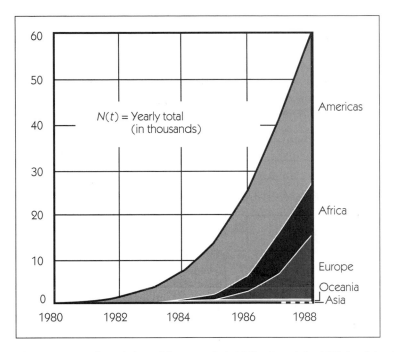

60

50

40    $N(t)$ = Yearly total
           (in thousands)

30

20

10

0

1980   1982   1984   1986   1988

Americas

Africa

Europe

Oceania

Asia

Figure 4.31 Adapted from Mann et al. (1988). Copyright 1988 by Scientific American, Incorporated. All rights reserved.

b. Estimate the year when the number of new AIDS cases will equal 1,000,000.

c. (Optional) Do library research to find out the actual increase in AIDS since 1989. Compare with the theoretical predictions based on exponential growth. Discuss any discrepancies between the actual data and the exponential growth model. Propose a more realistic theoretical model for the growth in the AIDS epidemic, if this is needed.

4.14 You can make yogurt by placing one tablespoon ($\frac{1}{2}$ ounce) of starter culture in 8 ounces of boiled skimmed milk and letting the culture stand for 12 hours at 27° C. At the end of 12 hours the concentration of yogurt cells is the same as in the starter culture. There are 10^6 cells in the initial one tablespoon of starter culture.

a. Assume there is exponential growth, $\frac{dx}{dt} = kx$. What value of k fits the data?

b. For the value of k found in part a, how long does it take for the population to double?

Parts c and d deal with fitting the yogurt growth kinetics to the Verhulst and Gompertz growth equations. To do this assume that the value of k in these equations is known, and that it is 20 percent larger than the value computed in part a.

c. Assume there is Gompertzian growth, $\frac{dx}{dt} = kxe^{-\alpha t}$. What value of α best fits the data? How many cells per tablespoon would be present when growth ceases?

d. Assume there is Verhulstian growth, $\frac{dx}{dt} = kx - \beta x^2$. What value of β best fits the data? For this value of β, after how many hours is the growth rate a maximum?

e. Graph the three growth curves for the parameters found in this question. Extend the time axis sufficiently far so that the asymptotic behavior in time is shown.

✐ **4.15** Consider the differential equation

$$\frac{dx}{dt} = f(x),$$

where

$$f(x) = -9x + 3x^3, \qquad -\infty < x < \infty.$$

a. Sketch $f(x)$. Be sure to show all maxima, minima, and inflection points.

b. Find all the steady states in the differential equation, and algebraically determine if they are stable or unstable. Starting from an initial condition of $x = 0.1$, what happens as $t \to \infty$?

✐ **4.16** For this exercise, only use geometric arguments. No algebra is required. The equation

$$\frac{dx}{dt} = \frac{A\theta^2}{\theta^2 + x^2} - \gamma x, \qquad x \geq 0,$$

where A, θ, and γ are positive constants, is a model of a negative feedback system. How many steady states are there in this system, and what is the stability of these states? Starting from an initial condition of $x = 100$, what happens in the limit $t \to \infty$?

✐ **4.17** Assume that the population density x of a species is determined by the equation

$$\frac{dx}{dt} = \frac{2x^2}{1 + x^3} - x, \qquad 0 \leq x.$$

a. Determine the fixed points for $x \geq 0$.

b. Determine the stability of each fixed point. (HINT: Algebraically compute the stability of the fixed points at $x = 0$ and $x = 1$. If there are additional fixed points, try to estimate their location and stability using geometric arguments.)

c. Discuss the behavior in the limit $t \to \infty$ for $x(0) = 0.001$, $x(0) = 0.8$, and $x(0) = 10.0$.

✏ **4.18** A theoretical ecologist is examining mathematical models for population dynamics. She considers the equation

$$\frac{dx}{dt} = f(x) = \frac{2x^m}{1 + x^4} - x, \qquad x \geq 0,$$

where x is the population density and m is a positive integer. Note that $x = 0$ and $x = 1$ are fixed points of the differential equation. This problem deals with analyzing the differences in the qualitative dynamics in this problem when $m = 1$ and $m = 2$.

a. For $m = 1$, determine the number and stability of all fixed points. Sketch $f(x)$.

b. For $m = 2$, determine the number and stability of all fixed points. Sketch $f(x)$.

c. Describe the dynamics as $t \to \infty$ for initial conditions of very small positive densities for the two cases described above.

d. Describe the dynamics as $t \to \infty$ for initial conditions of very large positive densities for the two cases described above.

✏ **4.19** Explain why the *area* under the spike, and not the spike's amplitude, describes the amount of the drug in a pill. (HINT: Set $\alpha = 0$ in Eq. 4.16 and solve for x to find the amount by which a single pill increases x.)

✏ **4.20** A patient in a hospital is being administered a drug in bolus intravenous doses every four hours. The size of each bolus is 100 mg. The drug has a half-life of four hours and decays exponentially. You can assume the system is linear.

a. After the patient has been on this regimen for ten days, drug administration is stopped. Give the equation for the decay of the drug following cessation of drug administration in terms of D_0, where D_0 is the amount of drug in the body immediately before the administration of the last dose.

b. Compute D_0 described in part a. Use any technique you wish. One technique (but not the simplest) uses the fact that for the geometric series

$$h_0 = a, \quad h_1 = ar, \quad h_2 = ar^2, \quad \ldots, h_n = ar^n,$$

$$\sum_{i=0}^{\infty} h_i = \frac{a}{1-r}.$$

4.21 The differential equation for a low-pass filter with input $f(t)$ and output $x(t)$ is

$$\frac{dx}{dt} = -\omega_0 x + f(t),$$

where ω_0 is a positive constant. Assume the input is $f(t) = A \sin \omega t$.

a. Show that the output after the initial transient has died out is

$$x(t) = B \sin(\omega t - \phi).$$

b. Determine approximate expressions for B in the limits (i) $0 < \omega \ll \omega_0$; and (ii) $\omega_0 \ll \omega$.

c. The graph shown in Figure 4.32 of $\ln B$ as a function of $\ln \omega$ is called the *Bode plot*. Determine c_1, c_2, and c_3 as a function of A and ω_0.

4.22 This problem concerns the economics of production and trade.

Assume that there are two producers of widgets, A and B. Each producer has a certain fraction of the total market for widgets. The cost of producing widgets depends on how many are produced, so the cost for each company depends on the fraction of the market that company captures.

Let the fractions of the market captured by company A be v. Company B fraction is therefore $1 - v$. Denote the average cost per widget for company A as $A(v)$ and likewise the cost for company B as $B(1 - v)$.

It has been traditional to assume that there are increasing marginal costs of production. This means that it costs more to produce an additional single widget if many widgets are already being produced than if few widgets are being

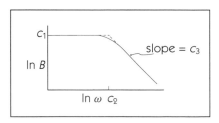

Figure 4.32

produced. An example of such an average cost function is

$$A_\uparrow(v) = 1.3 \frac{e^v - 1}{v}.$$

In some industries, however, the average cost decreases as production increases. For example, in the software industry, the main expense is in developing the software, and it costs virtually nothing to produce an extra copy of the software. An example of a cost function where this is the case is

$$A_\downarrow(v) = \frac{1 + 2(1 - e^{-v})}{v}.$$

Figure 4.33 shows graphs of both increasing and decreasing marginal costs. As a model of the free market, assume that $\frac{dv}{dt}$ is proportional to the difference in

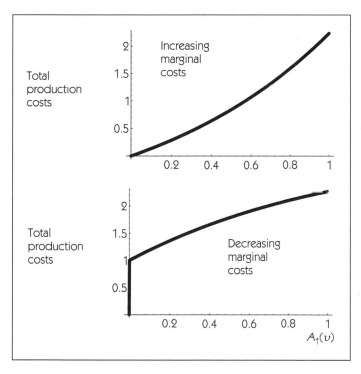

Figure 4.33 The total production costs $vA(v)$ for the average production function with increasing marginal costs, $A_\uparrow(v)$, and the function with decreasing marginal costs, $A_\downarrow(v)$.

production cost per widget between company B and company A. That is,

$$\frac{dv}{dt} = B(1 - v) - A(v),$$

so that if $A(v)$ is less than $B(1 - v)$, company's A market share will increase. Obviously if company A is more efficient than company B, we expect company A to capture a larger share of the market. For this example, though, we will assume that both companies are *identical* in terms of their production costs, so that $B(v) = A(v)$.

a. For the case of increasing marginal costs, the differential equation describing company A's market share is

$$\frac{dv}{dt} = A_\uparrow(1 - v) - A_\uparrow(v).$$

Show that the stable fixed point for this system is $v = 0.5$, that is, both companies split the market evenly.

b. For the case of decreasing marginal costs, write the differential equation for v in terms of $A_\downarrow$. Show that there is a fixed point at $v = 0.5$, but that it is unstable. Describe where the stable fixed points are. (Remember, since v is a fraction of the market, it is limited to the range 0 to 1.)

c. Discuss how initial conditions are related to the asymptotic value of v in the case of increasing marginal costs, and in the case of decreasing marginal costs.

✐ **4.23** Use geometric techniques to show that linear differential equations can have only one fixed point.

Explain graphically the difference between a linear differential equation (which gives exponential growth or decay) and an equation that produces linear growth or decay.

✐ **4.24** The spruce budworm is a caterpillar that infests the spruce and fir forests of eastern Canada and the northeastern US. The budworm will stay at a low population level for many years and then will dramatically increase in population when the trees in the forest have reached a certain maturity. This explosion of the caterpillar population can be devastating to the forest.

A simple differential equation describing the growth of the budworm is given by

$$\frac{dx}{dt} = R(1 - x/Q) - \frac{x}{1 + x^2} \tag{4.30}$$

where $x(t)$ is the number of budworms at any time, and Q is a parameter that stays fixed. R is a parameter that changes in time, and represents the food resources available to the budworm. As the forest grows and more food becomes available, R increases.

One way to think of Eq. 4.30 is as a balance between growth rates and death rates. We re-write Eq. 4.30 as

$$\frac{dx}{dt} = (f(x) - g(x))\, x. \qquad (4.31)$$

The term

$$f(x) = R(1 - x/Q)$$

is positive for small x, and reflects the birth of new budworms. As the forest grows, R increases and $f(x)$ changes accordingly. The term

$$g(x) = \frac{x}{1 + x^2}$$

reflects death, and does not change with R.

The figure shows $f(x)$ and $g(x)$ for $R = 0.3$ and $Q = 8$.

a. Using Figure 4.34, find any steady states of x and say whether they are stable or unstable. (You can give an approximate numerical value for x at the steady state.)

b. Find the x- and y-intercepts of $f(x)$ in terms of R and Q. In the parts c and d, keep in mind that $f(x)$ is a line drawn between these two points.

c. Graphically, find a value of R at which there are 3 steady states. Give approximate numerical values for the positions of these steady states, and say which ones are stable and which ones are unstable.

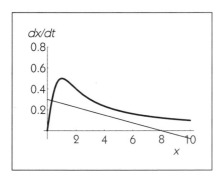

Figure 4.34

d. Graphically, find the smallest value for R at which there is only one steady state with value of $x > 3$. Is this steady state stable or not?

e. Imagine that the forest is immature, so that $R = 0.3$. The forest grows with time, so that R increases steadily. After 10 years, R reaches the value you found in part d. Q is held fixed at $Q = 8$.

Make a rough sketch of the budworm population versus time in years. (You can assume that the budworm reproduces with a short generation time, so that the population never takes more than a few weeks to reach its steady state value for a given Q and R.)

Continue your graph, using the fact that if the budworm reaches $x = 3$, then the forest is wiped out, and R returns to 0.3 within a few months. Mark when the population explosion begins, and explain why it occurs in terms of the stability of steady states.

✎ **4.25** Money in your bank account makes 5% interest per year, compounded daily. Write the finite-difference equation for this situation. What exponential equation gives the same growth rate?

✎ **4.26** Suppose that a herd of ten cows is introduced to a field with almost no vegetation, $V = 0.1$. Using the graphs in Figure 4.11, show that the vegetation grows faster than it is eaten, so that V increases. Seeing the growth of vegetation, a land manager decides to add ten more cows to the field. What is the smallest value of V at which this can be done in a way that will keep all the cows well fed? What happens if the new cows are introduced too early?

In the real world, it is difficult to make precise measurements of V. Growth and consumption curves are only approximations to real growth and consumption, which are affected by factors outside of the equations, such as the weather. Comment on how attempts to maximize the production of beef can lead to disaster.

✎ **4.27** What happens if Δ is too large in the Euler method? Use the original example of $\frac{dx}{dt} = 1.2(x - x^2)$ with $\Delta = 1$ and $\Delta = 0.5$.

✎ **4.28** Find the doubling time t_{DT} in terms of the constant of proportionality a in Eq. 4.5. In exponential growth, the doubling time is independent of the initial condition $x(0)$. Is this true for linear growth?

✎ **4.29** This problem deals with an alternative technique to solve Eq. 4.16 using an **integrating factor**. Let us rewrite Eq. 4.16 as

$$\frac{dx}{ds} - \alpha x = I(s).$$

HINT: to carry out the two parts of this problem multiply this equation by the integrating factor $e^{-\alpha s}$.

a. Integrate this equation for $I(s) = k$ between the limits $s = 0$ to $s = t$. This provides an alternative method to solve the equation in Example 4.3.

b. Integrate this equation for any $I(s)$. This provides an alternative derivation of Eq. 4.23.

COMPUTER PROJECTS

Project 1 A basic technique in the study of dynamical systems is to solve differential equations using numerical methods. Many different techniques are possible. The simplest is called the **Euler method.**

As we discussed in Section 4.6, the nonlinear differential equation Eq. 4.14,

$$\frac{dx}{dt} = f(x)$$

can be approximated by the finite-difference equation Eq. 4.15

$$x_{t+1} = f(x_t)\Delta + x_t.$$

The **Euler method** for the numerical integration of differential equations exploits this relationship to numerically integrate nonlinear ordinary equations. The accuracy of the approximation depends on Δ. As Δ decreases, the accuracy of the integration improves.

This project deals with numerical integration of Eq. 4.7. The analytical solution of this equation is given by Eq. 4.8. Use a computer to plot out the values of $x(t)$ in Eq. 4.8 for the case $\alpha = 1, k = 1$. Now integrate Eq. 4.7 using the Euler method. To do this you simply apply Eq. 4.15 with the appropriate form for $f(x)$. It is necessary to specify Δ. Carry out the integration using different values for Δ. Try to assess the accuracy of the approximation as a function of Δ. How small does Δ have to be in order to obtain agreement between the analytical solution and the numerical solution of 1%? At what value of Δ does the dynamics show oscillations as $t \to \infty$ rather than an approach to a steady state? The fact that this approximate method gives a qualitatively wrong answer if Δ is too large, should impress on you the necessity for testing for possible artifacts introduced by numerical integration. Testing routines for numerical integration by exercising the numerical method against an analytic solution, as you have done in this problem, is a practice that will help eliminate numerical errors when developing programs to carry out numerical integration.

Project 2 Write a computer program to use the Euler method to integrate one-variable delay-differential equations such as

$$\frac{dx}{dt} = P(x(t - \tau)) - \alpha x(t).$$

You will have to keep track of past values of x—this is easier if you select Δ to divide τ evenly, for instance $\Delta = \tau/100$. In specifying the initial condition, you will need to give not just $x(0)$, but also the previous values of x going as far back as $x(-\tau)$.

A very simple delay-differental equation is

$$\frac{dx}{dt} = h(x(t - \tau)),$$

where the function $h()$ is

$$h(x(t - \tau)) = \begin{cases} -1 & \text{if } x(t - \tau) > 0; \\ 1 & \text{otherwise.} \end{cases}$$

Integrate this equation numerically, to see if it produces regular or irregular oscillations, and how these oscillations depend on τ.

Another simple delay-differential equation is

$$\frac{dx}{dt} = -\alpha x(t - \tau)$$

which will produce oscillations that either increase or decrease in amplitude depending on the value of α relative to τ. Experiment with different values of α, and show that when α is such that the oscillations neither increase nor decrease in amplitude, the period of the oscillation is 4τ.

Project 3 This project deals with the numerical integration of the delay differential equation Eq. 4.26 proposed as a theoretical model for the production of red blood cells.

This equation can also be integrated using the Euler method. However, in specifying the initial condition it is necessary to specify the in the value of $x(t)$ over an initial time interval, rather than just at a single time. The reason for this is that the derivative at the current time t, depends on the value of x at time $(t - \tau)$ where τ is the time delay in the equation. This type of delay differential equation is not very well understood mathematically and there are many questions of research calibre that can easily be addressed.

One of the issues involves trying to analyze the bifurcations of this equation. Consider the following equation

$$\frac{dx}{dt} = \frac{2x(t - \tau)}{1 + x(t - \tau)^n} - x.$$

Assume that $\tau = 2$ and study the effect of varying n. Use the Euler method to integrate the equations. In using the Euler method, you have to pick a value for τ and the time delay, Δ such that τ is a multiple of Δ.

One research-level question involves studying the bifurcations in this problem and comparing them with bifurcations in one-dimensional finite-difference equations with a single hump. (See the Computer exercises following Chapter 1.) Mackey and Glass observed (1977), that the delay equation for blood cell control shows period-doubling bifurcations as well as chaotic dynamics, but it is not yet known if the same sequence of periodic orbits is observed in the delay differential equations and the one-dimensional finite-difference equations. One of the problems in studying the bifurcation sequence here is to compute the period of periodic orbits numerically. You will have to figure out a way to do this. Here is a hint for how to get started. Embed the trajectory in a two-dimensional plane in which the value $x(t - \tau)$ is plotted as a function of $x(t)$. Such a time-delay embedding (see Section 6.6) can be used to help identify periodic and chaotic orbits; see Glass and Mackey (1979).

Another class of projects involve determining if there are different asymptotic behaviors starting from a different initial condition. Start with different initial conditions. For example, you can set the value of x between $t = 0$ and $t = 2$ to be a modulated sine wave that is offset so that x is positive over this interval. Does the asymptotic behavior depend on the initial condition?

CHAPTER 5

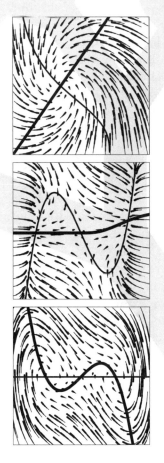

Two-Dimensional Differential Equations

In the previous chapter we studied differential equations in which quantities increased or decreased in a monotonic fashion, reaching a fixed point as time increased. We know that in the real world quantities can also oscillate up and down in a regular or irregular fashion. The one-dimensional differential equations in the previous chapter, which have a single variable and a first derivative, cannot produce oscillation. In this chapter we consider differential equations with either a pair of variables and their first derivatives, or a single variable and its first and second derivatives. These two classes of problems are equivalent and are called **second-order** or **two-dimensional ordinary differential equations**.

5.1 THE HARMONIC OSCILLATOR

This section introduces several important concepts by considering a familiar problem from elementary physics courses—a mass on a spring (see Figure 5.1). Although masses and springs are of interest mainly to mechanical

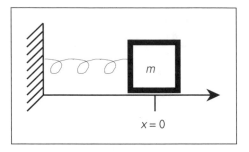

Figure 5.1
The mass on a spring: the archetypical harmonic oscillator.

engineers, the mathematics describing them are fundamental to understanding the dynamics of many other systems. Because the problem is of general interest, it has a general name: the **harmonic oscillator**.

Consider a mass, m, that is attached to a spring resting on a very smooth table so that there is no friction between the mass and the table. If the spring is neither stretched nor compressed, the mass will rest at a steady-state position. Call this position $x = 0$. If the spring is compressed, that is, if $x < 0$, there will be a force tending to increase x, if the spring is stretched, $x > 0$, there will be a force tending to decrease x. According to Hooke's law, familiar from elementary physics, the force, F, is proportional to the position

$$F = -kx,$$

where the constant k is called the **spring constant**. Note that Hooke's law says that there is a *linear* relationship between force and position. Newton's second law of motion says that the acceleration a of a particle of mass m is related to the force on the particle by the famous expression

$$F = ma.$$

In differential calculus, acceleration is simply the second derivative of the position with respect to time. This is because velocity is the rate of change of x with respect to time, $v = \frac{dx}{dt}$, and acceleration is the rate of change of velocity with respect to time, $a = \frac{dv}{dt} = \frac{d^2x}{dt^2}$. Using this fact along with Newton's second law of motion and Hooke's law, we find

$$m\frac{d^2x}{dt^2} = -kx. \tag{5.1}$$

This is a linear, second-order, ordinary differential equation. In general, we want to solve this equation given some initial values of the position and the velocity.

5.2 SOLUTIONS, TRAJECTORIES, AND FLOWS

Let us assume that at $t = 0$ the mass in Figure 5.1 is displaced to a position $x(0)$ and released from rest so that the initial velocity is $v(0) = 0$. We propose the following function as a solution to Eq. 5.1:

$$x(t) = x(0) \cos \omega t \quad \text{where} \quad \omega = \sqrt{\frac{k}{m}}. \tag{5.2}$$

Demonstrating that this is indeed a solution is straightforward: If we substitute this proposed solution into Eq. 5.1 and carry out the second derivative, we find that both sides of the equation are the same. A graph of this solution is shown in Figure 5.2. The solution oscillates without approaching a steady state. The time it takes to complete one cycle of the oscillation is $\frac{2\pi}{\omega}$.

What is the initial condition for this solution? By analogy to Chapter 4, we might say that it is $x(0)$. But this is only half the story. If we placed the mass at position $x(0)$, it might be moving either to the right, to the left, or not at all; to provide a complete description of the initial condition, we also need to specify $v(0)$. In the solution given in Eq. 5.2, we happened to set $v(0) = 0$, but we might ask what are the solutions for other values of $v(0)$.

One way to gain insight into the dynamics of the harmonic oscillator is to consider all the possible initial conditions. Each possible initial condition can be represented as a point on a plane—the (x, v)-plane. The **state** of the harmonic oscillator at time t is the pair of values $(x(t), v(t))$. We can plot out the state as time proceeds simply by plotting $(x(t), v(t))$ in the (x, v)-plane. The path traced out is called the **trajectory**. The (x, v)-plane is called the **phase plane**.

Note that given a solution $x(t)$, we can easily find the velocity $v(t)$ by differentiation:

$$v(t) = -\omega x(0) \sin \omega t. \tag{5.3}$$

From Equations 5.2 and 5.3, and using the trigonometric identity $\sin^2 \omega t +$

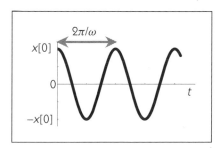

Figure 5.2
A solution $x(t)$ to Eq. 5.1.

$\cos^2 \omega t = 1$, we find

$$x^2(t) + \frac{v^2(t)}{\omega^2} = x^2(0). \qquad (5.4)$$

This is the equation for an ellipse in the (x, v)-plane (see Section A.8). An example of the trajectory for two different initial conditions is shown in Figure 5.3. Both initial conditions have $v(0) = 0$, but one has $x(0) = 0.5$ while the other has $x(0) = 1.0$. You can see that the two trajectories plotted in Figure 5.3 are both ellipses with the same shape but different sizes; the size is governed by the initial conditions $x(0)$ and $v(0)$.

Recall from physics that the **potential energy** of a mass on a spring is $\frac{1}{2}kx^2$ and the **kinetic energy** is $\frac{1}{2}mv^2$. It follows from Equation 5.4 and $\omega = \sqrt{\frac{k}{m}}$ that

$$\frac{1}{2}kx(t)^2 + \frac{1}{2}mv(t)^2 = \frac{1}{2}kx^2(0).$$

The sum of the potential and kinetic energies is the **total energy**, and we can see from the above equation that "energy is conserved," that is, the total energy does not change. In this case the conservation of energy holds because there is no friction and because nothing is putting energy into the system. The energy always stays at the same value it had originally. In many other systems, energy is not conserved. Later, we will study some such systems.

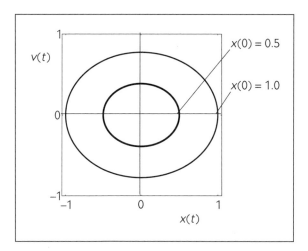

Figure 5.3   The trajectory of two solutions to Eq. 5.1, plotted in the phase plane. One solution has initial condition $x(0) = 0.5$, $v(0) = 0$; the other has initial condition $x(0) = 1.0$, $v(0) = 0$.

One of the consequences of the conservation of energy in the harmonic oscillator concerns the stability of the trajectories. We have already seen that all the trajectories are closed ellipses. These closed ellipses correspond to periodic cycles. Are these cycles stable? Just as in finite-difference equations, a stable cycle is a cycle that is reestablished following a small displacement from the cycle. In the current case, a small displacement leads to another closed ellipsoidal trajectory—the displaced trajectory will not find its way back to the original trajectory. Thus, the cycles in the harmonic oscillator are not stable.

The initial condition is a special case of the state: It is the state at time $t = 0$. So, given the trajectory from an initial condition, we also have the trajectory through many other possible initial conditions—any initial condition that lies on a given trajectory will follow that same trajectory.

A two-dimensional differential equation can be represented as a pattern in the phase plane. The equation can be thought of as a rule that tells us how any given state changes in time. In other words, the equation tells us how a trajectory passes through any point in the phase plane. For any given initial condition, there is only one trajectory; however, the differential equation tells us about all possible trajectories.

We could plot out this information by showing every possible trajectory. This would not be very practical, since the entire phase plane would be covered with ink. Instead, we will draw the trajectory through only a few points, indicating the direction of the trajectory by making the line thicker as time progresses. The entire pattern of trajectories in the phase plane is called the **flow** of the differential equation (analogous to the flow of water). A single trajectory is analogous to the path that would be followed by a (massless) particle if it had been placed in the water; the initial condition is analogous to the place the particle is first placed. Figure 5.4 shows the flow for the harmonic oscillator.

5.3 THE TWO-DIMENSIONAL LINEAR ORDINARY DIFFERENTIAL EQUATION

In the analysis of one-dimensional nonlinear finite-difference equations (Chapter 1) and differential equations (Chapter 4), the basis for the local stability analysis was a firm understanding of the linear system. Similarly, the analysis of two-dimensional nonlinear ordinary equations follows in a straightforward fashion once we understand the linear problem. The linear problem is also of interest in its own right, since many theoretical models in kinetics, mechanics, and electrical circuits are formulated as two-dimensional linear ordinary equations.

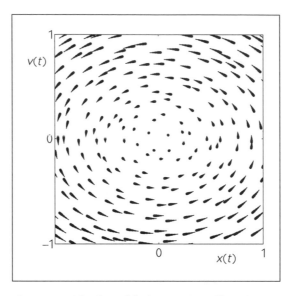

Figure 5.4   The flow of the harmonic oscillator in Eq. 5.1.

The two-dimensional linear ordinary differential equation is written as

$$a\frac{d^2x}{dt^2} + b\frac{dx}{dt} + cx = 0, \tag{5.5}$$

where a, b, and c are constants that we will assume are real numbers. In Chapter 4 we saw that the solution to the one-dimensional linear ordinary differential equation is an exponential. It is an amazing fact that an exponential is also often the solution to higher-dimensional ordinary differential equations—but of course there is a complex twist to the story.

In order to solve Eq. (5.5) we will substitute in a **trial solution**:

$$x(t) = Ce^{\lambda t}. \tag{5.6}$$

Here C and λ represent constants—we do not yet know their value, but we are hoping to be able to find them from the differential equation. We will be able to do so only if Eq. 5.6 is an appropriate form for a solution to Eq. 5.5. Substituting the trial solution into Eq. 5.5 and carrying out the derivatives, we find

$$aC\lambda^2 e^{\lambda t} + bC\lambda e^{\lambda t} + cCe^{\lambda t} = 0.$$

Dividing each term of this equation by $Ce^{\lambda t}$, we obtain an equation that is called the **characteristic equation**, or the **eigenvalue equation**:

$$a\lambda^2 + b\lambda + c = 0, \tag{5.7}$$

If we can find any values for λ that solve this equation, then we know that the trial solution is valid for those values of λ. Of course, Eq. 5.7 is a quadratic equation in λ. The solution for λ as a function of the parameters a, b, and c can be found from the quadratic formula:

$$\lambda_1 = \frac{-b + \sqrt{b^2 - 4ac}}{2a}, \qquad \lambda_2 = \frac{-b - \sqrt{b^2 - 4ac}}{2a}. \tag{5.8}$$

We call λ_1 and λ_2 the **characteristic values**, or **eigenvalues**, of Eq. 5.5.

Since there are two valid values of λ, we have found two solutions to the differential equation. Actually, there is an infinity of possible solutions, which have the general form

$$x(t) = C_1 e^{\lambda_1 t} + C_2 e^{\lambda_2 t}, \tag{5.9}$$

where C_1 and C_2 are constants. Note that the characteristic equation did not put any constraint on C in the trial solution, so any constant value of C gives a valid solution. The actual values of C_1 and C_2 for any given trajectory are set by the initial conditions.

❏ **EXAMPLE 5.1**

Verify that Eq. 5.9 is a solution to Eq. 5.5.

Solution: Taking the first and second derivative of $x(t)$ from Eq. 5.9 and substituting into Eq. 5.5, we find

$$a(C_1\lambda_1^2 e^{\lambda_1 t} + C_2\lambda_2^2 e^{\lambda_2 t}) + b(C_1\lambda_1 e^{\lambda_1 t} + C_2\lambda_2 e^{\lambda_2 t}) + c(C_1 e^{\lambda_1 t} + C_2 e^{\lambda_2 t}) = 0$$

Re-arranging terms gives

$$(a\lambda_1^2 + b\lambda_1 + c)C_1 e^{\lambda_1 t} + (a\lambda_2^2 + b\lambda_2 + c)C_2 e^{\lambda_2 t} = 0.$$

Eq. 5.9 is a solution to Eq. 5.5 only if the above equation is true. But, since the values of λ_1 and λ_2 are chosen to satisfy the characteristic equation (Eq. 5.7), we know that the terms in the parentheses are zero in the above equation, and so the left-hand side does indeed equal zero. This is true for any values of C_1 and C_2.

◻

Here's the twist in the story: If $b^2 < 4ac$, it follows from Eq. 5.8 that λ_1 and λ_2 are complex numbers. They can be written as

$$\lambda_1 = \alpha + \beta i, \qquad \lambda_2 = \alpha - \beta i,$$

where

$$\alpha = -\frac{b}{2a}, \qquad \beta = \frac{\sqrt{4ac - b^2}}{2a},$$

and of course the infamous $i = \sqrt{-1}$.

You may well be wondering, how can a differential equation that is supposed to describe the real world have a solution that involves imaginary numbers? The answer, in brief, is that C_1 and C_2 are also complex numbers, and that for any real initial conditions, C_1 and C_2 will cancel out the imaginary part of the solution, leaving only the real part.

Many people would feel more comfortable if the solution to Eq. 5.5 could be presented without any mention of imaginary numbers. This real solution is (at least, it's real as long as $b^2 < 4ac$)

$$x(t) = C_3 e^{\alpha t} \cos \beta t + C_4 e^{\alpha t} \sin \beta t, \tag{5.10}$$

where C_3 and C_4 are now *bona fide* real constants, which can be set from initial conditions. However, if $b^2 > 4ac$, then β in Eq. 5.10 is itself complex, and you have to start worrying about what the sine and cosine of a complex number are. In this case, go back to Eq. 5.9, which will now look like a perfectly ordinary solution in terms of exponential functions of real numbers.

For those readers who are interested in understanding the relationship between Eqs. 5.9 and 5.10, we offer the following information. If we have a complex number $\gamma + \delta i$, then

$$e^{\gamma + \delta i} = e^{\gamma} (\cos \delta + i \sin \delta).$$

(See Problem 5.3 for a derivation of this relationship.) Similarly,

$$\cos \omega t = \frac{1}{2} \left(e^{i\omega t} + e^{-i\omega t} \right)$$

and

$$\sin \omega t = \frac{1}{2i} \left(e^{i\omega t} - e^{-i\omega t} \right).$$

These identities lead to one of the most magical relationships in all of mathematics, which involves the seemingly unrelated irrational numbers e and π, along with $i = \sqrt{-1}$:

$$e^{i\pi} + 1 = 0.$$

❏ **EXAMPLE 5.2**

In the real world, a harmonic oscillator such as a spring does not swing forever; it eventually slows down due to friction and air resistance. This friction is called "damping," and the equation for a damped spring can be written as

$$\frac{d^2x}{dt^2} + \mu \frac{dx}{dt} + \omega^2 x = 0,$$

where μ is a number that describes how much damping there is. If μ were zero (i.e., no damping), then the solution to the equation would be a sinusoid with a period of oscillation of $\frac{2\pi}{\omega}$. Determine the solution of this equation in the presence of damping, starting from an initial condition of $x(0) = 5$ deg and $\frac{dx}{dt} = 0$ deg/sec.

Solution: The characteristic equation for this system is

$$\lambda^2 + \mu\lambda + \omega^2 = 0.$$

The eigenvalues of this are

$$\lambda_1 = \frac{1}{2} \left[-\mu + \sqrt{\mu^2 - 4\omega^2} \right] \quad \text{and} \quad \lambda_2 = \frac{1}{2} \left[-\mu - \sqrt{\mu^2 - 4\omega^2} \right].$$

If $\mu^2 > 4\omega^2$, both eigenvalues are negative. If $\mu^2 < 4\omega^2$, both eigenvalues are complex conjugates. These two cases are treated differently, as desribed below.

- When $\mu^2 > 4\omega^2$: Call $\alpha = \sqrt{\mu^2 - 4\omega^2}$. The solution can be written as

$$x(t) = C_1 e^{\frac{-\mu+\alpha}{2} t} + C_2 e^{\frac{-\mu-\alpha}{2} t}.$$

From the initial conditions ($x(0) = 5$ and $\frac{dx}{dt} = 0$) we find that

$$C_1 + C_2 = 5; \qquad \left(\frac{-\mu + \alpha}{2} \right) C_1 + \left(\frac{-\mu - \alpha}{2} \right) C_2 = 0.$$

Since there are two equations in the two unknowns, we can solve for C_1 and C_2:

$$C_1 = \frac{5}{2} \left(\frac{\alpha + \mu}{\alpha} \right) \quad \text{and} \quad C_2 = \frac{5}{2} \left(\frac{\alpha - \mu}{\alpha} \right).$$

Therefore, the solution of the equation is

$$x(t) = \frac{5}{2} \left(\frac{\alpha + \mu}{\alpha} \right) e^{\frac{-\mu + \alpha}{2} t} + \frac{5}{2} \left(\frac{\alpha - \mu}{\alpha} \right) e^{\frac{-\mu - \alpha}{2} t}.$$

Since $\mu > \alpha$, both eigenvalues are negative and there is a monotonic approach to $x = 0$. This is illustrated in Figure 5.5.

- When $\mu^2 < 4\omega^2$: Call $\alpha = \sqrt{4\omega^2 - \mu^2}$. Therefore, from Eq. 5.10 we know that the solution is

$$x(t) = C_3 e^{-\frac{\mu t}{2}} \cos \frac{\alpha t}{2} + C_4 e^{-\frac{\mu t}{2}} \sin \frac{\alpha t}{2}.$$

Now applying the initial conditions at $t = 0$, we find

$$C_3 = 5, \qquad \left(\frac{-\mu}{2} \right) C_3 + \left(\frac{\alpha}{2} \right) C_4 = 0.$$

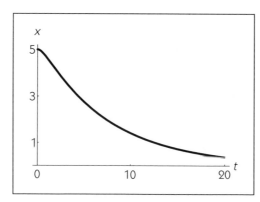

Figure 5.5
The solution of the differential equation for the damped pendulum with $\mu = 2, \omega = 0.5$.

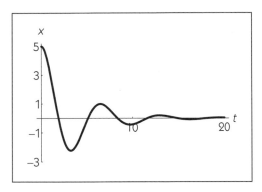

Figure 5.6
The solution to the differential equation for the damped pendulum with $\mu = 0.5, \omega = 1$.

Consequently, we have

$$C_3 = 5 \quad \text{and} \quad C_4 = \frac{5\mu}{\alpha}.$$

Therefore, the solution $x(t)$ is

$$x(t) = 5e^{-\frac{\mu t}{2}} \cos \frac{\alpha t}{2} + \frac{5\mu}{\alpha} e^{-\frac{\mu t}{2}} \sin \frac{\alpha t}{2}.$$

This is an oscillatory decay to $x = 0$, as illustrated in Figure 5.6. $\quad\square$

5.4 COUPLED FIRST-ORDER LINEAR EQUATIONS

In the case of the mass on a spring, there was one fundamental variable, position, from which the velocity and acceleration could be derived. In other systems there may be more than one fundamental variable, and the rate of change of each of the variables may be a function of the current values of all the variables. Here, we will consider the case where there are two such variables. The two variables might represent, for example, two interacting animal species in an ecological system, two different conductances of ion channels in a cell membrane, two different chemicals in a chemical reaction, or the concentration of a drug in two different organs.

Such systems can be represented by a pair of **coupled** ordinary differential equations. In a simple but important case, the derivatives are linear functions of the variables so that

$$\frac{dx}{dt} = Ax + By, \qquad \frac{dy}{dt} = Cx + Dy, \tag{5.11}$$

where A, B, C, and D are constants. Although Eqs. 5.5 and 5.11 and at first appear to be different, they are completely equivalent. Therefore, once you know how to solve one of them, you can solve the other.

In order to show the equivalence of both formulations, we first compute the second derivative $\frac{d^2x}{dt^2}$ in Eq. 5.11, to obtain

$$\frac{d^2x}{dt^2} = A\frac{dx}{dt} + B\frac{dy}{dt}.$$

Now substituting the value for $\frac{dy}{dt}$ from Eq. 5.11 into the above expression, we find

$$\frac{d^2x}{dt^2} = A\frac{dx}{dt} + BCx + BDy.$$

Finally, since from Eq. 5.11 we know that $By = \frac{dx}{dt} - Ax$, we can substitute this value to obtain finally the expression

$$\frac{d^2x}{dt^2} - (A + D)\frac{dx}{dt} + (AD - BC)x = 0.$$

Thus, Eq. 5.11 is equivalent to Eq. 5.5 as long as

$$-(A + D) = \frac{b}{a} \quad \text{and} \quad AD - BC = \frac{c}{a}.$$

For any a, b, and c, values of A, B, C, and D that satisfy this relationship can always be found, and vice versa.

We can find the solution to Eq. 5.11 in terms of A, B, C, and D by solving the characteristic equation. In the current case, following the same procedure as in the preceding section, the characteristic equation is

$$\lambda^2 - (A + D)\lambda + (AD - BC) = 0, \tag{5.12}$$

so that the eigenvalues are computed from the quadratic equation as

$$\lambda_1 = \frac{A + D}{2} + \frac{\sqrt{(A - D)^2 + 4BC}}{2}$$

$$\lambda_2 = \frac{A + D}{2} - \frac{\sqrt{(A - D)^2 + 4BC}}{2}. \tag{5.13}$$

Thus, the solution for $x(t)$ is given by

$$x(t) = C_1 e^{\lambda_1 t} + C_2 e^{\lambda_2 t}$$

which is real if λ_1 and λ_2 are real numbers. If $(A - D)^2 + 4BC < 0$, then λ_1 and λ_2 are complex numbers. Let

$$\alpha = \frac{A + D}{2} \quad \text{and} \quad i\beta = \frac{\sqrt{(A - D)^2 + 4BC}}{2}.$$

Then, $\lambda_1 = \alpha + i\beta$ and $\lambda_2 = \alpha - i\beta$ and the solution is

$$x(t) = e^{\alpha t}(C_3 \cos \beta t + C_4 \sin \beta t).$$

C_1 and C_2, or C_3 and C_4 can be found from the initial condition $x(0)$ and $\frac{dx}{dt}(0)$. If λ_1 and λ_2 are real, then

$$x(0) = C_1 + C_2$$
$$\frac{dx}{dt}(0) = \lambda_1 C_1 + \lambda_2 C_2,$$

which can be solved for C_1 and C_2. If λ_1 and λ_2 are complex, then

$$x(0) = C_3$$
$$\frac{dx}{dt}(0) = \alpha C_3 + \beta C_4.$$

DYNAMICS IN ACTION

14 METASTASIS OF MALIGNANT TUMORS

Metastasis of cancer is a process whereby cancer cells spread in the body. In some cases, the cancer cells spread through the bloodstream and are arrested in the capillary bed of an organ. Most of the arrested cells either die or are dislodged from the capillary bed, but some are able to traverse the capillary wall and initiate metastatic foci in the tissue of the organ. Liotta and DeLisi (1977) studied metastasis of radioactively labeled tumor cells to the lungs of laboratory mice. The cells were injected into the tail veins of mice and transported to the lung by the bloodstream. The radioactive labeling allowed the number of tumor cells in the mice's lungs to be measured.

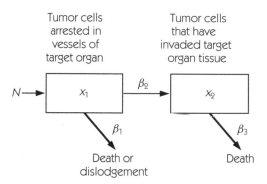

Compartmental model for metastatic spread of cancer cells. x_1 is the number of cancer cells arrested in the vessels of the target organ and x_2 is the number of tumor cells that have invade the target organ tissue. The cells pass between compartments following linear rate laws as described in the text. Adapted from Liotta and Delisi (1977).

The figure on the facing page shows the number of tumor cells plotted on a semilogarithmic scale. If the data were described by an exponential decay, they would fall on a straight line, but this is not the case. Liotta and DeLisi proposed a more complicated theoretical model accounting for the idea that tumor cells are first arrested in the capillary bed of the lung ("compartment 1"), and then invade the lung tissue itself ("compartment 2").

By measuring the various rates from experimental data, it is possible to assess how effective treatments are in reducing metastasis. Based on their knowledge of the biology of metastasis, Liotta and DeLisi propose the following mathematical description of the kinetics of radioactively labeled cells:

$$\frac{dx_1}{dt} = -(\beta_1 + \beta_2)x_1,$$

$$\frac{dx_2}{dt} = \beta_2 x_1 - \beta_3 x_2.$$

The number of arrested cells is designated x_1 and the number that successfully invade the target tissue is designated x_2. Cells pass from compartment 1 to compartment 2 at a rate $\beta_2 x_1$. Cells are lost from compartment 1 by death or dislodgement at a rate $\beta_1 x_1$, and from compartment 2 at a rate $\beta_3 x_2$. These relationships are schematically represented in the upper figure. The initial conditions are $x_1(0) = N$ and $x_2(0) = 0$. N is the number of cells that are initially arrested in the target organ.

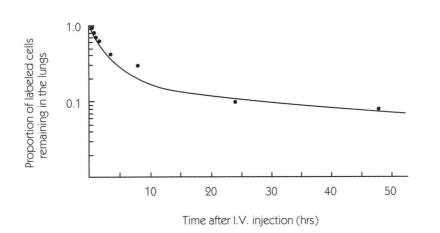

The proportion of labeled cells remaining in the lungs following intravenous injection in the tail veins of mice. The dots show the experimental data, and the line is a fitted solution to the model. Note the semilogarithmic axes. Adapted from Liotta and Delisi (1977) based on Proctor et al. (1976).

Experimentally, the total number of tumor cells in the lung, $x_1(t) + x_2(t)$, is measured. The model can be used to calculate $x_1(t) + x_2(t)$, and the experimental measurement of this number can then be used to estimate the rates in the model.

Since the variable x_1 follows the kinetics of exponential decay, we can use the methods in Chapter 3 to find

$$x_1(t) = Ne^{-(\beta_1 + \beta_2)t}.$$

To find the solution for $x_2(t)$, we notice that the pair of differential equations looks just like Eq. 5.11 with $x_2 = x$ and $x_1 = y$, and

$$A = -\beta_3, B = -\beta_2, C = 0, \text{ and } D = -(\beta_1 + \beta_2).$$

We can sustitute these values for A, B, C, and D into Eq. 5.13 to find

$$\lambda = -\frac{\beta_1 + \beta_2 + \beta_3}{2} \pm \frac{\sqrt{(\beta_1 + \beta_2 - \beta_3)^2}}{2}$$

so that we find the two eigenvalues

$$\lambda_1 = -\beta_3, \qquad \lambda_2 = -(\beta_1 + \beta_2).$$

Therefore, we obtain

$$x_2(t) = C_1 e^{-\beta_3 t} + C_2 e^{-(\beta_1 + \beta_2)t},$$

where C_1 and C_2 are constants that still need to be set from the initial conditions.

At $t = 0$, from the initial conditions stated in the problem we know that $x_2(0) = 0$ and $\frac{dx_2}{dt}(0) = \beta_2 N$. Equating the expression for $x_2(t)$ equal to 0, we find

$$C_1 + C_2 = 0.$$

Taking the derivative of the expression for $x_2(t)$ and equating it to $\beta_2 N$, we find

$$-\beta_3 C_1 - (\beta_1 + \beta_2)C_2 = \beta_2 N.$$

Thus, from the two initial conditions, we have been able to derive two equations that can be solved simultaneously to obtain values for the two unknowns, C_1 and C_2. Carrying out the algebra, we find

$$C_1 = -\phi N, \qquad C_2 = \phi N,$$

where

$$\phi = \frac{\beta_2}{\beta_3 - (\beta_1 + \beta_2)}.$$

Therefore,

$$x_2(t) = \phi N \left[-e^{-\beta_3 t} + e^{-(\beta_1 + \beta_2)t} \right].$$

Consequently, the total amount of radioactive label in the lung as a function of time is

$$x_1(t) + x_2(t) = N \left[(\phi + 1)e^{-(\beta_1 + \beta_2)t} - \phi e^{-\beta_3 t} \right].$$

In the graph on page 223, the solid curve shows the fit to the data with $\beta_1 = 0.32$ hr^{-1}, $\beta_2 = 0.072$ hr^{-1}, and $\beta_3 = 0.02$ hr^{-1}. Therefore, for t sufficiently large that $(\beta_1 + \beta_2)t \gg 1$, we find that the cells have disappeared from compartment 1, and the long time behavior is dominated by the destruction of cells remaining in compartment 2 at a rate β_3.

DETERMINANTS AND EIGENVALUES*

The characteristic equation for a pair of coupled first-order linear differential equations (Eq. 5.11) can also be expressed in terms of **determinants**. The basic idea is simple, but it requires some linear algebra. If you haven't studied linear algebra, keep in mind that you already know the solution to Eq. 5.11 as given by Eq. 5.9 or, equivalently, Eq. 5.10.

Equation (5.11) can be written as a **matrix** equation:

$$
\begin{pmatrix} \dfrac{dx}{dt} \\ \dfrac{dy}{dt} \end{pmatrix} = \begin{pmatrix} A & B \\ C & D \end{pmatrix} \begin{pmatrix} x \\ y \end{pmatrix}. \tag{5.14}
$$

Suppose we could define two variables, ξ and η such that for some constants α, β, γ, and δ,

$$
x = \alpha\xi + \beta\eta,
$$
$$
y = \gamma\xi + \delta\eta, \tag{5.15}
$$

and such that

$$
\begin{pmatrix} \dfrac{d\xi}{dt} \\ \dfrac{d\eta}{dt} \end{pmatrix} = \begin{pmatrix} \lambda_1 & 0 \\ 0 & \lambda_2 \end{pmatrix} \begin{pmatrix} \xi \\ \eta \end{pmatrix}. \tag{5.16}
$$

This equation is much easier to solve, because it is two uncoupled equations:

$$
\frac{d\xi}{dt} = \lambda_1\xi \quad \text{and} \quad \frac{d\eta}{dt} = \lambda_2\eta.
$$

From the previous chapter, we know that these two equations have the solution $\xi(t) = \xi(0)e^{\lambda_1 t}$ and $\eta(t) = \eta(0)e^{\lambda_2 t}$. Now it would be easy to find $x(t)$ and $y(t)$ simply by applying Eq. 5.15.

The problem of finding ξ and η that satisfy Eq. 5.15 and Eq. 5.16 is well known in linear algebra as the **eigenvalue** problem. The solution is routine once one knows the technique. It involves solving the equation

$$
\det \begin{vmatrix} A - \lambda & B \\ C & D - \lambda \end{vmatrix} = 0, \tag{5.17}
$$

---

*This section employs linear algebra. It gives an alternative and more elegant method to show that the eigenvalues of Eq. 5.11 are those given in Eq. 5.13. Using this method facilitates computations, but it is not essential.

where $\det| \cdot |$ denotes the determinant of the matrix. The determinant of a matrix with two rows and two columns is defined as

$$\det \begin{vmatrix} a & b \\ c & d \end{vmatrix} = ad - bc.$$

Applying the definition of the determinant to Eq. 5.17, we find that it is exactly the same as Eq. 5.12.

5.5   THE PHASE PLANE

Two-dimensional *nonlinear* ordinary differential equations are often written in the form

$$\frac{dx}{dt} = f(x, y),$$

$$\frac{dy}{dt} = g(x, y), \tag{5.18}$$

where $f(x, y)$ and $g(x, y)$ are nonlinear functions of x and y. Just as we saw in Chapter 1, the introduction of nonlinear functions can make it difficult, if not impossible, to find an analytic form for the solution.

A *qualitative* understanding of two-dimensional nonlinear ordinary differential equations can often be gained from studying the **phase plane** of the system. This can provide information about multiple stable and unstable fixed points that is not given by numerical integration. In this section we will describe geometric methods of studying the phase plane. In the following section, we will return to the algebraic method for the analysis of the stability of fixed points. Later, we will describe a numerical method for finding approximate solutions to nonlinear ordinary differential equations.

As an example of the use of geometric phase-plane techniques, consider the interaction of a predator and a prey species. Let x be the population of a prey species and y be the population of a predator species. We assume that if there were no predator, the prey would increase exponentially, and that if there were no prey, the predator would decrease exponentially. By eating the prey, the predator increases its own population and, obviously, decreases the population of the prey. The rate at which predator and prey meet (and therefore the rate at which the prey disappears and the predator thrives) is assumed to be proportional to the product of the populations of the predator and the prey. The justification for this is that if the population of either predator or prey is zero, the meeting rate is zero.

The equations are written as

$$\frac{dx}{dt} = \alpha x - \beta xy,$$

$$\frac{dy}{dt} = \gamma xy - \delta y, \qquad (5.19)$$

where $x, y \geq 0$ and α, β, γ, and δ are positive constants. These are the **Lotka-Volterra equations**. The equations were proposed independently by Volterra, who was a mathematician interested in ecology, and Lotka, a chemist interested in oscillatory chemical reactions.

The first step in examining the geometry of the dynamics involves looking at the **isoclines** of the flow. The **x-isocline** is the locus of points in (x, y)-plane along which $\frac{dx}{dt} = 0$. The **y-isocline** is, similarly, the locus of points along which $\frac{dy}{dt} = 0$. Fixed points are values at which both $\frac{dx}{dt} = 0$ and $\frac{dy}{dt} = 0$. Fixed points occur at the points of intersection of the x- and y-isoclines.

Let us now consider the Lotka-Volterra equation as an example of geometrical analysis of the phase plane. Figure 5.7 shows the flow, as well as the x- and y-isoclines. The x-isocline is defined by the expression

$$f(x, y) = \alpha x - \beta xy = 0.$$

This will be satisfied if

$$x = 0 \quad \text{or} \quad \alpha - \beta y = 0,$$

which describes two perpendicular lines in Figure 5.7. Similarly, the y-isocline is found from

$$g(x, y) = \gamma xy - \delta y = 0.$$

This expression is satisfied if

$$y = 0 \quad \text{or} \quad \gamma x - \delta = 0,$$

again, two perpendicular lines.

There are two points of intersections of the x- and y-isoclines, and hence two fixed points. The fixed point at $x = y = 0$ has an obvious biological interpretation: There are no predators and no prey, and therefore nothing would ever change in time. The second fixed point, $y = \frac{\alpha}{\beta}$, $x = \frac{\delta}{\gamma}$, is a point where the populations of predator and prey are exactly balanced. Away from the x- and y-isoclines there will be changes in the population levels of x and y.

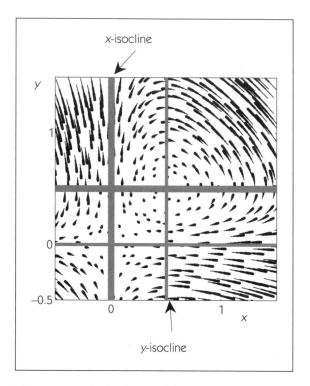

Figure 5.7   The isoclines and flow of the Lotka-Volterra system (Eq. 5.19 with $\beta = \gamma = 2$ and $\alpha = \delta = 1$.) The x-isocline (thick lines) and the y-isocline (thin lines) intersect at the two fixed points of the dynamics.

In order to examine the dynamics away from the isocline, one looks at the flow imposed by the differential equations. This can easily be done. In a short time interval Δ there will be a displacement in the x direction of approximately $x = f(x, y)\Delta$. The displacement in the y direction is approximately $y = g(x, y)\Delta$. The local trajectory through x, y can be found by taking the vector sum of the x and y displacements. For detailed pictures of the sort shown in Figure 5.7, it is convenient to use a computer to draw the picture of the flow in the phase plane.

For understanding the dynamics of a system, a quick, "back-of-the-envelope" picture of the dynamics is often sufficient. This can be drawn as follows:

1. Draw the x- and y-isoclines.

2. On one side of the x-isocline the flow will be to the left and on the other side, the flow will be to the right. Use the equations to decide which side is which, and draw many arrows showing the flow in the x direction. This is shown in Figure 5.8.

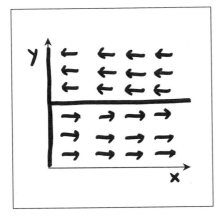

Figure 5.8
The x-isocline and arrows showing the direction of flow in the x direction on each side of the isocline.

3. Similarly, on one side of the y-isocline the flow will be downwards, and on the other side the flow will be up. Draw many arrows showing the flow in the y direction (see Figure 5.9).

4. Combine the x and y arrows to give the vector flow field. This is shown in Figure 5.10.

Of course, it is possible, either by hand or using a computer, to draw a detailed picture of the flow. In the Lotka-Volterra system, by tracing a trajectory through the flow, we see that starting from any point with positive populations, we will cycle around the fixed point, producing oscillations of predator and prey. It is not possible with this geometric method to tell if the cycling will be periodic or will spiral in to the fixed point or away from it. However, additional analysis using a quantity analogous to the energy in the harmonic oscillator shows that in this problem the trajectories are closed paths, just as we found in the ideal

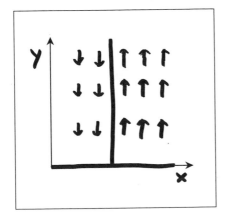

Figure 5.9
The y-isocline and arrows showing the direction of flow in the y direction.

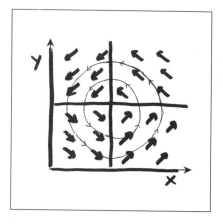

Figure 5.10
Combining the x and y flow gives an idea of what the trajectories look like.

harmonic oscillator. Therefore, the Lotka-Volterra system gives rise to periodic cycles in population. (See Problem 5.28.)

5.6 LOCAL STABILITY ANALYSIS OF TWO-DIMENSIONAL, NONLINEAR DIFFERENTIAL EQUATIONS

The local stability analysis of fixed points in two-dimensional nonlinear ordinary differential equations such as Eq. 5.18 is based on approximating the nonlinear equation by a linear equation in the neighborhood of fixed points of the equation. We can then make use of our understanding of two-dimensional linear equations to determine the dynamics in the neighborhood of the fixed points.

Assume that we are given the nonlinear Eq. 5.18. Let us assume that there is a fixed point (x^*, y^*) for which $f(x^*, y^*) = g(x^*, y^*) = 0$. The linear analysis involves carrying out a Taylor expansion of the nonlinear functions $f(x, y)$ and $g(x, y)$ in the neighborhood of (x^*, y^*). The Taylor expansion of a function $f(x, y)$ is

$$f(x, y) = f(x^*, y^*) + \left.\frac{\partial f}{\partial x}\right|_{x^*, y^*} (x - x^*) + \left.\frac{\partial f}{\partial y}\right|_{x^*, y^*} (y - y^*) + \cdots, \quad (5.20)$$

where the dots represent terms with higher-order derivatives such as $\frac{1}{2} \frac{\partial^2 x}{\partial t^2} (x - x^*)^2$. If we now let

$$X = x - x^*, \qquad Y = y - y^*, \quad (5.21)$$

We can expand Eq. 5.18 to obtain

$$\frac{dX}{dt} = AX + BY + \cdots ,$$

$$\frac{dY}{dt} = CX + DY + \cdots , \qquad (5.22)$$

where

$$A = \left.\frac{\partial f}{\partial x}\right|_{x^*, y^*} \qquad B = \left.\frac{\partial f}{\partial y}\right|_{x^*, y^*}$$

$$C = \left.\frac{\partial g}{\partial x}\right|_{x^*, y^*} \qquad D = \left.\frac{\partial g}{\partial y}\right|_{x^*, y^*}. \qquad (5.23)$$

In the neighborhood of the fixed point, the higher-order terms are negligible in comparison with the linear terms in Eq. 5.22. Consequently, in the neighborhood of the fixed point, the nonlinear equation can be approximated by a linear equation:

$$\frac{dX}{dt} = AX + BY,$$

$$\frac{dY}{dt} = CX + DY. \qquad (5.24)$$

The process of approximating a nonlinear differential equation by equations of the form of Eq. 5.24 is called **linearization**.

The geometry of the vector field in the neighborhood of the fixed points in the phase-plane representation can be classified based on the eigenvalues of the linear approximation given in Eq. 5.24. We have already determined the eigenvalues of the linear equation in Eq. 5.13. We found that the eigenvalues, λ_1 and λ_2, are

$$\lambda_1 = \frac{A + D}{2} + \frac{\sqrt{(A - D)^2 + 4BC}}{2},$$

$$\lambda_2 = \frac{A + D}{2} - \frac{\sqrt{(A - D)^2 + 4BC}}{2}.$$

Several different cases can be distinguished. The flows for three different cases are illustrated in Figures 5.11, 5.12, and 5.13.

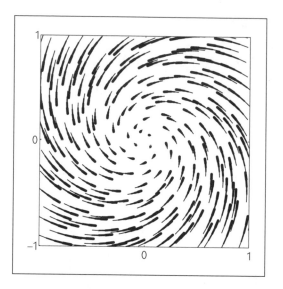

Figure 5.11   A stable focus. $A = -1$, $B = -1.9$, $C = 1.9$, and $D = -1$.

Focus $(A - D)^2 + 4BC < 0$. In this case, the eigenvalues are complex numbers. This means that the flow winds around the fixed point (see Figure 5.11). The size of the imaginary part tells how fast the winding occurs. The real part is $\frac{A+D}{2}$. If $\frac{A+D}{2} < 0$ the focus is stable, and if $\frac{A+D}{2} > 0$ the focus is unstable. The special case where $\frac{A+D}{2} = 0$ is called a center.

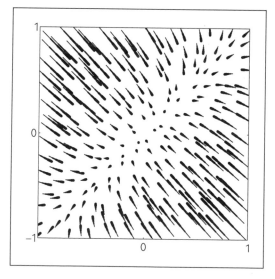

Figure 5.12   A stable node. $A = -1.5$, $B = 1$, $C = 1$, and $D = -1.5$.

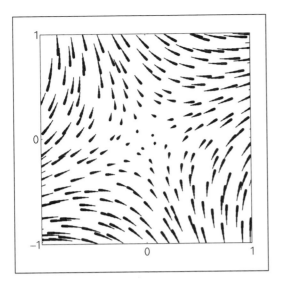

Figure 5.13 A saddle point. $A = 1$, $B = 1$, $C = 1$, and $D = -1$.

Node $(A - D)^2 + 4BC > 0$ and $|A + D| > \left| \sqrt{(A - D)^2 + 4BC} \right|$.
In this case the eigenvalues are both real and the same sign. If $\frac{A+D}{2} < 0$ the node is stable (see Figure 5.12), and if $\frac{A+D}{2} > 0$ the node is unstable.

Saddle point

$$(A - D)^2 + 4BC > 0 \text{ and } |A + D| < \left| \sqrt{(A - D)^2 + 4BC} \right|.$$

In this case the eigenvalues are both real, but with different signs. The trajectories of the vector field in the neighborhood of the saddle point are similar to the way water would flow on a horse's saddle (see Figure 5.13).

❑ **EXAMPLE 5.3**

Characterize the dynamics of the Lotka-Volterra equations (Eq. 5.19) near the fixed points.

Solution: We found in Section 5.5 that the fixed points occur at $x^* = 0$, $y^* = 0$, and at $x^* = \delta/\gamma$, $y^* = \alpha/\beta$. We will consider each of these fixed points in turn.

Near a fixed point, the dynamics are well approximated by a linear system

$$\frac{dz}{dt} = Az + Bw, \qquad \frac{dw}{dt} = Cz + Dw$$

where $z = x - x^*$ and $w = y - y^*$. The constants A, B, C, and D are found by evaluating the partial derivatives at (x^*, y^*):

$$A = \left.\frac{\partial f}{\partial x}\right|_{(x^*, y^*)} = \alpha - \beta y^* \qquad B = \left.\frac{\partial f}{\partial y}\right|_{(x^*, y^*)} = -\beta x^*$$

$$C = \left.\frac{\partial g}{\partial x}\right|_{(x^*, y^*)} = \gamma y^* \qquad D = \left.\frac{\partial g}{\partial y}\right|_{(x^*, y^*)} = \gamma x^* - \delta$$

The fixed point at the origin ($x^* = 0, y^* = 0$) is especially important, because it corresponds to extinction of both predator and prey. If this fixed point were stable, then even if both populations were non-zero, the predator-prey dynamics might lead to extinction. At the origin, we have $A = \alpha$, $B = 0$, $C = 0$, and $D = -\delta$. The eigenvalues are therefore

$$\lambda = \frac{\alpha - \delta}{2} \pm \frac{\sqrt{(\alpha + \delta)^2}}{2}$$

or, simplifying,

$$\lambda_1 = \alpha \qquad \lambda_2 = -\delta.$$

Since in the Lotka-Volterra equations, α and δ are both positive, λ_1 is positive and λ_2 is negative. Thus, the fixed point at the origin is a saddle.

The other fixed point occurs at $x^* = \delta/\gamma$ and $y^* = \alpha/\beta$, which gives $A = 0$, $B = -\beta\delta/\gamma$, $C = \gamma\alpha/\beta$, $D = 0$. The eigenvalues are therefore

$$\lambda = \pm\sqrt{-\alpha\delta}.$$

These eigenvalues are purely imaginary, meaning that the populations of predators and prey oscillate around the fixed point. Since $(A + D)/2 = 0$, the focus is a center, but this would be meaningful only if the linearized system were exactly faithful to the full nonlinear system. Using an argument analogous to the conservation of energy, it is possible to show that the trajectory consists of closed curves around the fixed point. (See Problem 5.28.)

Since the fixed point at $x^* = 0, y^* = 0$ is a saddle, it is unstable in the sense that for almost any nonzero level of predator and prey population near extinction, the system will eventually lead to an increase in both populations. (The "almost any" is intended to exclude the case where the prey population is set to exactly zero. In this case, the predator population will die out exponentially, whatever is its initial value.) This might suggest that predator-prey systems are robust to disturbances; that extinction is difficult. Notice, though, that the seeming robustness is sensitive to details in the model construction. If the model were changed slightly so that the predator did not depend for sustenance solely on the prey, then extinction is a real possibility for the prey. ❑

❏ EXAMPLE 5.4

In mutual inhibition, there are two variables, each of which inhibits the other. For example, in the lambda bacteriophage (see *Dynamics in Action 2*), the lambda repressor and the cro protein mutually inhibit each other. Here, we shall see how the Boolean network model for the lambda bacteriophage translates into a differential equation model.

A theoretical model for mutual inhibition is

$$\frac{dx}{dt} = f(x) = \frac{\left(\frac{1}{2}\right)^n}{\left(\frac{1}{2}\right)^n + y^n} - x,$$

$$\frac{dy}{dt} = g(x) = \frac{\left(\frac{1}{2}\right)^n}{\left(\frac{1}{2}\right)^n + x^n} - y,$$

where x and y are positive variables and n is a positive constant greater than two. There is a steady state at $x^* = y^* = \frac{1}{2}$. Discuss the bifurcations and sketch the flows in the (x, y)-plane as n varies.

Solution: We linearize around the fixed point at $x^* = \frac{1}{2}$, $y^* = \frac{1}{2}$

$$A = \left.\frac{\partial f}{\partial x}\right|_{(x^*,y^*)} = -1$$

$$B = \left.\frac{\partial f}{\partial y}\right|_{(x^*,y^*)} = -\left.\frac{\left(\frac{1}{2}\right)^n}{\left(\left(\frac{1}{2}\right)^n + y^n\right)^2} ny^{n-1}\right| = -\frac{n}{2}$$

$$C = \left.\frac{\partial g}{\partial x}\right|_{(x^*,y^*)} = -\left.\frac{\left(\frac{1}{2}\right)^n}{\left(\left(\frac{1}{2}\right)^n + x^n\right)^2} nx^{n-1}\right|_{(x^*,y^*)} = -\frac{n}{2}$$

$$D = \left.\frac{\partial g}{\partial y}\right|_{(x^*,y^*)} = -1$$

Using Eq. 5.13, the eigenvalues are $-\frac{2}{2} \pm \frac{\sqrt{4-4+\sqrt{n}}}{2}$, or

$$\lambda_1 = -1 + \frac{n}{2} \qquad \lambda_2 = -1 - \frac{n}{2}.$$

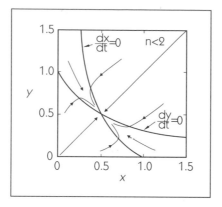

Figure 5.14
Phase plane for mutual inhibition showing a stable node.

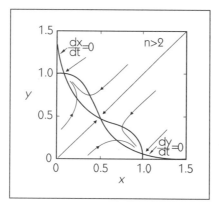

Figure 5.15
Phase plane for mutual inhibition showing a saddle point plus two stable nodes.

The steady state is therefore a stable node for $n \leq 2$ and a saddle point for $n > 2$. The trajectories in the (x, y)-plane can be sketched; see Figures 5.14 and 5.15.

The sketches show that for $n > 2$ there are two additional stable nodes. This is a typical bifurcation in two-dimensional ordinary differential equations in which a stable node splits into a saddle point plus two stable nodes. The biological interpretation is as follows. The larger the value of n, the stronger the inhibitory interactions will be. At strong interactions, one of the variables wins out and reaches a high value, whereas the other variable is at a low value. Such a model captures the essence of mutual inhibition and as such may be important in the analysis of competition of manufacturing production or of ecological species. ❒

The quantitative analysis of fixed points using linearization and the calculation of eigenvalues provides exact information about the stability of fixed points. For heuristic purposes, the isocline method can also be used to provide qualitative understanding of the behavior near a fixed point. The procedure is quite simple. First, draw the x- and y-isoclines in the region of their intersection. If the isoclines are not parallel where they intersect, the two isoclines divide the plane into four quadrants. Now, choose one of the quadrants (it doesn't matter which one) and calculate $\frac{dx}{dt}$ and $\frac{dy}{dt}$ in that quadrant. The vector ($\frac{dx}{dt}$, $\frac{dy}{dt}$) indicates the direction of flow in that quadrant.

Repeat this procedure for the other three quadrants. Or, you might note that if ($\frac{dx}{dt}$, $\frac{dy}{dt}$) points in the $(+, +)$ direction in one quadrant, then in the quadrant across the y-isocline, it will point in the $(+, -)$ direction; in the quadrant across the x-isocline, it will point in the $(-, +)$ direction; and in the remaining quadrant it will point in the $(-, -)$ direction. Three cases are shown in Figures 5.16, 5.17, and 5.18.

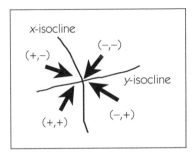

Figure 5.16
The geometry of a node. Flow near the intersection of the x- and y-isoclines. In each quadrant, the sign of $\frac{dx}{dt}$ and $\frac{dy}{dt}$ is shown (for example, $(-, -)$ in the upper-right quadrant) and the corresponding rough direction of the flow in that quadrant is indicated by an arrow.

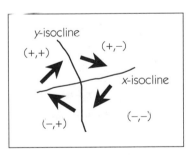

Figure 5.17
The geometry of a focus.

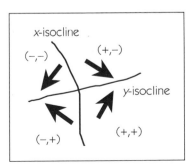

Figure 5.18
The geometry of a saddle.

FLOWS AND VISUAL PERCEPTION

The human visual system is particularly effective at perceiving flow fields. This allows us to experiment with some of the concepts contained in the previous mathematical material without doing any algebra.

We saw in Section 5.5 how the flow field can be sketched by drawing arrows at many places in the phase plane. The eye is capable of seeing flow patterns even when the whole arrow is not sketched. Just putting dots at the positions of the head and tail of the arrow will suffice.

A useful method for generating the visual appearance of a flow field is provided by the superimposition of dot patterns. Figure 5.19 shows three related dot patterns composed of random dots. On the top is a random pattern (A). The pattern in the center (B) is an expanded version of these same random dots (the x- and y-coordinates of all points in A are multiplied by 1.05). Pattern C is formed by multiplying the x coordinate of all points in pattern A by 1.05 and multiplying the y coordinate by 0.95.

Each of the three patterns looks random and shows no sign of a flow field. By placing one pattern over another one, and by rotating the overlaid patterns slightly, it is easy to perceive the geometries of flow fields in the neighborhood of fixed points. By superimposing pattern A on itself, but rotating slightly, there is a circular image; superimposing pattern A on pattern B without rotation gives rise to the geometry of a node; superimposing pattern A on pattern B with rotation gives the geometry of a focus (see Figure 5.20); finally, superimposing pattern A on pattern C gives rise to a saddle point geometry (see Figure 5.21). This shows how simple expansions, contractions, and rotations underlie the various geometries in the neighborhoods of steady states in nonlinear ordinary differential equations. These images, originally described by one of us (Glass) and colleagues, are being studied by scientists who are interested in evaluating the types of computation the brain performs during visual perception.

The best way to explore how contractions and rotations create different sorts of flow fields is to make two photocopies of the random dot patterns in Figure 5.19, one on ordinary paper and the other on transparent film. By aligning the two copies of the different dot patterns with one another (use the square brackets in the top right corner and along the left edge), and rotating them, you will see different flow patterns appear. If you make just one copy and match it up to the printed copies in the book, you may observe that your photocopier rescales the image slightly.

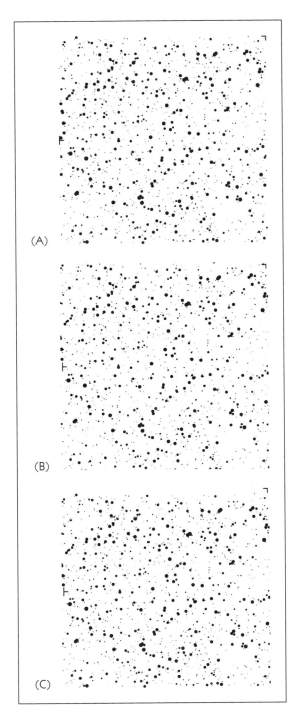

Figure 5.19 The pattern of random dots in (A) is enlarged in both directions in (B) and enlarged in one direction and shrunken in the other in (C).

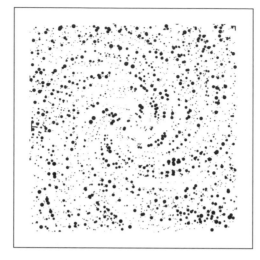

Figure 5.20
Superimposing pattern A on pattern B with a rotation of 0.1 radians creates the flow near a focus.

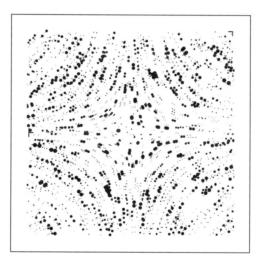

Figure 5.21
Superimposing pattern A on pattern C, with no rotation, creates the flow near a saddle.

5.7 LIMIT CYCLES AND THE VAN DER POL OSCILLATOR

So far we have considered two differential equations that display oscillations—the ideal harmonic oscillator and the Lotka-Volterra equations. In both of these, if some outside disturbance moves the state off of its original trajectory, the new trajectory after the disturbance will be different in amplitude and will never rejoin the original trajectory (unless another outside disturbance happens to do the job). Most biological oscillations show a different behavior. If there is a small outside disturbance, then after sufficient time (i.e., as $t \rightarrow \infty$) the original trajectory is established. This type of behavior is called a **stable limit cycle**. The French mathematician Henri Poincaré (1854–1912) was the first to realize that this type of behavior could arise in differential equations. You have already seen this type of behavior in *Dynamics in Action* 1.

Figure 5.22, repeated from *Dynamics in Action* 1, gives an example of an electrical shock delivered to oscillating cardiac tissue. The reestablishment of the oscillation with the same period and amplitude as before the shock is an indication that a theoretical formulation for the oscillation should have a stable limit cycle oscillation. Probably the first and simplest theoretical model for cardiac oscillations was proposed by B. van der Pol, an electrical engineer, and his collaborator, J. van der Mark.

The **van der Pol equations** are

$$\frac{dx}{dt} = f(x, y) = \frac{1}{\epsilon}\left(y - \frac{x^3}{3} + x\right),$$

$$\frac{dy}{dt} = g(x) = -\epsilon x, \tag{5.25}$$

where it is usual to assume that $0 < \epsilon \ll 1$.

Even though it is not possible to find an analytic solution of the van der Pol equations, the properties of this equation can be determined using the qualitative methods introduced in the previous two sections. We first sketch the flow in the (x, y) plane, as shown in Figure 5.23. The x-isocline, found by setting $\frac{dx}{dt} = 0$,

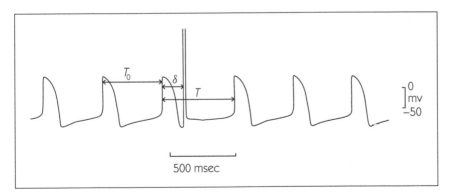

Figure 5.22 Recording of transmembrane voltage from spontaneously beating aggregates of embryonic chick heart cells. The intrinsic cycle length is T_0. A stimulus delivered at a time δ following the start of the third action potential leads to a phase resetting so that the subsequent action potential occurs after time T. After this, the aggregate returns to its intrinsic cycle length. Adapted from Guevara et al. (1981).

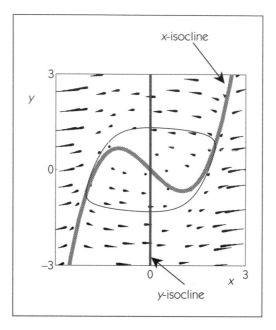

Figure 5.23 The flow and isoclines of the van der Pol equations (Eq. 5.25, $\epsilon = 0.1$). The limit cycle is shown as a thin line.

is the cubic function

$$y = \frac{x^3}{3} - x.$$

Similarly, the y-isocline, found by setting $\frac{dy}{dt} = 0$, is

$$x = 0.$$

There is only one intersection of the x- and y-isoclines, and therefore only one fixed point, which is at $x = y = 0$.

The flow vectors plotted in Figure 5.23, suggest the flow is mostly horizontal, toward the x-isocline. However, there is also a slight vertical component to the flow. Since we are assuming $0 < \epsilon \ll 1$, any initial condition that is not on the x-isocline will lead to relatively rapid changes in the value of x until the state is in the neighborhood of the x-isocline, whereas the vertical component of flow, $\frac{dy}{dt}$, is small. Near the x-isocline $\frac{dx}{dt}$ is small, so there is not much flow in the horizontal direction. In this region, the small vertical component to the flow becomes significant, causing motion along the x-isocline. This motion is either up or down, depending on whether the state is on the left or right limb of the isocline. Once the vertical flow has carried the state near the local extremum of the x-isocline, the horizontal flow again dominates, producing a jump to the other limb of the x-isocline. Since the fixed point at the origin is unstable (see Example 5.5), we know that trajectories do not spiral into the origin. Instead, there is a stable limit cycle, which is approached no matter what the initial condition.

Figure 5.24 shows x as a function of time. The various segments are labeled to correspond with the region of the phase-plane plot. Note that the oscillation, with its slow drifts in the value of x, interrupted by sudden changes in the value of x, is similar to the recording of cardiac electrical activity. Modifications to the van der Pol equation proposed by several researchers form the basis for theoretical studies of oscillations in cardiac tissue even 70 years after the equations were proposed.

❏ EXAMPLE 5.5

Consider the van der Pol equations with $\epsilon > 0$. Evaluate the stability of the fixed point $x^* = y^* = 0$.

Solution: In order to determine the eigenvalues of Eq. 5.25 at the fixed point, we compute

$$A = \left.\frac{\partial f}{\partial x}\right|_{0,0} = \frac{1}{\epsilon}, \qquad B = \left.\frac{\partial f}{\partial y}\right|_{0,0} = \frac{1}{\epsilon},$$

$$C = \left.\frac{\partial g}{\partial x}\right|_{0,0} = -\epsilon, \qquad D = \left.\frac{\partial g}{\partial y}\right|_{0,0} = 0.$$

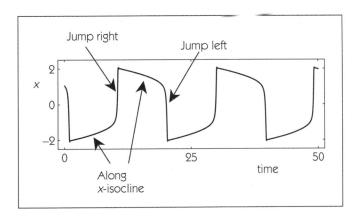

Figure 5.24 x measured from the van der Pol system with $\epsilon = 0.1$.

Using Eq. 5.13, we find the eigenvalues are $\lambda = \frac{1}{2\epsilon} \pm \frac{\sqrt{\frac{1}{\epsilon^2} - 4}}{2}$ or, simplifying,

$$\lambda = \frac{1}{2\epsilon}(1 \pm \sqrt{1 - 4\epsilon^2}).$$

Consequently, for $0 < \epsilon < \frac{1}{2}$ there is an unstable node, and for $\frac{1}{2} < \epsilon$ there is an unstable focus. Notice that the stability analysis gives us a better understanding of the dynamics in the neighborhood of the fixed point than is possible with the phase-plane analysis, but the analysis does not give information about the dynamics in the limit $t \to \infty$.

5.8   FINDING SOLUTIONS TO NONLINEAR DIFFERENTIAL EQUATIONS

We have seen how to use isoclines to understand qualitatively the dynamics of nonlinear differential equations, and how to use linearization and eigenvalues to calculate quantitatively the stability of fixed points. We have not yet seen any general method for calculating solutions to nonlinear differential equations. The reason is that it is generally difficult or impossible to find such solutions algebraically. In Chapter 1, we used the procedure of iteration to find numerical solutions to the nonlinear finite-difference equations we wanted to study. In this section, we shall present an analogous method for finding approximate numerical solutions to nonlinear differential equations. This method can be used to find the trajectory from any given initial condition.

The method for numerical integration of differential equations, called the **Euler method**, is based on the same approximation of the derivative $\frac{dx}{dt}$ that we made in Section 4.6. As there, we define a discrete-time variable $x_t = x(t)$ for $t = 0, \Delta, 2\Delta, \ldots$. Then we have

$$\frac{dx}{dt} = \lim_{\Delta \to 0} \frac{x_{t+1} - x_t}{\Delta}. \tag{5.26}$$

Applying this definition of the derivative in Eq. 5.18, we get the equations

$$x_{t+1} - x_t = f(x_t, y_t)\Delta,$$
$$y_{t+1} - y_t = g(x_t, y_t)\Delta, \tag{5.27}$$

or

$$x_{t+1} = f(x_t, y_t)\Delta + x_t,$$
$$y_{t+1} = g(x_t, y_t)\Delta + y_t. \tag{5.28}$$

Equation 5.28 is a pair of coupled finite-difference equations, and they can be iterated to find the solution from any initial condition $x(0)$, $y(0)$.

DYNAMICS IN ACTION

15 ACTION POTENTIALS IN NERVE CELLS

To illustrate numerical integration, we will consider a mathematical model of the nerve cell. Nerve cells have a long branch called an axon, which transmits electrical impulses. The axon is an example of an excitable medium (see Section 2.5). Under normal conditions it rests quiescently. Given a small stimulus, it will return to rest almost immediately. However, a sufficiently large stimulus will cause the axon to "fire," after which time it is refractory and returns to rest. The sequence of firing and returning to rest is called an **action potential**.

The first detailed and accurate description of the mechanics of the axon was given in a complicated set of equations by A. L. Hodgkin and A. F. Huxley in 1952. This work won them the Nobel prize. A caricature of the Hodgkin-Huxley equations, which nonetheless conveys important aspects of the dynamics, is given by the **Fitzhugh-Nagumo** equation:

$$\frac{dv}{dt} = I - v(v - a)(v - 1) - w,$$

$$\frac{dw}{dt} = \epsilon(v - \gamma w). \tag{5.29}$$

γ, ϵ, and a are parameters, and v and w are the dynamical variables. v is the voltage across the cell membrane, and w is a recovery variable. I is the stimulus current that is injected into the cell.

Like the real axon, the equations have a quiescent resting state, and a small stimulus current does not produce an action potential. In our case, we want to see how large a current pulse is needed to generate an action potential when the cell is quiescent.

As you might have anticipated, the quiescent resting state corresponds to a stable fixed point in the differential equations. The figure on the next page shows the isoclines and the flow field when $I = 0$. There is a fixed point at $v = 0$, $w = 0$.

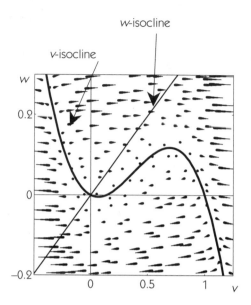

The isoclines and flow field for the Fitzhugh-Nagumo equations of nerve cell dynamics ($I = 0$).

Linearizing the equations around this fixed point, we find

$$\frac{dv}{dt} = -av - w$$

$$\frac{dw}{dt} = \epsilon v - \epsilon \gamma w.$$

The eigenvalues are

$$\lambda = -\frac{a + \epsilon \gamma}{2} \pm \frac{\sqrt{(\epsilon \gamma - a)^2 - 4\epsilon}}{2}.$$

For the resting state to be quiescent, we clearly want to set a, γ, and ϵ to give stable eigenvalues. Here, we will use the parameters suggested by Rinzel (1977) and set $\epsilon = 0.008$, $a = 0.139$, and $\gamma = 2.54$. This gives the eigenvalues $\gamma = -0797 \pm 0.067i$. This means that the fixed point is a focus, and since the real part of both eigenvalues is less than 0, we know that the fixed point is stable. Physically, the stable fixed point means that the axon is quiescent; it will stay near the fixed point until a large enough disturbance moves it away. The current stimulus pulse provides this disturbance. What the stability analysis does not tell is us how large the current pulse needs to be to cause an action potential.

The first step in integrating these equations, after picking the parameters ϵ, a, and γ, is to select a value for the size of the time step, Δ. In order for Eq. 5.28 to be a good approximation to Eq. 5.18, we need to pick Δ to be as small as possible. On the other hand, in order to keep the amount of computation small, we want to set Δ to be as large as possible. One way is to set the value for Δ to be some starting value, say $\Delta = 0.5$. We carry out the iteration according to Eq. 5.28. Then, we reduce Δ by half and repeat the iteration. If we find that the results of the two iterations are approximately the same, then Δ is small enough. Otherwise, reduce Δ by half again, and repeat. Keep in mind that setting Δ too large can have nasty effects; for example, fixed points that are stable in the differential equation can be unstable in the finite-difference approximation if Δ is too large.

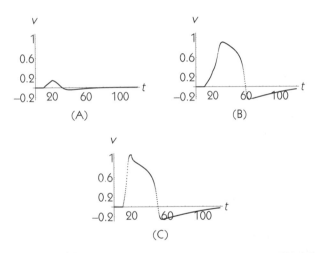

v versus time in the Fitzhugh-Nagumo model of electrical activity in the nerve cell. Current of amplitude I is turned on at time $t = 10$ and turned off at $t = 20$. (A) $I = 0.02$. No action potential occurs. (B) $I = 0.03$. An action potential. (C) $I = 0.10$. An action potential.

The iteration according to Eq. 5.28 can be carried out on a computer, or with a calculator, or simply with paper and pencil. Hodgkin and Huxley did their numerical calculations from much more complicated equations using 1950s-era mechanical hand calculators.

In our numerical experiment, we will start the cell at the stable fixed point $v = 0$, $w = 0$. At time $t = 10$, we will inject current of amplitude I for 10 time units. Then we will turn off the current and allow the system to evolve autonomously. We want to find what amplitude I is needed to trigger an action potential.

We will start with a current pulse of amplitude $I = 0.02$. The current is turned on at $t = 10$ and turned off at $t = 20$. The figure on the previous page shows transmembrane voltage v versus time; there is a small deflection in the voltage, which returns to its resting value by $t = 80$. In contrast, when a slightly larger current is given, $I = 0.03$, the voltage deflection is much larger and lasts much longer. This is an action potential. Increasing the current further to $I = 0.10$ does not change the amplitude of the action potential by very much.

Equation (5.26) is true only in the limit $\Delta \to 0$. For $\Delta > 0$, the equation is only an approximation. One way to make the approximation good is to use very small Δ. Another way, beyond the scope of this text, is to use more accurate methods for numerical integration, such as the Runge-Kutta method (Press et al. 1992), instead of the simple Euler method.

5.9 ADVANCED TOPIC: DYNAMICS IN THREE OR MORE DIMENSIONS

In the real world, it is unusual to have only a small number of interacting elements. Rather, there are complex networks of interactions. For example, consider the food webs in ecological systems, the multiple synaptic connections in neural networks, or the competition between several businesses in economic systems. In all these circumstances, theoretical models formulated as linear and nonlinear differential equations with more than two variables have been proposed to account for the complex interactions. Even though a great deal of effort has been expended in trying to understand such systems, there remain huge gaps in our mathematical understanding of the dynamics in nonlinear differential equations with three or more interacting variables.

Although much is known about the dynamics in the neighborhood of steady states, and about the bifurcations that arise as a consequence of parametric changes, fundamental mathematical questions involving the classification and the geometry of asymptotic behaviors in the limit $t \to \infty$ are still open. In the absence of a complete mathematical theory, there has been a lot of attention on the analysis of particular nonlinear equations. In this section we first give examples of some three-dimensional equations that display chaotic dynamics. Then we show how results concerning analysis of stability in first- and second-order differential equations generalize to higher-dimensional systems.

THE LORENZ AND ROSSLER EQUATIONS

In order to see the kinds of dynamics that can be found in nonlinear differential equations in more than two dimensions, we first consider equations initially studied by the meterologist E. N. Lorenz in 1963. Lorenz was interested in basic issues of why it might be so hard to predict weather. His approach was to consider simplified equations representing fluid flow in thermal gradients. Such equations are believed to play a role in the development of weather patterns since there are temperature gradients acting on the atmosphere (but, as Lorenz knew, the real situation is much more complicated than the problems studied by Lorenz). After several approximations, he came down to a set of three coupled nonlinear differential equations:

$$\frac{dx}{dt} = 10(y - x),$$

$$\frac{dy}{dt} = x(28 - z) - y, \tag{5.30}$$

$$\frac{dz}{dt} = xy - \frac{8}{3}z.$$

These equations look innocuous enough, but the dynamics the equations display have been a source of wonder and intense mathematical study. Figure 5.25 shows a trajectory in three dimensions. The dynamics here do not

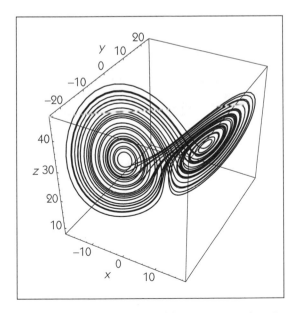

Figure 5.25   The trajectory of the Lorenz equations Eq. 5.30.

approach a steady state, or limit cycle, but rather display deterministic chaos. A plot of the trajectory is shown in Figure 5.25. Just as in the other examples that we studied that showed chaos, the dynamics here have sensitive dependence to initial conditions so that two initial conditions that are arbitrarily close will diverge as time proceeds. Lorenz discovered this using numerical integration on the primitive computers in use circa 1963. Figure 5.26 shows results of computer calculations of the sort Lorenz carried out. Starting at two initial conditions that are close to each other eventually leads to different dynamics. Without carrying out the numerical integration of Eq. 5.30, Lorenz would have been unable to make this important discovery, since mathematical methods of that time (or now!) cannot be used to predict dynamic behavior for most nonlinear equations without numerical integration.

Lorenz coined the term **butterfly effect** to describe the extreme sensitivity of nonlinear systems to the initial conditions. Lorenz suggested that although the flapping of butterfly's wings is a minute perturbation, it may nevertheless be adequate to change the weather in distant locations several days hence. Notice that this is different from saying that if a butterfly flaps its wings in Beijing this means it will rain in Montreal in five days. We have seen this type of distortion in our local newspapers; Chinese butterflies do not have this mystical power.

Another beautiful example in equations that are also deceptively simple was carried out by Otto Rossler, who was interested in chemical kinetics. Since chemical-reaction mechanisms that involve two compounds typically proceed at a rate governed by the two concentrations multiplied together, Rossler explored equations that contained products between two variables. He discovered many

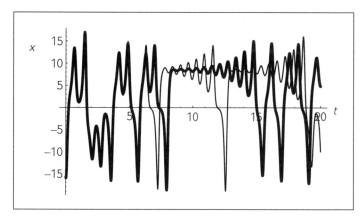

Figure 5.26 The x-component found by numerical integration of the Lorenz equations for two different initial conditions. Heavy line, $x(0) = -15.80$, $y(0) = -17.48$, and $z(0) = 35.64$. For the thin line, $y(0)$ and $z(0)$ are the same, but $x(0) = -15.79$.

equations that showed chaos, but the best-known example is now called the **Rossler** equation:

$$\frac{dx}{dt} = -(y + z),$$

$$\frac{dy}{dt} = x + 0.2y, \tag{5.31}$$

$$\frac{dz}{dt} = 0.2 + z(x - 5.7).$$

A plot of the trajectory in these equations is shown in Figure 5.27. Once again, a system that looks deceptively simple has remarkably complicated dynamics.

Since the study of the mathematics in higher-dimensional nonlinear systems is a matter for graduate studies and mathematics research, the reader must consult more-advanced sources to continue studying these problems.

LINEAR STABILITY ANALYSIS

Just as in the analysis of finite-difference equations and low-order differential equations, an understanding of the dynamics in linear systems is essential. Indeed, the dynamics in first- and second-order linear differential equations generalizes in a remarkable way to higher-order systems.

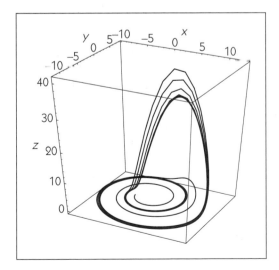

Figure 5.27 The trajectory of the Rossler equation, Eq. 5.31.

A linear differential of order N can be written as

$$\frac{dx_1}{dt} = a_{11}x_1 + a_{12}x_2 + \cdots + a_{1N}x_N,$$

$$\frac{dx_2}{dt} = a_{21}x_1 + a_{22}x_2 + \cdots + a_{2N}x_N,$$

$$\vdots$$

$$\frac{dx_N}{dt} = a_{N1}x_1 + a_{N2}x_2 + \cdots + a_{NN}x_N, \tag{5.32}$$

where the a_{ij} represent real constants. There are two alternative ways in which such equations can be written. One way is as a single differential equation in which the highest order of the derivative is N:

$$\alpha_N \frac{d^N x}{dt^N} + \alpha_{N-1} \frac{d^{N-1} x}{dt^{N-1}} + \cdots + \alpha_1 \frac{dx}{dt} + \alpha_0 x = 0, \tag{5.33}$$

where the α_i are constants that can be calculated in principle by the reduction of Eq. 5.32 in a manner similar to the reduction of the two-variable linear differential equation. A more compact representation of the same equation is

$$\frac{d\mathbf{x}}{dt} = \mathbf{Ax}, \tag{5.34}$$

where $\mathbf{A}$ is the $N \times N$ matrix of coefficients of Eq. 5.32, and $\mathbf{x}$ is the N-vector $(x_1, x_2, \cdots, x_N)$.

In almost all circumstances the solution of this equation can be written as

$$x_i(t) = C_{i1}e^{\lambda_1 t} + C_{i2}e^{\lambda_2 t} + \cdots + C_{N1}e^{\lambda_N t}, \tag{5.35}$$

where the C_{ij} are constants set by the initial conditions, and the λ_i are the eigenvalues of $\mathbf{A}$. The constants and eigenvalues can be real or complex, but a basic result in algebra asserts that complex roots must occur in pairs of complex conjugates. Thus, the important thing to remember is that the solution to linear differential equations is a sum of exponential functions.

In exact analogy to the two-dimensional case, the eigenvalues are determined from the characteristic equation, which is either

$$\alpha_N \lambda^N + \alpha_{N-1} \lambda^{N-1} + \cdots \alpha_1 \lambda + \alpha_0 = 0, \tag{5.36}$$

or, in matrix notation,

$$|\mathbf{A} - \lambda \mathbf{I}| = 0, \tag{5.37}$$

where **I** is the diagonal unit matrix. There is one situation where the above results are not true: if two or more eigenvalues are identical. Since this is a special situation that will only occur for certain choices of coefficients in the original equation, we do not consider it further.

The behavior of the linear differential equation in N dimensions in the limit $t \to \infty$ is determined by the eigenvalues. If all the eigenvalues have negative real parts, then in the limit $t \to \infty$ all variables will decay to 0. The origin is locally stable. The decay will be monotonic if all the eigenvalues are negative real numbers, or will be oscillatory if some of the eigenvalues are complex conjugates with negative real parts. If the real parts of some of the eigenvalues are positive, then the origin is not locally stable, and usually the dynamics will diverge in the limit $t \to \infty$. If the real parts of some of the eigenvalues are zero, then these are special cases. Small changes in the coefficients will generally lead to nonzero real parts of all the eigenvalues. However, if we think of the equations arising in realistic situations in which the coefficients depend on parameters, then parameter values at which the real parts pass through zero are associated with qualitative changes in the dynamics (bifurcations), and as such are important mathematically.

The analysis of the linear equations sets the stage for the analysis of the nonlinear equations:

$$\frac{dx_i}{dt} = f_i(x_1, x_2, \cdots, x_N), \qquad i = 1, 2, \cdots, N. \tag{5.38}$$

In perfect analogy to the two-dimensional case, the fixed points are found by finding values for which all the derivatives equal 0. In the neighborhood of a steady state, we can evaluate the stability from a consideration of the eigenvalues of Eq. 5.37 where the elements a_{ij} of the stability matrix **A** are determined from

$$a_{ij} = \left. \frac{\partial f_i}{\partial x_j} \right|_{\text{fixed point}}$$

where the evaluation of the partial derivatives is carried out at the fixed point. Since there are more variables now, the simple classification scheme for the two-dimensional differential equations is no longer applicable, but you can still visualize the geometry of the flows in the neighborhood of a steady state from the eigenvalues at that steady state.

5.10 ADVANCED TOPIC: POINCARÉ INDEX THEOREM

In this chapter, we have analyzed many theoretical models for dynamics in physical and biological systems. The different examples had different numbers of fixed points, with different stability characteristics. For example, the van der Pol oscillator has a single unstable state that is either a node or a focus. The model for mutual inhibition has either one stable node, or a saddle point and two stable nodes. It may be surprising, but there are mathematical results that enable one to place restrictions on the numbers and types of fixed points that can be found in differential equations.

The mathematical work dates to the end of the nineteenth century, when Henri Poincaré discovered a remarkable result concerning the geometry of vector fields of differential equations. This result is considered an advanced topic in mathematics; it is rarely presented in advanced courses at the undergraduate or even graduate level. Yet Poincaré's development of this result uses only elementary arguments that can be appreciated by students with no advanced mathematics. Because of the beauty and importance of this result, we give the main ideas. In the development we reconstruct Poincaré's central argument, which can be found in his collected works [1954]. John Harper, of the University of Rochester, provided us with ideas about how to present some of this material.

A little bit of terminology is necessary. A **manifold** is a space in which the local geometry of each point is identical and looks like a little piece of Euclidean space. For example, the circumference of a circle is a one-dimensional manifold. The surface of a sphere is a two-dimensional manifold since locally each point is surrounded by a two-dimensional region. **Topology** is a branch of mathematics that deals with properties of geometric spaces that do not change as the space is stretched or distorted, without cutting.

Two geometrical objects are called **topologically equivalent** if they can be transformed from one to another by streching only without any cutting or pasting. For example, the surface of a cube, the surface of a pyramid in Eqypt, and the surface of a sphere are all topologically equivalent. **Convex polyhedra** are solid objects whose surfaces are topologically equivalent to a sphere. Convex polyhedra are composed of faces (polygons), edges (where two faces meet), and vertices (where three or more edges meet). We designate the number of faces, edges, and vertices of a convex polyhedron by F, E, and V, respectively. For example, for a cube we have $F = 6$, $E = 12$, and $V = 8$, and for an Egyptian pyramid we have $F = 5$, $E = 8$, and $V = 5$, see Figure 5.28.

A remarkable topological theorem, discovered by Euler relates the number of faces, edges and vertices of a convex polyhedron. **Euler's theorem** states that

$$F - E + V = 2 \qquad (5.39)$$

We give a plausibility argument for this result.

Imagine a convex polyhedron drawn on a balloon. If a hole is made in one face of the polyhedron, the graph of the polyhedron can be laid out flat on a planar surface so that no two edges intersect. For example, for a cube we have

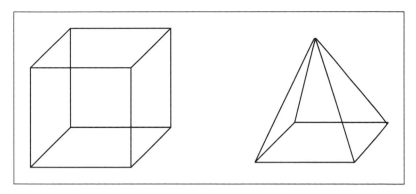

Figure 5.28 A cube (left) and a pyramid (right). For both we have $F - E + V = 2$.

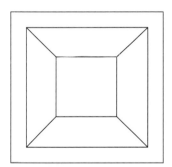

Figure 5.29
$F = 6, E = 12, V = 8.$

the situation shown in Figure 5.29. The face in which the hole was initially made is now an external face of the graph embedded on the plane. If any number of the edges bounding the external face is removed, $F - E + V$ remains invariant since the removal of each of these edges decreases both the number of faces and the number of edges by 1. In Figure 5.30 we show how the object looks after all the edges bounding the external face in Figure 5.29 are removed. It is now

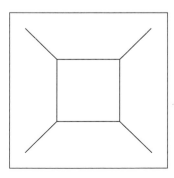

Figure 5.30
$F = 2, E = 8, V = 8.$

Figure 5.31
$F = 2, E = 4, V = 4$.

possible to remove in turn the edges and vertices which jut out into the external face. Since this operation decreases the number of both edges and vertices by 1 simultaneously, once again $F - E + V$ remains invariant. This process can be continued, with only minor differences for *any* initial polyhedron until a single polygon, as in Figure 5.31, is produced. In the polygon $E = V$. Since there are two faces, an internal and an external face, we obtain Eq. 5.39.

Eq. 5.39 is true for any polyhedron that is topologically equivalent to a sphere.

A **torus** is a two-dimensional manifold that is topologically equivalent to the surface of a standard donut. It is *not* topologically equivalent to a sphere. Let us build a torus from a convex polyhedron that has two different faces with the same number of edges n, but the two faces do not share a common edge. We assume that the numbers of faces, edges, and vertices of the convex polyhedron are designated F_0, E_0, and V_0. Let us now paste together the two faces with same number of edges to form a torus. Call F', E', and V' the numbers of faces, edges, and vertices, respectively, of the toroidal polyhedron. By construction we have

$$F' = F_0 - 2,$$

$$E' = E_0 - n,$$

$$V' = V_0 - n,$$

so that

$$F' - E' + V' = 0.$$

Doing similar surgery to construct a torus with γ holes, we find that

$$F - E + V = 2 - 2\gamma. \tag{5.40}$$

The torus with γ holes is called a surface of **genus** γ. It is a two-dimensional manifold since each point of the surface locally looks like a two-dimensional surface. The number $2 - 2\gamma$ is called the **Euler-Poincaré characteristic** of this manifold.

Poincaré used this earlier result from Euler in a fundamental way. Assume that we have a vector field generated by a nonlinear differential equation that is defined on a surface of genus γ, with a finite number of fixed points of the vector field. We construct a polyhedron of genus γ on the surface where each fixed point is isolated in a single face of the polyhedron. Calling F, E, and V the number of faces, edges, and vertices of this polyhedron we obtain Eq. 5.40.

The trajectories of the dynamical system will in general cut across the edges of the polyhedron. However, some of the trajectories may be tangent to the edges of the polyhedron. If a trajectory is tangent to an edge, in the neighborhood of the tangency it will be located on one side of the edge. A tangent is called an **internal tangent** or **external tangent** to a face depending on if it is inside or outside the face at its point of tangency. For each fixed point the **index**, I, is defined as

$$I = 1 - \frac{\text{Ext} - \text{Int}}{2}, \tag{5.41}$$

where Ext and Int designate the numbers of external and internal tangents, respectively, to the face in which the fixed point is located. (Poincaré actually defined the index as -1 times the index defined here, but our definition conforms to modern usage). This definition for the index is invariant to smooth transformations of the vector field inside of the face in which a fixed point is located, provided no new fixed points are generated inside the face. Using this definition, the indices of the fixed points discussed in Section 5.6 is $+1$ for nodes and foci, and -1 for saddles Figure 5.32.

The **Poincaré index theorem** asserts that for a dynamical system embedded on a surface of genus γ with a finite number of isolated fixed points,

$$\sum_{\text{fp}} I = 2 - 2\gamma, \tag{5.42}$$

where the sum is taken over all the fixed points. Since by construction each fixed points is located in a single face, by substituting Eq. 5.41 in Eq. 5.42 we find

$$\sum_{\text{fp}} I = F - \sum_{F} \frac{\text{Ext} - \text{Int}}{2}.$$

Here is the key insight. Except at the vertices, a tangent that is internal to one face is external to its neighboring face. Therefore, the summation over faces can be taken over vertices. A single trajectory passes through each vertex. The **degree** of the vertex i, designated E_i, is equal to the number of edges terminating at it. The trajectory through the ith vertex will be an external tangent to $E_i - 2$ faces and

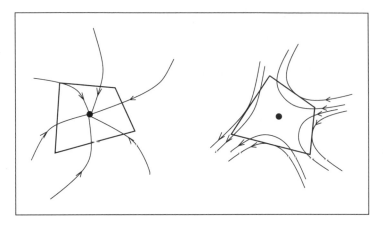

Figure 5.32 A node (left) and a saddle point (right). For the node there are no external or internal tangents of the flow to the face bounding the fixed point so $I = 1$ (from Eq. 5.41). For, the saddle point, there are four external tangents but no internal tangents so that $I = -1$. Figure provided by G. Bub.

will not be an internal tangent to any faces see Figure 5.33. Therefore, the summation can be rewritten as

$$\sum_{\text{fp}} I = F + V - \sum_V \frac{E_i}{2}.$$

Since each edge terminates at two vertices, $\sum_V \frac{E_i}{2} = E$, and the Poincaré index theorem Eq. 5.42 follows.

Call $\mathcal{N}$, $\mathcal{F}$, and $\mathcal{S}$ the numbers of nodes, foci, and saddle points, respectively, of a vector field embedded on a surface of genus γ, and assume these are the only fixed points present. Since the index of nodes and foci is $+1$, and the index of saddle points is -1, we find that

$$\mathcal{N} + \mathcal{F} - \mathcal{S} = 2 - 2\gamma.$$

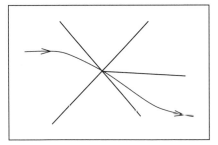

Figure 5.33
A vertex with degree 5, since 5 edges terminate at it. The trajectory through the vertex is an external tangent to three faces. Figure provided by G. Bub.

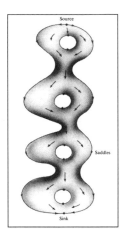

Figure 5.34
A donut with γ holes. Adapted from Guillemin and
Pollack (1974).

An unbelievable consequence of this result occurs in geography. Imagine a
globe in which there are mountain tops (peaks), depressions (pits), and passes.
If we think of water flowing on the surface of the globe, then the peaks and pits
would correspond to either foci or nodes of a vector field, and the passes would
correspond to saddle points. Then, we find that

$$\text{peaks} + \text{pits} - \text{passes} = 2.$$

In meteorology we can also make assertions concerning the numbers of high-
pressure areas, low-pressure areas, and "saddles" on a global barometric weather
map.

The "tastiest" method of computing the Euler-Poincaré characteristic of a
surface is to prepare a chocolate covered donut with γ holes (see Figure 5.34) in
the manner of Guillemin and Pollack (1974). Place this out in the sun until the
chocolate starts to melt, and examine the vector field formed by the flowing
chocolate on the surface. There will be two nodes and 2γ saddle points, so once
again the Euler-Poincaré characteristic is equal to $2 - 2\gamma$.

Surprisingly, there is an application of this result to theoretical models
of two-dimensional nonlinear dynamical systems. We are usually interested in
problems in which there is a two-dimensional region. On the boundary of the
region there are no critical points, and all trajectories point into the region.
Then it follows that inside the region $\mathcal{N} + \mathcal{F} - \mathcal{S} = 1$. Therefore, systems
with either a single node or focus are possible—such a situation arises in the
van der Pol equations. Alternatively, we can also have a phase plane with two
stable nodes and a saddle point such as we saw in Example 5.4 on mutual
inhibition.

SOURCES AND NOTES

A very nice elementary book on differential equations with lots of interesting historical notes is Simmons (1991). Readers interested in a more rigorous mathematical treatment, but still at an elementary level should consult Hirsch and Smale (1974). Glantz (1979) provides an excellent introduction to linear differential equations and compartmental analysis with special reference to biomedical applications such as pharmacokinetics. A fine presentation of the applications of nonlinear differential equations to biology that covers much of the material here at a bit higher level is Edelstein-Keshet (1988). Finally, Murray (1989) provides an excellent advanced text in mathematical biology that treats two-dimensional differential equations with biological applications.

The three dimensional equations presented by Rossler (1976) and Lorenz (1964b) are two important examples of simple nonlinear ordinary differential equations that display chaotic dynamics. A legitimate mathematical analysis of these equations is hard, and a complete analysis is not possible, but see Guckenheimer and Holmes (1983) for ideas of how to start.

The random dot patterns were discovered by Glass (1969) with demonstrations of the varied geometries of the vector fields in the neighborhoods of critical points given in Glass and Perez (1973). Marr (1982) called these images "Glass patterns". The patterns are still being used in the study of mechansims of visual perception, for example see (Kóvacs and Julesz, 1992). These patterns provide a dramatic illustration of the local stretching and rotation that generates the different geometries of the vector fields in the neighborhood of critical points and complement the algebraic analysis of critical points based on the eigenvalues of the linearized equations.

The Poincaré Index Theorem is considered an advanced topic in mathematics and is never presented at an elementary level. Surprisingly, Poincaré uses simple geometrical ideas. The notions underlying Poincaré's proof can be appreciated by undergraduate students with little mathematical background and this result is often a memorable feature of the course. A legitimate proof of this theorem is given in Guillemin and Pollack (1974), whose many-holed-hot-fudge-covered donuts are a wonderful didactic and gedunkin' device. See Glass (1975) for more information and references to the Poincaré Index Theorem and extension to higher dimensions.

✐ EXERCISES

✐ **5.1** The solution to the linear two-dimensional ordinary differential equation is given by Eq. 5.10, which involves two constants, C_3 and C_4. Physically, we might measure the initial condition in terms of the initial position $x(0)$ and the initial velocity $v(0)$. Find the values of C_3 and C_4 in terms of the initial condition $x(0)$ and $v(0)$.

✐   **5.2** An electrical circuit is composed of an inductance of magnitude L, a resistance of magnitude R, and a capacitance of magnitude C connected in a loop. At $t = 0$, there is an initial charge of q_0 across the capacitance and the current $\frac{dq}{dt} = 0$. The dynamics for this system is described by the following second-order linear differential equation:

$$L\frac{d^2q}{dt^2} + R\frac{dq}{dt} + \frac{1}{C}q = 0.$$

As time proceeds the charge is lost from the capacitor and is dissipated as heat is produced as the current passes through the resistor. Under what circumstances is the system oscillatory?

✐   **5.3** Use the Taylor series expansion of the exponential, sine, and cosine functions to show that

$$e^{\gamma + \delta i} = e^{\gamma}\left(\cos \delta + i \sin \delta\right).$$

✐   **5.4** Gatewood et al. (1968) proposed that glucose–insulin interaction could be modeled by the equation

$$\frac{dg}{dt} = -m_1 g - m_2 h,$$

$$\frac{dh}{dt} = m_4 g - m_3 h,$$

where $m_1, m_2, m_3,$ and m_4 are positive constants, g is the displacement of the glucose concentration from its basal value, and h is the displacement of the insulin concentration from its basal value.

a. What is the value of g as $t \to \infty$?

b. Under what conditions will g show an oscillatory approach to the steady state?

c. Sketch the flows in the (g, h) phase plane.

✐   **5.5** This problem is based on a mathematical model for the passage of food through the digestive tract in ruminants (e.g., deer) presented by Blaxter et al. (1956). Let $r(t)$ be the amount of food in the rumen and $\mu(t)$ the amount of food in the abomasum. The passage of food in the rumen and abomasum is described by the linear differential equations

$$\frac{dr}{dt} = -k_1 r,$$

$$\frac{d\mu}{dt} = k_1 r - k_2 \mu,$$

where k_1 and k_2 are positive constants and r and μ are greater than or equal to 0 for all times $t \geq 0$.

a. Give a diagram with two compartments that can serve to illustrate the passage of food through the rumen and abomasum, indicating with arrows the direction of the passage of food and the associated rates.

b. Sketch the flows in the positive quadrant of the (r, μ) phase plane.

c. Using this sketch, describe the dynamics of both variables starting from an initial condition $r(0) = r_0$, $\mu(0) = 0$. Be sure to indicate where the variables pass through extrema and what happens in the limit $t \to \infty$.

d. Write the original equations as a single second-order differential equation in μ.

e. Solve the equation in part d and give algebraic expressions for $r(t)$ and $\mu(t)$ starting from the initial condition $r(0) = r_0$, $\mu(0) = 0$. Confirm that the qualitative description of the dynamics in part c is correct.

✎ **5.6** This problem is based on an example discussed at length in Glantz (1979). An intravenous administration of a drug can be described by a two-compartment model, with compartment 1 representing the blood plasma and compartment 2 representing body tissue. The dynamics of evolution of the system are given by the differential equations

$$\frac{dC_1}{dt} = -(K_1 + K_2)C_1 + K_3 C_2$$

$$\frac{dC_2}{dt} = K_1 C_1 - K_3 C_2, \qquad C_1 \geq 0, \qquad C_2 \geq 0$$

a. Draw a schematic diagram that shows the compartments and the flows into and out of them.

b. Write the differential equations above as a single, linear second-order differential equation for C_1.

c. Solve this equation starting from an initial condition $C_1 = N$, $C_2 = 0$ for the special case $K_1 = 0.5$, $K_2 = K_3 = 1$.

d. Sketch the flows in the phase plane for the special case in which $K_1 = 0.5$, $K_2 = K_3 = 1$. What happens in the limit $t \to \infty$ starting from the initial condition in part c?

✏ **5.7** A chemotherapeutic agent is being used to treat an intracranial tumor. Let x be the number of molecules of the agent in the blood and y the number of molecules that have crossed the blood–brain barrier. At $t = 0$, $x = N$ and $y = 0$. The dynamics are described by the differential equations

$$\frac{dx}{dt} = \alpha(y - x) - \gamma x,$$

$$\frac{dy}{dt} = \alpha(x - y).$$

a. Write a second-order differential equation for y.

b. Find the characteristic equation. Show that if γ is much larger than α, the roots of the characteristic equation are approximately $-\gamma$ and $-\alpha$.

c. Use the result from part b to solve the equation for y as a function of time for $\alpha = 10^{-3}$ hr^{-1} and $\gamma = 1$ hr^{-1}.

d. For the values of α and γ in part c, compute the time when y is a maximum. What is the approximate value of y at this time?

e. For the values of α and γ in part c, compute approximately (to within 10 percent) the time when x is one half of its initial value.

✏ **5.8** A chemotherapeutic drug is administered intravenously. Assume that x is the concentration of the drug in the bloodstream, and y is the concentration of the drug in a target organ. Assume that the dynamics can be represented by

$$\frac{dx}{dt} = -k_1 x + k_2(y - x),$$

$$\frac{dy}{dt} = k_2(x - y),$$

where k_1 and k_2 are positive constants and $x \geq 0$, $y \geq 0$. At $t = 0$, a single large injection of the drug is given such that $x(0) = 250$ mg, and $y(0) = 0$.

a. Sketch the flows in the (x, y) plane.

b. Based on this sketch, give graphs showing x and y as a function of time starting from initial conditions of $x = 250$, $y = 0$. This can be a very rough sketch.

c. Find a single second-order linear ordinary differential equation for x in which all terms containing y have been eliminated.

d. Solve the equation found in part c starting with an initial condition of $x = 250$, $y = 0$, with $k_1 = 2$ hr^{-1}, $k_2 = 0.5$ hr^{-1}.

5.9 This problem is based on data in Phang et al. (1971). Rat tissue is incubated in a medium containing radioactive carbon. The kinetics for the accumulation of radioactive label in the rat tissue are:

$$\frac{dN_1}{dt} = \alpha \left(\frac{N_2}{V_2} - \frac{N_1}{V_1} \right),$$

$$\frac{dN_2}{dt} = \alpha \left(\frac{N_1}{V_1} - \frac{N_2}{V_2} \right),$$

where α is a positive rate constant, N_1 and N_2 are the number of molecules of radioactive label in the medium and tissue, respectively, and V_1 and V_2 are the volume of medium and tissue, repectively. Assume that the system is closed and at $t = 0$ there are M molecules which are present only in the medium and not in the tissue.

a. What is the rate of change of $(N_1 + N_2)$? What is $N_1 + N_2$ as a function of time?

b. At equilibrium, what is the value of N_1? What is the value of N_2?

c. Derive a second-order linear differential equation for N_2.

d. Derive the characteristic equation and use it to solve for $N_2(t)$.

e. If you have done parts c and d correctly, you will find

$$N_2(t) = K(1 - e^{-\gamma t}).$$

Express K and γ in terms of M, N_1, V_1, N_2, and V_2.

f. The graph in Figure 5.35, from Phang et al. (1971), shows the fraction of initial radioactivity per 100 mg of tissue as a function of time. This is

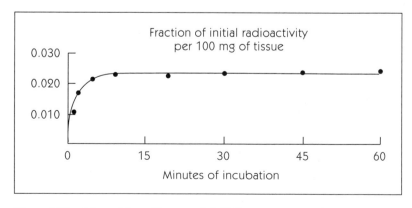

Figure 5.35   Adapted from Phang et al. (1971).

proportional to $N_2(t)$. Using any technique you wish estimate the value of γ in part e.

g. Sketch the flow in the N_2, N_1 phase plane ($N_1 \geq 0$, $N_2 \geq 0$).

By now you may realize that you have already done an equivalent problem using a different method, Example 4.3.

5.10 A chemical compound undergoes the transformation

$$A \xrightarrow{K_1} B \xrightarrow{K_2} C.$$

This process is described by the kinetic equations

$$\frac{dA}{dt} = -K_1 A,$$

$$\frac{dB}{dt} = K_1 A - K_2 B,$$

$$\frac{dC}{dt} = K_2 B,$$

for $0 \leq A$, $0 \leq B$, $0 \leq C$, where K_1 and K_2 are positive constants and A, B, and C represent the concentrations of each chemical species. When $t = 0$, $A(0) = N$, $B(0) = 0$, $C(0) = 0$.

a. Determine A as a function of time.

b. Give a single second-order linear differential equation in which only B and its derivatives appear. Solve this equation for $B(t)$.

c. If $K_1 = 2K_2$, at what time is B a maximum?

d. Use your answer to part b to determine $C(t)$.

e. What are the values of A, B, and C as $t \to \infty$? This can be answered without doing any algebra if you understand what is happening.

5.11 An ionic channel can exist in three states: S_1, S_2, and S_3. S_1 and S_3 represent closed states (no ions can pass through the channel), and S_2 is an open state. On a given cell there are a large number of channels, and the fractions of channels in states S_1, S_2, and S_3 are designated x, y, and z, respectively.
Transitions between the states follow the schematic diagram

$$S_1 \underset{k_3}{\overset{k_1}{\rightleftharpoons}} S_2 \overset{k_2}{\rightarrow} S_3,$$

where k_1, k_2, and k_3 are positive rate constants. A differential equation for this system is

$$\frac{dx}{dt} = -k_1 x + k_3 y,$$

$$\frac{dy}{dt} = k_1 x - (k_2 + k_3)y,$$

$$\frac{dz}{dt} = k_2 y,$$

where $1 \geq x \geq 0$, $1 \geq y \geq 0$, and $1 \geq z \geq 0$.

a. Sketch the flow in the x, y plane.

b. Based on this sketch, give graphs showing x and y as a function of time starting from initial conditions of (i) $x = 1$, $y = 0$, $z = 0$; (ii) $x = 0$, $y = 1$, $z = 0$. Note: The graphs may be approximations.

c. Find a single second-order linear ordinary differential equation for y in which all terms containing x and z have been eliminated.

d. Solve the equation found in part c starting with an initial condition of $x = 0$, $y = 1$, and $z = 0$.

e. Disregard the solution found above, and assume an initial condition of $x = 0$, $y = 1$, and $z = 0$. Solve for y as a function of time assuming: (i) $k_1 = 0$ and the other rate constants are positive; (ii) $k_3 = 0$ and the other rate constants are positive. HINT: This can be done with minimal computation if you understand the kinetic scheme above and the associated differential equations.

✎ **5.12** The graph in Figure 5.36 shows the results of an experiment in which the percentage of a tracer remaining in the blood is followed over 300 hours. Note that the ordinate is not linear. On this logarithmic scale, an exponential function is plotted as a straight line. The solid curve is the function

$$x(t) = c_1 e^{-\lambda_1 t} + c_2 e^{-\lambda_2 t},$$

where $\lambda_2 < \lambda_1$ and all constants are positive.

a. Give a rough estimate of the values of c_1, c_2, λ_1, and λ_2. (HINT: Figure out first what the dashed line and the dash-dot line represent.)

b. What is an approximate expression (using a single exponential) for $x(t)$ for long times (i.e., $t > 200$ hrs)?

c. Write a second-order linear differential equation for $x(t)$, expressing all constants in terms of c_1, c_2, λ_1, and λ_2.

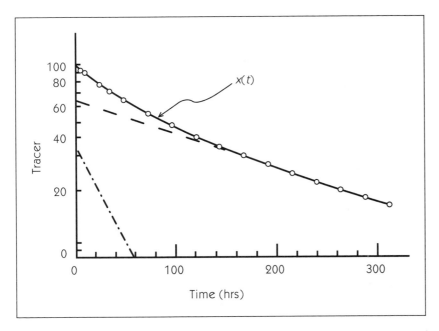

Figure 5.36 Adapted from Edelstein-Keshet (1988): Mathematical Models in Biology, Random House, copyright 1988. Reproduced with permission of McGraw-Hill, Inc.

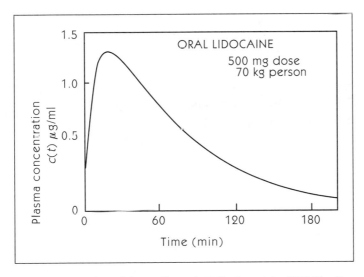

Figure 5.37 Adapted from Glantz (1979). Copyright 1979 The Regents of the University of California.

📎 **5.13** Following a 500 mg oral dose of the antiarrhythmic drug lidocaine, the plasma concentration of lidocaine is as shown in Figure 5.37, reproduced from (Glantz, 1979, p. 174). The concentration profile is well described by the equation

$$c(t) = 92.8 \left(-0.129 e^{-\frac{t}{6.55}} + 0.218 e^{-\frac{t}{65.7}} - 0.089 e^{-\frac{t}{13.3}} \right),$$

where the time units are in minutes and the concentration is in $\mu g/ml$.

a. This is the solution to a linear differential equation. What is the order of this differential equation?

b. Estimate the time at which the plasma concentration is one half its value at 180 min.

c. With what physiological processes is the time constant of 65.7 min associated?

📎 **5.14** This problem is motivated by an advertisement for Dalmane (a sleeping pill) that appeared in the *J.A.M.A.* **250**, 1136–1138, 1983. A sleeping pill will be most effective if the active substances appear rapidly in the bloodstream and have a half-life such that they are at negligible levels by morning. The upper panel in Figure 5.38 is a retracing of the graph shown in the advertisement, and the lower panel is experimental data following a single 30 mg oral drug dose in one subject taken from de Silva et al. (1974). The tracing in the advertisement appears to be based on this experimental graph. The advertising copy states there are "two short-half-life elements that appear rapidly and are rapidly eliminated," and "N_1-hydroxyethyl-flurazepam . . . has a serum half-life of 2 to 3 hours."

Blood concentration was measured at 1, 3, 6, 12, and 24 hours after the dose was administered by two different techniques (the "scanner" and "elution" techniques). For this question consider the data for N_1-hydroxyethyl-flurazepam (HEF) (which is apparently the basis for the graph in the advertisement). Calling $x(t)$ the concentration of HEF as a function of time, assume

$$x(t) = c_1 e^{-\alpha t} + c_2 e^{-\beta t},$$

where α and β are positive constants.

a. Assume that this system is described by a linear differential equation. What is the order of the differential equation?

b. Assume that $x(0) = 0$, $\frac{dx}{dt}\big|_{t=0} > 0$, and $\beta > \alpha$. What can you say about c_1 and c_2? Which is positive?

c. Determine the time when x is a maximum in terms of α and β. (Assume that the extremum is a maximum—it is not necessary to do the second derivative test.)

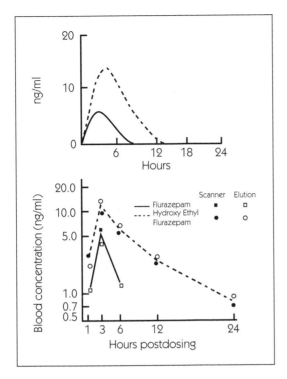

Figure 5.38   Top panel adapted from an advertisement that appeared in *J.A.M.A.* **250**, 1136–38 (1983). Bottom panel adapted from de Silva et al. (1974). Reproduced with permission of the American Pharmaceutical Association.

d. From the data in the lower graph determine the half-life of HEF.

e. Assume $\beta = 8\alpha$. Use the data for the subject, found in the lower panel of Figure 5.38, to compute β and α using the half-life computed in part d.

f. Assume that $\frac{dx}{dt}\big|_{t=0} = \frac{12\,\text{ng/ml}}{\text{hr}}$. Use this and the results in parts b and e to find c_1 and c_2.

g. Use the values computed to determine the time when HEF is a maximum and the concentration at that time.

h. Discuss whether the claims in the advertisement are substantiated by the data.

5.15 A modification of the Lotka-Volterra predator–prey equations is

$$\frac{dx}{dt} = ax - bx^2 - xy,$$

$$\frac{dy}{dt} = mxy - ny,$$

where a, b, m, and n are positive constants and x and y are positive variables.

 a. Which variable represents the predator (e.g., foxes) and which the prey (e.g., rabbits)?

 b. Suppose $y = 0$ and $x > 0$ at $t = 0$. What is the value of x as $t \to \infty$? What is the value of y as $t \to \infty$?

 c. Sketch the flows in the (x, y) phase plane for $x > 0$, $y > 0$. Assume $\frac{a}{b} > \frac{n}{m}$.

 d. On the basis of your analysis can you tell whether or not there are limit cycles?

✏ **5.16** Limpets and seaweed live in a tidepool. The dynamics of this system are given by the differential equations

$$\frac{ds}{dt} = s - s^2 - sl,$$

$$\frac{dl}{dt} = sl - \frac{l}{2} - l^2, \qquad l \geq 0, \quad s \geq 0,$$

where the densities of seaweed and limpets are given by s and l, respectively.

 a. Determine all steady states in this system.

 b. For each nonzero steady state determined in part a, evaluate the stability and classify it as a node, focus, or saddle point.

 c. Sketch the flows in the phase plane.

 d. What will the dynamics be in the limit as $t \to \infty$ for initial conditions:
  (i) $s(0) = 0$, $l(0) = 0$?
  (ii) $s(0) = 0$, $l(0) = 15$?
  (iii) $s(0) = 2$, $l(0) = 0$?
  (iv) $s(0) = 2$, $l(0) = 15$?

✏ **5.17** The "Brusselator" is a mathematical model for chemical oscillations. The equations for the Brusselator are

$$\frac{du}{dt} = 1 - (b + 1)u + au^2v,$$

$$\frac{dv}{dt} = bu - au^2v,$$

where $u \geq 0$, $v \geq 0$, and a and b are positive constants.

 a. Determine the values of u and v in terms of a and b at the steady state.

 b. Find the characteristic equation that can be used to determine the stability of the steady states.

c. Solve this characteristic equation.

d. Try to find parameter values of a and b that give a (i) stable node; (ii) stable focus; (iii) unstable node; (iv) unstable focus; (v) saddle point. Not all of these are possible in this equation; indicate those that are possible and explain why.

e. If u is held constant at some nonzero value, what will be the behavior of v starting at different initial conditions?

5.18 The following equations arise in the analysis of nonlinear equations in population biology (Edelstein-Keshet, 1988). Your problem here is to consider the dynamics determined by these equations.

$$\frac{dP}{dt} = -S,$$

$$\frac{dS}{dt} = \alpha P(1 - P) - S,$$

where $-\infty < P < \infty$, $-\infty < S < \infty$, and $\alpha > 0$.

a. Determine the steady states.

b. Find the characteristic equation that can be used to determine the stability of the steady states.

c. Solve this characteristic equation and classify each steady state (e.g., as a stable focus, unstable node, saddle point, etc).

d. Sketch the flows in the (P, S) plane, being sure to show the evolution starting from different initial conditions. What happens in the limit $t \rightarrow \infty$ from different initial conditions?

5.19 The following two-dimensional nonlinear ordinary differential equation has been proposed as a model for cell differentiation. Your problem here is to consider the dynamics determined by this equation.

$$\frac{dx}{dt} = y - x,$$

$$\frac{dy}{dt} = \frac{5x^2}{4 + x^2} - y,$$

where $0 \leq x < \infty, 0 \leq y < \infty$.

a. Determine the steady states.

b. Determine the characteristic equation in the neighborhood of each steady state, and solve this characteristic equation to classify each steady state (e.g., as a stable focus, unstable node, saddle point, etc).

c. Sketch the trajectories in the (x, y) plane, being sure to show the evolution starting from different initial conditions.

d. What happens in the limit $t \to \infty$ from different initial conditions, and why might this be appropriate to model cell differentiation?

5.20 Assume that the densities of circulating blood cells (density x) is controlled by a hormonal agent (y) produced by the blood cells. The dynamics are determined by the differential equations

$$\frac{dx}{dt} = \frac{2y}{1 + y^2} - x,$$

$$\frac{dy}{dt} = x - y.$$

a. Determine the steady states for $x, y \geq 0$.

b. Sketch the flows in the (x, y)-phase plane for $x, y \geq 0$.

c. For an initial condition of $x = 10$, $y = 0.1$, what will happen in the limit $t \to \infty$?

5.21 In an article on periodic enzyme synthesis, Tyson (1979) analyzes a mathematical model for feedback inhibition of enzyme synthesis. This problem deals with an equation from Tyson's paper. Let x_1 and x_2 represent the concentrations of biochemicals. Assume that

$$\frac{dx_1}{dt} = \frac{1}{x_2^n + 1} - Kx_1,$$

$$\frac{dx_2}{dt} = x_1 - Kx_2,$$

where n is a positive integer and $x_1 \geq 0$, $x_2 \geq 0$. Consider this equation for $K^2 = \frac{1}{2}$.

a. There is a steady state in this equation when $x_2 = 1$. Find the value of x_1 at this steady state.

b. Determine the stability of the steady state computed in part a. Show that the stability of the steady state does not depend on the value of n.

c. Sketch the flows to the above equation in the $(x_1 - x_2)$ phase plane for $n > 1$, indicating the behavior as $t \to \infty$.

5.22 A model for feedback inhibition is

$$\frac{dx}{dt} = \frac{0.5^n}{0.5^n + y^n} - x,$$

$$\frac{dy}{dt} = \frac{x^n}{0.5^n + x^n} - y,$$

where x and y are positive variables and n is a positive constant greater than 2.

   a. Sketch the flows in the (x, y) phase plane $(x > 0, y > 0)$.

   b. There is one steady state, at $x = y$. By inspection, find the values of x and y at this steady state.

   c. Compute the eigenvalues at the steady state. Is the steady state stable or unstable? What type of steady state is this (node, focus, or saddle point)?

5.23 The Duffing equation is

$$\frac{dx}{dt} = y,$$

$$\frac{dy}{dt} = -y + x - x^3. \qquad (5.43)$$

Assume that $-\infty < x < +\infty, \quad -\infty < y < +\infty$.

   a. Determine the steady states.

   b. For each steady state algebraically determine the stability and specify if it is a node, a saddle point, or a focus.

   c. Sketch the flows in the $(x - y)$-plane.

   d. Describe the dynamics starting from $x = 0, y > 0$, in the limit $t \to \infty$.

5.24 In an excitable system such as a neuron, a small deviation from a stable steady state can lead to a large excursion before the steady state is reestablished. As we discussed in *Dynamics in Action* 15, the Fitzhugh-Nagumo equation can be used as a model for a neuron. This problem also deals with the Fitzhugh-Nagumo equation using a different set of parameters. Consider the differential equation

$$\frac{dx}{dt} = \frac{1}{\epsilon}\left(y - \frac{x^3}{12} + x\right),$$

$$\frac{dy}{dt} = -\epsilon\left(2x + y - \frac{8}{3}\right), \qquad 1 \gg \epsilon > 0.$$

There is one steady state at $x = 2, y = -\frac{4}{3}$.

   a. Determine the x-isocline. For this curve determine the maxima, minima, and inflection points, using appropriate algebraic tests. Find the values of x and y for each of these points. Sketch the curve.

   b. Algebraically determine the stability of the steady state and classify it as node, focus, or saddle point.

   c. Sketch the flows in the (x, y) phase plane, assuming $1 \gg \epsilon > 0$.

d. Suppose there is a small displacement from the steady state to $x = 1$, $y = -\frac{4}{3}$ for $1 \gg \epsilon > 0$. Sketch the graph that shows x as a function of time. It is not necessary to put any units on the time axis, but try to estimate values on the x-axis.

✎ **5.25** The following equations arise in the analysis of nonlinear dynamics in neurobiology. Your problem here is to consider the dynamics determined by these equations.

$$\frac{dx}{dt} = y - \frac{5x^3}{8} + \frac{9x}{4},$$

$$\frac{dy}{dt} = -y, \qquad \text{for } x < 0,$$

$$\frac{dy}{dt} = -y + \frac{x^3}{8 + x^3}, \qquad \text{for } x \geq 0.$$

where $-\infty < x < \infty, -\infty < y < \infty$.

a. Sketch the x- and y-isoclines.

b. There is one steady state at $x = 2$, $y = \frac{1}{2}$. From examination of the graphs of the x- and y-isoclines, determine the values of x and y at the other steady states. HINT: There are a total of three steady states in this problem.

c. Sketch the flows in the (x, y)-plane, being sure to show the dynamics starting from different initial conditions. Based on this sketch, classify the steady states (e.g., as a stable focus, unstable node, saddle point, etc.) that are present in the phase-plane sketch. What happens in the limit $t \to \infty$ from the initial condition $x = 0.5$, $y = 0$?

d. Find the characteristic equation that can be used to determine the stability of the steady states. Solve this characteristic equation to classify each steady state. HINT: In doing this it is easy to make mistakes in the algebra, so try to work carefully. Use your sketch to help eliminate algebraic errors.

✎ **5.26** This problem deals with the van der Pol oscillator, Eq. 5.25.

a. Show that the van der Pol equation can also be written as a single second-order differential equation

$$\epsilon \frac{d^2 x}{dt^2} + (x^2 - 1)\frac{dx}{dt} + \epsilon x = 0.$$

b. For $|x| \ll 1$, the above equation can be approximated by the linear equation

$$\epsilon \frac{d^2 x}{dt^2} - \frac{dx}{dt} + \epsilon x = 0.$$

Solve this equation for $\epsilon = 0.6$ and initial conditions $x(0) = 0$, $\frac{dx}{dt}\big|_{t=0} = 1$.

c. What is the behavior of the solution to part b in the limit $t \to \infty$?

d. Compare the dynamics in the linear equation and in the original nonlinear van der Pol equation in the limit $t \to \infty$.

 5.27

a. Draw three different vector fields on the surface of a sphere in which there are two nodes.

b. Draw three different vector fields on a torus in which there are no steady states.

5.28 When we linearized the Lotka-Volterra equations about the fixed point at $x^* = \frac{\delta}{\gamma}$, $y^* = \frac{\alpha}{\beta}$, we found that the real part of the eigenvalues was zero. In order to show that the trajectory really is that of a center, closed loops around the fixed point, we consider the following quantity, analogous to energy:

$$E = \alpha \ln y + \delta \ln x - \beta y - \gamma x.$$

a. Show that $\alpha \ln y - \beta y$ has a minimum at $y = \alpha/\beta$. Similarly, show that $\delta \ln x - \gamma x$ has a minimum at $x = \frac{\delta}{\gamma}$. Since E is these two terms added together, E also has a minimum at the fixed point, and has a bowl-like shape; curves of constant E are closed curves around the fixed point.

b. Show that $\frac{dE}{dt} = 0$ for the trajectories of the Lotka-Volterra system. You can do this by finding $\frac{dE}{dt}$ in terms of $\frac{dx}{dt}$ and $\frac{dy}{dt}$, and substituting in the values for $\frac{dx}{dt}$ and $\frac{dy}{dt}$ from the Lotka-Volterra equations.

Since x and y move along curves of constant E, the trajectory consists of closed curves around the fixed point: periodic cycles.

COMPUTER PROJECTS

Project 1 Write a computer program that does Euler integration of two-dimensional ordinary differential equations. Test it on the Lotka-Volterra equations (or other equations that are presented in the exercises in this chapter).

Project 2 Write a computer program to integrate the Lorenz equations using the Euler method.

1. Start with $\Delta = 0.05$ and make a plot of $x(t)$. Then reduce Δ to 0.01, and see if $x(t)$ changes substantially. The changes become more dramatic as time increases. Repeat this process to find a satisfactory value of Δ.

2. Once you have settled on a value for Δ, integrate the Lorenz equations starting from an initial condition that is very close to the attractor. You can find such an initial condition by starting at another arbitrary initial condition and integrating the equations until you are on the attractor. Then, pick off the last x, y, and z values to use as your new initial condition.

3. Change the initial condition by a small amount, and see how long it takes for the sensitive dependence on initial conditions to create a very large change in $x(t)$ compared to that found in (2). Do this again for other initial conditions that are even closer to that in (2), and describe how the time that it takes for $x(t)$ to deviate dramatically from the $x(t)$ calculated in (2) depends on the difference in initial conditions.

Project 3 In Section 5.8 we introduced the Fitzhugh-Nagumo equations,

$$\frac{dv}{dt} = I - v(v - a)(v - 1) - w,$$

$$\frac{dw}{dt} = \epsilon(v - \gamma w). \tag{5.44}$$

These models show a current pulse injected into an axon can generate an action potential. By injecting current steadily, it is possible to generate repeated action potentials. Part I. Use linear stability analysis to figure out how large the current I needs to be to destabilize the fixed point in the model. The sequence of steps you will need to follow is:

1. Find the fixed point as a function of I. It is actually possible to solve algebraically the cubic equation for v. Symbolic calculation packages like Mathematica® or Maple® will do this automatically, but you can also find the solution to the cubic in many mathematics handbooks. Alternatively, you could find the fixed point numerically using Newton's method.

2. Linearize the equations about the fixed point.

3. Find the eigenvalues of the linear equations. If the real part of the eigenvalues is less than 0 for a given value of I, then the fixed point is stable.

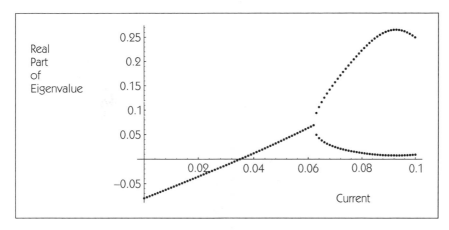

Figure 5.39   The real part of the eigenvalues of the linearized dynamics at the fixed point versus the current I injected into the axon.

Figure 5.39 shows a graph of the real part of the eigenvalues versus I, found using Mathematica. For $I < 0.03508$, the real part of the eigenvectors is negative, meaning that the fixed point is stable. For larger values of the current, the fixed point is unstable.

Part II. Use the Euler method to show the trajectory for $I = 0.1$, where the fixed point is unstable.

CHAPTER 6

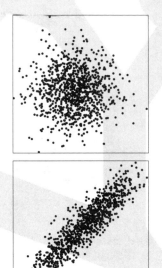

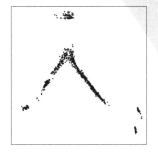

Time-Series Analysis

6.1 STARTING WITH DATA

Up until now we have examined mathematical descriptions of dynamical systems and seen how different types of behavior can be generated, such as fixed points, limit cycles, and chaos. The goal of applied dynamics is to relate these mathematical systems to physical or biological systems of interest. The approach we have taken so far is model building—we use our understanding of the physical system to write dynamical equations. For example, we used our understanding of the interaction of predators and prey to motivate the Lotka-Volterra equations. These equations then suggested the types of dynamics we were likely to observe in the field, such as population oscillations around a fixed point, or extinction.

In this chapter, we shall take the opposite approach. Starting with a sequence of measurements—a **time series**—we want to see what the data themselves can tell us about the dynamics. In particular, we will introduce some tools from time-series analysis (often termed **signal processing**) that can sometimes be used to suggest what types of equations are appropriate, or to compare the predictions made by mathematical models to measurements made in the field.

The ultimate goal for time-series analysis might be to construct a computer program that, without any knowledge of the physical system from which the data come, can take the measured data as input and provide as output a mathematical model describing the data. This can be done with current technology (see Section 6.7), but the method has a severe shortcoming: The resulting mathematical model generally does not have identifiable components that can be given physical meaning. Thus, it is not possible to use such data-generated mathematical models to determine the effect of changing some aspect of the physical system, which is often the motivation for studying dynamics in the first place.

In practice, the approach that is taken is a combination of model building and time-series analysis. Model building based on our knowledge of the physical system is used to suggest what features to look for in the data; time-series analysis is used to detect and quantify these features or to refute their existence, thus motivating changes in the model.

In this chapter, we shall mimic this process; a series of models will be proposed, data will be generated from these models, and time-series analysis techniques will be introduced to show how the models and data can be related to one another. The choice of models here is intended to illustrate various aspects of time-series analysis and does not include the physical and biological information that would motivate realistic models of specific phenomena.

6.2 DYNAMICS, MEASUREMENTS, AND NOISE

In the previous sections of this book, we have dealt extensively with dynamics. By now, we are familiar with equations of the form

$$x_{t+1} = f(x_t)$$

and

$$\frac{dx}{dt} = g(x, y)$$
$$\frac{dy}{dt} = h(x, y).$$

The functions $f(\ )$, $g(\ )$, and $h(\ )$ govern the dynamics of the systems, and given the functions, we know how to look for dynamical behavior such as fixed points, cycles, and chaos.

When dealing with data, we need to introduce two new concepts: **measurement** and **noise**.

In conducting an experiment or making measurements in the field, we can measure only a limited set of quantities and are able to make those measurements with limited precision. For example, an ecologist studying predator–prey dynamics might be able to count the population of the predator only, even though it is clear from models such as the Lotka-Volterra equations that both the predator and prey play a role in the system dynamics.

When constructing a mathematical model of observed dynamics, it is essential to include an equation that describes how the actual measurements are related to the dynamical variables. For instance, in the Fitzhugh-Nagumo model of nerve cell dynamics (Eq. 5.29), the transmembrane voltage v is usually measured in experiments, while the recovery variable w cannot be measured directly. In this chapter, an additional equation will be added to dynamical models, describing how the measurement at time t, denoted as D_t or $D(t)$, is related to the variables in the dynamical system.

The measurements approximate the true dynamical variables; the difference between the two is called the **measurement error**. The measurement error arises from several factors: systematic bias, measurement noise, and dynamical noise.

Systematic bias results from a flaw in the measurement process. For instance, suppose one tried to measure the use of a university's library by counting the number of students in the library just before exams at the end of the semester. Such a count would probably seriously overestimate library usage over the course of a year. Such systematic bias will not be discussed further here.

Measurement noise refers to fluctuations in measurements that arise from chance. Even if there were a well-defined average level of library use, the number of students at any particular moment would likely differ from this average.

Dynamical noise is another important source of noise in data. Real-world systems do not exist in isolation. They are affected by outside influences. For example, the population of prey depends not just on the population of predators, but also on environmental variables such as the temperature and precipitation, which themselves fluctuate. One would like to include such outside influences in dynamical models. This is often done by regarding the outside influences as random noise that affects the dynamical variables.

DYNAMICS IN ACTION

16 FLUCTUATIONS IN MARINE POPULATIONS

In order to study the dynamics of phytoplankton, marine biologist W. E. Allen made daily measurements from 1920 to 1939 of the total number of diatoms per liter of water off of two piers in California, at the Scripps Institute of Oceanography and Point Hueneme. These impressive data sets are displayed in the figure. Like all measurements, there are flaws and shortcomings in this data. There is certainly a component of measurement noise here: Not every liter of water contains the same number of diatoms. Systematic biases in the measurements may also exist. Important dynamical variables, such as the number of organisms that eat phytoplankton, were not measured.

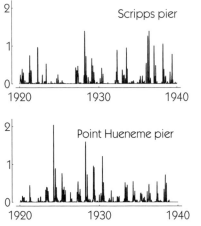

Weekly averages of daily counts of total number of diatoms (phytoplankton) (millions of cells per liter) at the Scripps and Point Hueneme piers, California, 1920–1939, collected by W. E. Allen. Data from Tont (1986).

There are many outside influences that affect the dynamics: the amount of sunlight, the water temperature, and the amount of nutrients in the water. These were not measured. Even if these variables had been measured at the piers, the fact that ocean currents carry phytoplankton from place to place makes it unclear how to interpret measurements made in a single place.

GAUSSIAN WHITE NOISE

A source of random numbers with which everyone is familiar is a deck of cards. Imagine that you have a very large deck of cards and that each card has a number from −1 to 1 written on it. The deck has been thoroughly shuffled so that the cards are in random order. Each card that you draw from the deck tells you virtually nothing about either the previous cards that were drawn or the subsequent cards yet to be drawn. In this situation, the drawn cards are said to be **independent** of one another. The resulting numbers are said to be "drawn from a distribution" of numbers. Here the distribution is the set of all the numbers in the deck.

It is easy to imagine a situation in which numbers drawn from a distribution would not be independent of one another. Suppose the cards in the deck were sorted in ascending order. Then each card would give you a good idea of what the value on the following card would be. When the random numbers drawn from the deck are independent of one another—when the deck is shuffled randomly—the numbers form a source of **white noise**.

White noise is often a good model of measurement and dynamical noise. But what is the distribution from which the white noise is drawn? It might seem that the distribution will depend on details of the system being studied, but for reasons described ahead, it happens that a very commonly encountered distribution in practice is the **Gaussian distribution**.

The random variability in a measurement or a random outside influence is often the sum of many different types of random variability. For example, in measuring the population of flies in a field, there are many potentially random events: the number of flies that happen to be near the capturing net, the temperature and wind velocity at the time the measurement was made (which influences the number of flies who are up and about), and so on. Careful experimental design can minimize the influence of such factors, but whichever ones remain often tend to add up.

In terms of the deck-of-cards analogy, this means that each measurement error or outside perturbation is not a single card drawn from a deck, but instead results from drawing several cards at once and adding up the numbers on the cards. *Dynamics in Action* 7 describes a **random walk**, a process in which independently drawn random numbers are added up to give a final result. As seen in Appendix A, the probability distribution for a random walk is the bell-shaped **Gaussian distribution** shown in Figure 6.1.

$$p(x)dx = \frac{1}{\sqrt{2\pi\sigma^2}} \exp \frac{-(x - M)^2}{2\sigma^2} dx. \tag{6.1}$$

M and σ are constants: M is the **mean** value, and σ is called the **standard deviation**.

Equation 6.1 is to be interpreted in the following way: The probability that a value drawn from a Gaussian distribution will fall into the range x to $x + dx$ is $p(x)dx$ when dx is small. $p(x)$ is called the probability density. If we want to know the probability of noise falling in a larger range, it is necessary to calculate the integral—the probability that the noise is in the range $a \leq x \leq b$ is

$$\int_a^b p(x)dx. \tag{6.2}$$

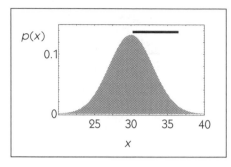

Figure 6.1
A Gaussian probability density, Eq. 6.1, with mean $M = 30$ and standard deviation $\sigma = 3$. The black bar has length 2σ.

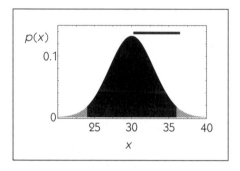

Figure 6.2   The probability of a single measurement falling into a specified range is the integral of the probability density over that range. The probability of the measurement falling in the range $[M - 2\sigma, M + 2\sigma]$ is the area shown in black, which is approximately 0.95.

Table 6.1   The probability that a single measurement, drawn from a Gaussian distribution with mean M and standard deviation σ, falls into the indicated interval.

Interval			Prob.
$M - 0.5\sigma$	to	$M + 0.5\sigma$	0.383
$M - \sigma$	to	$M + \sigma$	0.683
$M - 1.5\sigma$	to	$M + 1.5\sigma$	0.866
$M - 2\sigma$	to	$M + 2\sigma$	0.954
$M - 2.5\sigma$	to	$M + 2.5\sigma$	0.988
$M - 3\sigma$	to	$M + 3\sigma$	0.997

The integral in Eq. 6.2 is so important in practice that tables of its values are widely published. Using one of these tables, such as Table 6.1, we can see that the probability of the noise falling into the range $M - 2\sigma$ to $M + 2\sigma$ is roughly 0.954, or about 95 percent. See Figure 6.2.

✈ MODEL ONE

The behavior of the finite-difference equation

$$x_{t+1} = A + \rho x_t \qquad (6.3)$$

is easily studied with the methods presented in Chapter 1. There is a steady state at

$$x^\star = A/(1 - \rho) = M$$

that is stable if $|\rho| < 1$, which is the case we shall assume here. (We use the variable M as shorthand for $\frac{A}{(1-\rho)}$.) The solution to the finite-difference equation is exponential decay to the steady state: After the transient passes, we have steady-state behavior $x_t = M$.

For simplicity, we will assume that a direct measurement of the dynamical variable x_t is made, but since there is measurement noise the measurement at time t is

$$D_t = x_t + W_t, \qquad (6.4)$$

where W_t is a random number drawn independently at each t from a Gaussian probability distribution with a mean of zero and standard deviation σ.

Figure 6.3 shows data D_t generated from this model, with $A = 4, \rho = 0.95$, and consequently $M = \frac{A}{(1-\rho)} = 80$. W_t is Gaussian white measurement noise with a standard deviation of $\sigma = 2$.

This model might serve as a description of a system where there is some quantity (e.g., population level or amount of a circulating hormone) that is maintained at a steady level. The model assumes that no outside perturbation affects x_t—the dynamics of the model are completely trivial once the transient has died out: steady state.

Using the model as a motivation in interpreting measured data, we might ask the following questions:

- What is the value of the steady state in the data?
- What is the level of measurement noise in the data?

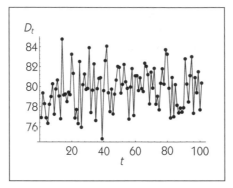

Figure 6.3
Data D_t from the model
$x_{t+1} = A + \rho x_t$ with
measurement $D_t = x_t + W_t$.
$A = 4$, $\rho = 0.95$, and the
standard deviation of W_t is
$\sigma = 2$.

We also might want to decide if the model is good for describing the measured data:

- Is there evidence that there really is a steady state?

- Is there evidence that there is only measurement noise and no outside perturbations to the state x_t?

6.3 THE MEAN AND STANDARD DEVIATION

We make a series of measurements, as in Figure 6.3 and we have a model in mind such as Model One, which suggests that the system is at a stable steady state. How do we estimate the value M of this steady state from the measurements? Intuition tells us that we should **average** all the N measurements $D_1, D_2, \ldots, D_N$ rather than take just a single measurement, say D_7, as our estimate of M. Because we cannot measure M directly, but rather estimate it from D_t, we will denote the quantity we estimate as M_{est}. Although M depends only on the dynamical equation 6.3 and—according to the model—is constant, M_{est} may vary depending on how many data points D_t we collect and on when they are collected.

To see where the idea of averaging comes from, consider trying to find the value M_{est} that is closest to all of the measurements $D_1, \ldots, D_N$. We take the separation between M_{est} and D_t to be $(D_t - M_{\text{est}})^2$. To make M_{est} as close as possible to all the measurements, we minimize the total separation E,

$$E = \sum_{t=1}^{N} (D_t - M_{\text{est}})^2. \tag{6.5}$$

To perform the minimization, take $\frac{dE}{dM_{\text{est}}}$ and set it equal to zero (remember, we're trying to find the value of M_{est} that gives the smallest value of E):

$$\frac{dE}{dM_{\text{est}}} = 0 = 2 \sum_{t=1}^{N}(D_t - M_{\text{est}}). \tag{6.6}$$

Rearranging the right-hand side of Eq. 6.6, we find

$$M_{\text{est}} = \frac{1}{N} \sum_{t=1}^{N} D_t. \tag{6.7}$$

This is the familiar formula for averaging. M_{est} is termed the **sample mean** of the set of measurements D_t.

STANDARD DEVIATION

By calculating the mean of the measured data, we now have an estimate, M_{est}, of the value of the steady state M. We are now interested in the fluctuations V_t of the measurements around the mean,

$$V_t = D_t - M_{\text{est}}.$$

Model One interprets these fluctuations as noise. One of the goals of time-series analysis of the Model One data is to assess the validity of this interpretation.

As a first step, we want to characterize the size of the fluctuations. One way (which will turn out not to be very useful) is to consider the mean value of the fluctuations:

$$\frac{1}{N} \sum_{t=1}^{N} V_t = \frac{1}{N} \sum_{t=1}^{N}(D_t - M_{\text{est}}) = \left(\frac{1}{N} \sum_{t=1}^{N} D_t \right) - M_{\text{est}} = M_{\text{est}} - M_{\text{est}} = 0$$

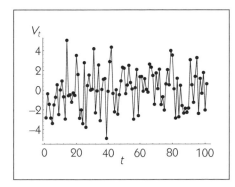

Figure 6.4
The sample mean M_{est} of the data shown in Figure 6.3 is 79.74. Subtracting this value from each data point D_t gives the fluctuations about the mean, $V_t = D_t - M_{\text{est}}$, as plotted here. The standard deviation of these fluctuations is 2.06.

The mean value of the fluctuations is always zero! This isn't so remarkable when we remember that the fluctuations are defined to be the difference between each measurement D_t and the mean $M_{est} = \sum_{t=1}^{N} \frac{D_t}{N}$. (The fact that the mean of the fluctuations around M_{est} is *always* zero, even though the fluctuations are hypothesized to be random, points out that M_{est} is only an *estimate* of the fixed point M—the fluctuations around M are unlikely to average out to be exactly zero.)

More useful is the mean value of the square of the fluctuations:

$$\sigma^2 = \frac{1}{N} \sum_{t=1}^{N} V_t^2 = \frac{1}{N} \sum_{t=1}^{N} (M_{est} - D_t)^2. \tag{6.8}$$

σ^2 is called the **variance**. The square root of the variance, σ, is the **standard deviation**. Note that $N\sigma^2$ is the same quantity that we minimized in Eq. 6.6 in order to find the mean, so the mean might be defined as "the value that minimizes the variance."

STANDARD ERROR OF THE MEAN

Although M_{est} is easy to calculate, it is only an estimate of the true mean M. Why only an estimate? Consider the limiting case where only a single measurement D_1 is made. In this case, $M_{est} = D_1$, and clearly any noise in D_1 is duplicated in M_{est}. With two measurements, D_1 and D_2, there is some chance that the noise will cancel out, but it probably will not cancel out exactly.

Intuition tells us that the more measurements we use in averaging, the better our estimate M_{est} will be. We can quantify this intuition. A good way to interpret M_{est} is that it is the sum of the true value M plus some uncertainty,

$$M_{est} = M + \text{uncertainty}. \tag{6.9}$$

The uncertainty in M_{est} comes from averaging the noisy components of the individual measurements. Very often the amplitude of the uncertainty is well described by a Gaussian probability distribution. The standard deviation of this uncertainty is

$$\frac{\sigma}{\sqrt{N}}, \tag{6.10}$$

which is called the **standard error of the mean**. Note that the $\frac{1}{\sqrt{N}}$ dependence of the standard error of the mean implies that taking more measurements reduces the uncertainty in the estimate of M, but that in order to reduce the uncertainty by a factor of 2, one needs to collect four times as much data.

An important assumption that goes into the derivation of the formula for the standard error of the mean given in 6.10 is that the measurements are independent of one another. In the next several sections, we will see various ways to test for such independence. When measurements are not independent, the uncertainty in the estimate of the mean may vary with N in different ways. An extreme case is that of $\frac{1}{f}$ noise, described in *Dynamics in Action* 6. For $\frac{1}{f}$ noise, the variance increases as N increases, and so the uncertainty in the estimate of the mean increases as more data are collected!

☐ Example 6.1

Are the data plotted in Figure 6.3 consistent with Model One? More specifically, does the mean of the data correspond to the theoretical value of the steady state for the parameters used in Model One?

Solution: The mean of the 100 data points plotted in Figure 6.3 is found to be $M_{est} = 79.74$, and the standard deviation is 2.06. The theoretical value of the steady state for the parameters used is $M = \frac{A}{(1-\rho)} = 80$. So now the question is whether 79.74 is close enough to 80 for us to conclude that the data and the model are consistent.

Since there are 100 data points, the standard error of the mean is $\frac{2.06}{\sqrt{100}} = 0.206$. This standard error describes the uncertainty in the estimate of the mean—how much estimated mean might deviate from the true mean just because of chance fluctuations in the data. As a rule of thumb, the difference between a number and M_{est} is only statistically significant if the difference is greater than twice the standard error of the mean. (This is only a guideline. A more accurate and precise statement of the meaning of statistical significance is given in statistics textbooks such as Snedecor and Cochran (1989).) In this case, the difference between M, the theoretical value of the steady state, and M_{est} is $|79.74 - 80| = 0.26$, which is less than twice the standard error of the mean. Therefore, we conclude that the difference between M_{est} and M is statistically insignificant: The data are consistent with the model.

☐

✈ Model Two

A possible deficiency with Model One is that it does not include any outside influences on the state variable x_t. For this reason, all the observed variability is modeled as measurement noise.

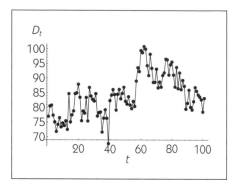

Figure 6.5
Data D_t from the model $x_{t+1} = A + \rho x_t + v_t$ with measurement $D_t = x_t + W_t$. $A = 4$, $\rho = 0.95$. The standard deviation of W_t is $\sigma = 2$ and that of v_t is 3.

A simple way to modify Model One to include outside influences is to write the finite-difference equation

$$x_{t+1} = A + \rho x_t + v_t. \tag{6.11}$$

This incorporates a random influence v_t on the state variable. As before, the measurement function D_t will be taken, for simplicity, to be the state variable x_t itself, plus random measurement noise W_t,

$$D_t = x_t + W_t. \tag{6.12}$$

We now have two different sources of noise in the model. We will assume that these two sources are completely independent and that each has its own mean and standard deviation.

Some simulated data from this model, with $A = 4$, $\rho = 0.95$ (i.e., $M = 80$, as in Model One) are shown in Figure 6.5. Here we again take the standard deviation of W_t to be 2, and we will assume that the standard deviation of v_t is 3. The mean of each of the random influences is assumed to be zero.

Some differences between the data from Model One and Model Two can be seen: Model Two produces a much greater range of variability than Model One and shows slow trends, whereas Model One does not.

In interpreting the measured data according to Model Two, we might ask:

- What are the dynamics of movement toward the stable fixed point after an outside perturbation? In particular, can we estimate the time constant of exponential decay, ρ, from the data?

- How much of the variability in the data is due to measurement error, and how much is due to outside perturbation?

6.4 LINEAR CORRELATIONS

One of the assumptions in Model One is that the observed fluctuations around the steady state are a result of white measurement noise; that is, the noise in each measurement is independent of the noise in every other measurement. How can we test the validity of this assumption in the data? If the fluctuations were not independent, how could we quantify their dependence?

So far, we have characterized fluctuations by their mean and standard deviation. These two statistics have an important property: They do not depend on the order in which the data occur. That is, if each measurement was written on its own card, and the stack of cards was shuffled, sorted, or rearranged in any way whatsoever, the mean and standard deviation would remain exactly the same.

As we discussed in Section 6.2, a randomly shuffled deck of cards generates values that are independent of one another. Since the mean and standard deviation are not influenced by the order of cards in the deck, they are of no use in deciding whether fluctuations are independent of each other.

In order to quantify the degree of dependence or independence, consider two limiting cases. Recall that the fluctuations around the mean are denoted V_t. If the fluctuations are white noise—this is the case of complete independence—then we can model them as

$$V_t = \mathcal{W}_t, \tag{6.13}$$

where $\mathcal{W}_t$ is white noise. (We write $\mathcal{W}_t$ instead of W_t in order to distinguish this model of V_t from the white noise used in Models One and Two that affected the variable D_t. You can think of W_t and $\mathcal{W}_t$ as different decks of cards.)

At the other extreme, V_{t+1} might be completely dependent on V_t, that is,

$$V_{t+1} = f(V_t).$$

Before moving on to nonlinear forms of the function $f(V_t)$, we will start here with the simplifying assumption that $f(V_t)$ is *linear*:

$$V_{t+1} = \rho V_t. \tag{6.14}$$

Combining these two extreme cases of Eqs. 6.13 and 6.14 into one model of the fluctuations, we can write

$$V_{t+1} = \rho V_t + \mathcal{W}_t. \tag{6.15}$$

Note that Eq. 6.15 hasn't been derived from any calculation; it is just a convenient way of writing a model having a parameter ρ that indicates the degree of dependence (with the assumption of linearity) between V_{t+1} and V_t. When $\rho = 0$, V_{t+1} is independent of V_t. If ρ is close to 1, then V_{t+1} is almost the same as V_t; if ρ is close to -1, then V_{t+1} is again almost the same as V_t, but with a value of the opposite sign. Remember that if $|\rho| > 1$, the steady state at $V = 0$ in Eq. 6.14 is unstable. If the data are not blowing up to ∞, then the model of Eq. 6.14 must have $|\rho| < 1$.

How can we estimate ρ from measured data? We can take the following approach: Look for a value ρ_{est} that makes the square of the difference between V_{t+1} and ρV_t as small as possible—a value that fits the equation $V_{t+1} = \rho_{est} V_t$ as closely as possible. We will do this using a least-squares criterion:

$$E = \sum_{t=1}^{N-1} (V_{t+1} - \rho_{est} V_t)^2. \tag{6.16}$$

Finding the minimum by taking the derivative of E with respect to ρ_{est} and setting this equal to zero, we get

$$\frac{dE}{d\rho_{est}} = 0 = \sum_{t=1}^{N-1} (V_{t+1} - \rho_{est} V_t) V_t, \tag{6.17}$$

which implies

$$\rho_{est} = \frac{\sum_{t=1}^{N-1} V_{t+1} V_t}{\sum_{t=1}^{N-1} V_t V_t}. \tag{6.18}$$

ρ_{est} is called the **correlation coefficient**.

❑ EXAMPLE 6.2

In the data from Models One and Two, are the fluctuations around the fixed point consistent with the assumption that they are due to white measurement noise?

Solution: We have already found the mean of the data D_t from Model One to be $M_{est} = 79.74$. The fluctuations around the mean are therefore

$$V_t = D_t - 79.74.$$

Using measured data in the formula for the correlation coefficient in Eq. 6.18, we find that $\rho_{est} = -0.0026$, which is close to zero and therefore consistent with

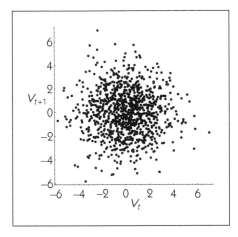

Figure 6.6
A scatter plot of the fluctuations around the mean: V_{t+1} versus V_t from Model One. (One thousand data points are shown.)

a claim that V_{t+1} is independent of V_t. (More advanced texts on statistics give a precise meaning of "close to zero" in terms of the uncertainty in the estimate ρ_{est}. See, for example, Box and Jenkins (1976).) Figure 6.6 shows V_{t+1} plotted against V_t for the Model One data. The round cloud of points is typical of a lack of correlation between the two variables.

The mean of the measurements from Model Two is $M_{est} = 84.10$. Calculating the correlation coefficient by applying Eq. 6.18, we find $\rho_{est} = 0.786$. This indicates a substantial degree of correlation between V_{t+1} and V_t, as shown by the cigar-shaped cloud of Figure 6.7. This leads us to conclude that the fluctuations from the mean in Model Two are not entirely the result of white noise measurement error.

The measurement noise W_t and the dynamical noise v_t in Model Two are both Gaussian white noise, but they play different roles. The measurement noise

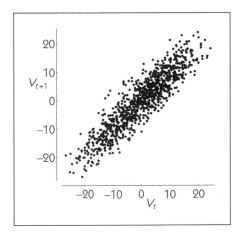

Figure 6.7
A scatter plot of the fluctuations around the mean: V_{t+1} versus V_t from Model Two. (One thousand data points are shown.)

is completely forgotten from one time step to the next—D_{t+1} contains no information about the measurement noise at time t. The dynamical noise v_t, however, changes the value of the state variable x_t. Imagine that after time t the dynamical noise v_t were turned off. The noise at time t would be remembered while the state variable moved back exponentially to its fixed point. This "memory" of past dynamical noise, which can be characterized by the **impulse response function** studied in Section 4.7 creates the correlation between V_t and V_{t+1}. In contrast, there is no mechanism to preserve memory of the measurement noise from one time to another.

The calculated value of the correlation coefficient, $\rho_{est} = 0.786$, tells us that consecutive measurements are not independent of one another. We might want to go further, and use ρ_{est} as an estimate of the value of ρ in the Model Two dynamics (Eq. 6.11), which we know to be $\rho = 0.95$. The difference between ρ_{est} and ρ arises mostly from the influence of the measurement noise W_t in Eq. 6.12. Since the measurement noise is incorporated in ρ_{est}, ρ_{est} cannot be used by itself to estimate ρ. In Example 6.3 we will see one way to estimate ρ from the measurements. ☐

✈ MODEL THREE

Models One and Two display fixed points and exponential decay to a fixed point, respectively. Another type of behavior frequently encountered is oscillations. For example, consider the two coupled differential equations

$$\frac{dx}{dt} = y + v(t), \qquad \frac{dy}{dt} = -ay - bx, \qquad (6.19)$$

where $v(t)$ is random noise. If we neglect the dynamical noise $v(t)$, we can use the tools from Chapter 5 and write down the characteristic equation for this differential equation, and then find the eigenvalues. They are

$$\lambda = \frac{-a}{2} \pm \frac{\sqrt{a^2 - 4b}}{2}, \qquad (6.20)$$

so for $a > 0$ and $b > \frac{a^2}{4}$ the equation produces oscillations of exponentially decaying amplitude. The frequency of the oscillations are $\omega = \frac{\sqrt{a^2-4b}}{2}$ and the time constant of the exponential decay is $\frac{2}{a}$.

In this case, we have two dynamical variables, $x(t)$ and $y(t)$. We shall assume that we measure only one of them, $x(t)$, along with Gaussian white measurement noise W_i. The measurements D_i are made at discrete times, every T time units,

$$D_i = x(iT) + W_i. \qquad (6.21)$$

Figure 6.8 shows a measured time series from Model Three with $a = 0.5$, $b = 3$, and $T = 0.1$. We set the standard deviation of the dynamical noise $v(t)$ to be 3 and that of the measurement noise W_i to be 1.

Although there are ups and downs in the data, it would be hard to claim from Figure 6.8 that the dynamics have much to do with an exponential decay in the amplitude of the oscillations. Nonetheless, motivated by the model we might ask

- What are the dynamics of movement toward the stable fixed point after an outside perturbation? In particular, what is the intrinsic frequency of the oscillation and the time constant of exponential decay?

- How much of the variability in the data is due to measurement error, and how much is due to outside perturbation?

To evaluate whether the model is appropriate for describing the data, ask:

- What is the evidence that there are oscillations in the dynamics, as opposed to random perturbations and exponential decay as in Model Two?

THE AUTOCORRELATION FUNCTION

The dynamics of Model Two involve exponential approach to the fixed point. The dynamics of Model Three involve sine-wave oscillations with an amplitude that decays exponentially. The data generated from the models do not show these dynamics very clearly but do indeed contain within them information about the exponential decay and sine-wave oscillations. We can use coefficients of correlation to reveal the dynamics obscured by noise.

Recall that V_t denotes fluctuations of the measured values around the mean, $V_t = D_t - M_{est}$. The correlation coefficient fits the relationship between V_{t+1}

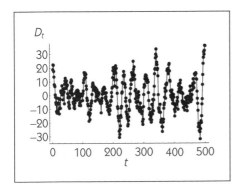

Figure 6.8
A time series from Model Three, with $a = 0.5, b = 3$, and $T = 0.1$. The differential equations were integrated numerically using the Euler method with a time step $\Delta = 0.1$. The standard deviation of the dynamical noise $v(t)$ is 3; that of the measurement noise $W(t)$ is 1.

and V_t to the equation $V_{t+1} = \rho V_t + W_t$. We can easily generalize the correlation coefficient to describe the relationship between V_{t+k} and V_t, giving us the **autocorrelation function** $R(k)$,

$$R(k) = \frac{\sum_{t=1}^{N-k} V_{t+k} V_t}{\sum_{t=1}^{N-k} V_t V_t}. \tag{6.22}$$

k is called the **lag** between the variables V_t and V_{t+k}. Note that the variable t is a "dummy variable"—it is used purely as an accounting device in the summations. $R(k)$ is quite simple to calculate from data: One repeats basically the same calculation for several different values of k.

❑ EXAMPLE 6.3

Use the autocorrelation function to show that the measured data from Models One, Two, and Three show distinct dynamics for the three models.

Solution: Figure 6.9 shows the autocorrelation function $R(k)$ for the data from Model One. The autocorrelation function for this data, and for all data, takes the value 1 at $k = 0$, that is, $R(0) = 1$. The reason for this can be seen by inspecting Eq. 6.22; when $k = 0$, the numerator is the same as the denominator.

For the Model One data, $R(k)$ is approximately zero for $k > 0$. (The deviations from zero are due to the finite length of the data used in calculating $R(k)$. See Exercise 6.5.) This is consistent with the model of the fluctuations as resulting from white measurement noise. In fact, this shape for $R(k)$ is often taken as the definition of white noise, especially in older textbooks written before the current appreciation of nonlinear dynamics and chaos.

For the Model Two data, $R(k)$ has a different shape, as Figure 6.10 shows. From its value of 1 at $k = 0$, $R(k)$ falls off sharply to approximately 0.8 at $k = 1$. For $k \geq 1$, $R(k)$ falls off exponentially. From the parameters used in Model Two, we know that the exponential dynamics in the absence of noise have the form

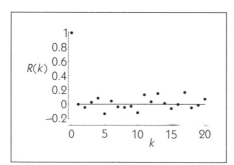

Figure 6.9
The autocorrelation function $R(k)$ versus k for the data from Model One.

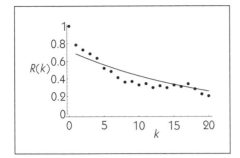

Figure 6.10
The autocorrelation function
$R(k)$ versus k for the data from
Model Two.

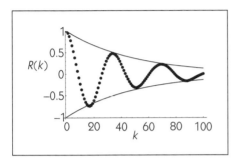

Figure 6.11
The autocorrelation function
$R(k)$ versus k for the data from
Model Three.

$x_t = 0.95^t x_0$. The thin line in Figure 6.10 plots this theoretical exponential decay and as can be seen, it fits the autocorrelation function very closely.

The sharp fall-off in $R(k)$ from $k = 0$ to $k = 1$ reflects the white measurement noise in Model Two. This fall-off can be used to estimate the variance of the measurement noise. Without going into detail, we note that the fall-off has an amplitude of roughly 0.2. This means that 20 percent of the total variance of the Model Two data can be ascribed to white measurement noise. Since the total variance can be calculated from Eq. 6.8 to be 50.1, the variance of the measurement noise is estimated to be roughly $50.1 \times 0.2 \approx 10$. This gives an estimated standard deviation of 3.2, consistent with the theoretical value of 3 used in generating the data.

The autocorrelation function for the Model Three data is shown in Figure 6.11. It consists of a sine wave of exponentially decaying amplitude. From the figure, the period of the sine wave is easily found to be roughly 36 time units. The thin lines show an exponentially decaying envelope of the form 0.98^t. This compares well with the theoretical form for the noiseless dynamics as $0.975^t \sin\left(\frac{2\pi t}{36.6}\right) + \cos\left(\frac{2\pi t}{36.6}\right)$, where A and B are set by the initial conditions. ⌐

6.5 POWER SPECTRUM ANALYSIS

Consider a slight modification of Model Three: The dynamics and measurement process are the same, except that in addition to measuring D_t, let us also measure the dynamical noise v_t. Perhaps in this situation it is impolite to call v_t "noise" since we know what it is. Thus we will now call v_t the **input** to the system, and we'll call D_t the **output**. We are interested in the input/output relationship.

THE FOURIER TRANSFORM

In Section 4.7, we saw how a signal could be broken down, or **decomposed**, into the sum of simpler signals. For instance, the signal shown Figure 4.17 can be decomposed into the four simpler signals shown in Figure 4.18. This type of decomposition can be performed in any number of ways.

One incredibly powerful decomposition is into sine waves of different frequencies. Recall from Section 4.7 the following facts for linear systems:

1. The output that results from a sine-wave input of frequency ω is a sine wave of the same frequency ω but perhaps of different amplitude and phase. The amplitude of the output sine wave $A_{\text{output}}(\omega)$ is proportional to the amplitude of the input sine wave $A_{\text{input}}(\omega)$:

$$A_{\text{output}}(\omega) = G(\omega)A_{\text{input}}(\omega).$$

For any input phase $\phi_{\text{input}}(\omega)$, the output phase $\phi_{\text{output}}(\omega)$ is shifted by a fixed amount at each frequency,

$$\Phi(\omega) = \phi_{\text{output}}(\omega) - \phi_{\text{input}}(\omega).$$

$G(\omega)$ is called the **gain** of the system, and it may be different at different frequencies. $\Phi(\omega)$ is called the **phase shift** and may also differ at different frequencies.

2. **Linear superposition of inputs** says that if the input can be written as a sum of sine waves of different frequencies, then the output is the sum of sine waves of those same frequencies. The amplitude and phase of the sine wave at each frequency in the output are exactly the same as if the input had been purely the single corresponding sine wave in the input.

The method for decomposing a signal into sine waves of different frequencies is called the **Fourier transform**. The details of how this is done are covered in many texts (see Press et al. (1992)). Here we simply point out that any signal can be decomposed into sine waves and that the result is an amplitude and phase at each frequency.

An especially important case is when the input is white noise. For white noise, $A_{input}(\omega)$ is a constant for all ω. The constant is proportional to the standard deviation of the white noise. The phase $\phi_{input}(\omega)$ varies from one frequency to another, and is generally regarded as random. Since $A_{input}(\omega)$ is constant, white noise can be considered as a sum of signals of all different frequencies. This is where the name "white" comes from, by analogy to the fact that white light is a mixture of equal parts of many different frequencies of light.

THE TRANSFER FUNCTION

Having measured the input and output signals from Model Three, we use the Fourier transform to decompose each of the two signals into a sum of sine waves of different frequencies. At each frequency ω, we have amplitudes $A_{input}(\omega)$ and $A_{output}(\omega)$ and phases $\phi_{input}(\omega)$ and $\phi_{output}(\omega)$. We can easily calculate

$$G(\omega) = \frac{A_{output}(\omega)}{A_{input}(\omega)} \quad \text{and} \quad \Phi(\omega) = \phi_{output}(\omega) - \phi_{input}(\omega).$$

Note that $G(\omega)$ and $\Phi(\omega)$ are functions of frequency ω. This pair of functions is called the **transfer function** of the system. If we know the transfer function for a linear system, then we can calculate the output for any given input, or vice versa (as long as $G(\omega) \neq 0$).

You may recall from Section 4.7 that an input/output system is described by its **impulse response**. The transfer function and impulse response are different ways of looking at exactly the same thing. In fact, the transfer function is the Fourier transform of the impulse response.

THE POWER SPECTRUM

Suppose that we do not actually measure the input but that we know or assume that it is white noise. This tells us that $A_{input}(\omega)$ is constant. Knowing this, we can calculate the gain $G(\omega)$ to within a constant of proportionality, even without having measured the input:

$$G(\omega) = \text{const } A_{output}(\omega).$$

However, since we don't know anything about $\phi_{input}(\omega)$, we cannot calculate $\Phi(\omega)$. The square of $G(\omega)$ is called the **power spectrum**.

The power spectrum contains exactly the same information as the auto-correlation function—the power spectrum is in fact the Fourier transform of the autocorrelation function. Although the information is the same, the different format of the information sometimes makes it advantageous to use the power spectrum rather than the autocorrelation function for analyzing data.

DYNAMICS IN ACTION

17 DAILY OSCILLATIONS IN ZOOPLANKTON

The top figure here shows hourly measurements of zooplankton density. The power spectrum, shown in the bottom figure, displays the square of the amplitude of the oscillations at each frequency. Here, instead of measuring frequency in units of cycles/second (Hertz), we use cycles/day to reflect the time scale over which zooplankton density changes significantly.

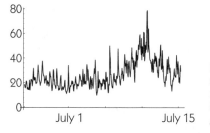

Hourly measurements of zooplankton density (in g/m^3) measured in the Middle Atlantic Bight starting on 25 June 1988. (See Ascioti et al., 1993)

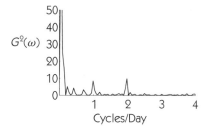

The power spectrum $G^2(\omega)$ of the data from the above figure.

The power spectrum $G^2(\omega)$ from this data shows a peak at 1 cycle per day. This peak corresponds to the daily changes in zooplankton density that come from the day/night cycle. (There is also a peak in $G^2(\omega)$ at 2 cycles per day. This suggests that the daily cycle is not a simple sine wave, but that each cycle has some other shape.)

In addition to the daily changes at 1 and 2 cycles per day, the zooplankton data contain other variations. For instance, there is a week-long buildup that reaches to a maximum on July 10. Such slow variability in the zooplankton density appears as the large values of $G^2(\omega)$ for low frequencies ($\ll$ 1 cycle/day). The power spectrum is often used, as in this case, to display periodic variability at a given frequency that might be hidden by other forms of variability.

✈ MODEL FOUR

Models One, Two, and Three have linear dynamics. The parameters used in the models have been set so that, in the absence of dynamical noise, the stable fixed point is approached asymptotically. Nonlinear models can have nonfixed asymptotic behavior. As we saw in Chapter 1, the quadratic map

$$x_{t+1} = \mu x_t (1 - x_t) \tag{6.23}$$

can show a variety of behaviors from stable fixed points, to stable periodic cycles, to chaos. In particular, for $\mu = 4.0$ the dynamics are chaotic, while for $\mu = 3.52$ there is a stable cycle of period 4. Equation 6.23 involves no dynamical noise.

In order to emphasize the difference between the chaotic dynamics of Model Four and the noisy linear dynamics of Models One, Two, and Three, we shall assume that there is no measurement noise:

$$D_t = x_t. \tag{6.24}$$

Figure 6.12 shows a time series taken from Model Four.

Since there is neither dynamical nor measurement noise, the model is completely **deterministic**. This means that, in principle, if we know the initial condition we can calculate all future values. Of course, if the model is chaotic, there may be practical limitations on our ability to do this.

With this model as a hypothesis, we might ask the following questions about our data:

1. What evidence is there that a deterministic process generates the data?

2. What evidence is there that the data involve a nonlinear process?

3. If the data are indeed chaotic, how large is the sensitive dependence on initial conditions?

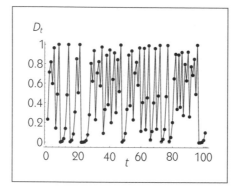

Figure 6.12
A simulated time series from
Model Four, with $\mu = 4.0$. There
is no measurement noise.

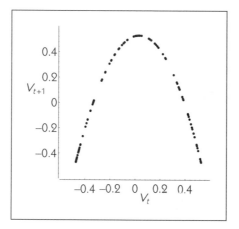

Figure 6.13
A scatter plot of fluctuations
around the mean: V_{t+1} versus V_t
from Model Four.

We can start the data analysis with the tools already at our disposal. The
mean of the data in Figure 6.12 is $M_{est} = 0.471$. The fluctuations about the mean
$V_t = D_t - M_{est}$ can be used to calculate the correlation coefficient between V_{t+1}
and V_t. This is $\rho_{est} = 0.054$, close to zero even though a scatter plot of V_{t+1} versus
V_t does not look like a ball. (Compare Figure 6.13 with Figure 6.6. Both scatter

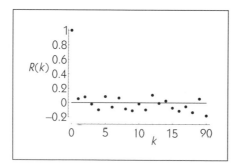

Figure 6.14
The autocorrelation function
$R(k)$ calculated from the data in
Model Four.

plots produce ρ_{est} near zero.) In fact, the autocorrelation function for the data is very similar to that found for the data from Model One (compare Figure 6.9 to Figure 6.14). This suggests that the data from Model Four are white noise, apparently contradicting the fact that the data are from a deterministic model.

The resolution to this paradox can be seen if we remember that the correlation coefficient and the autocorrelation function measure linear correlations in the data. The scatter plot of V_{t+1} versus V_t shows a very strong relationship, but the relationship is nonlinear and hence not accurately represented by the correlation coefficient and autocorrelation function.

❑

6.6   NONLINEAR DYNAMICS AND DATA ANALYSIS

In the previous section we saw that statistics such as the correlation coefficient and the autocorrelation function are not able to distinguish between the data from the linear Model One and those from the nonlinear Model Four. In this section we will describe data-analysis methods that are appropriate for nonlinear systems. Nearly all of the techniques have been developed since 1980, and new developments are made on an almost daily basis.

Most techniques for nonlinear data analysis involve two steps. In the first step, the data are used to **reconstruct** the dynamics of the system. This is the subject of the present section. The second step involves **characterization** of the reconstructed dynamics and will be the subject of Sections 6.7 and 6.8.

RECONSTRUCTING FINITE-DIFFERENCE EQUATIONS: RETURN MAPS

Model Four is a finite-difference equation (the quadratic map that we studied in Chapter 1). Compare Figure 6.13 to Figure 1.16. The scatter plot derived from data reproduces the parabolic form of the graph drawn from the finite-difference equation. This shouldn't be surprising. A finite-difference equation like $x_{t+1} = f(x_t)$ describes the relationship between x_{t+1} and x_t. A scatter plot of the measured data, D_{t+1} versus D_t, describes exactly the same relationship. Since in Model Four we defined $D_t = x_t$, each of the dots in the scatter plot falls on the function $f(\cdot)$, and the dots do a good job of indicating the parabolic geometry of $f(\cdot)$. (In Figure 6.13 we plot V_{t+1} versus V_t. This is this is the same thing as plotting D_{t+1} versus D_t but translating both axes by the mean M_{est}.)

The idea of using a scatter plot to display the relationship between successive measurements is fundamental to the analysis of data from nonlinear systems. We will call the scatter plot a **return plot**, but other names found in the technical literature for this type of scatter plot are *first-return plot, Poincaré return map,* and *return map.*

DYNAMICS IN ACTION

18 RECONSTRUCTING NERVE CELL DYNAMICS

The top figure shows a recording of the voltage across the membrane of a giant axon (the axon is a part of a nerve cell) from a squid. These data were collected by Alvin Shrier and John Clay at the Marine Biological Laboratory in Woods Hole, MA.

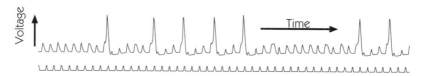

Transmembrane voltage from a periodically stimulated squid giant axon. The times of the stimuli are also indicated. The bottom trace shows the stimulation current. Stimuli were applied every 10 msec. These data were provided by Drs. A. Shrier and J. Clay.

An electrode has been inserted into the cell, and a periodic stimulus has been applied. In response to each stimulation, the axon has either a small response (a "subthreshold response") or a big one (an "action potential"). The transmembrane voltage has been sampled by a computer 10,000 times per second. Since the voltage does not change much over 0.0001 seconds, a return plot of the voltage x_{t+1} versus x_t stays very close to the line of identity, and there is no evidence in this plot for a single-valued nonlinear function (see the next figure).

One technique for generating a return plot appropriate for the squid axon data is to reduce the time series into a set of discrete measurements made at a time interval having a relationship to the systems's dynamics. In the squid axon case, a sensible time interval is the time between stimuli, rather than the time between successive voltage samples taken by the computer. Several types of measurements might be taken once per stimulus. For example, we might take a single measurement from the recording some fixed time (say, 20 msec) after each stimulus. Or we might choose to measure the recording only at the peak of the response to each stimulus

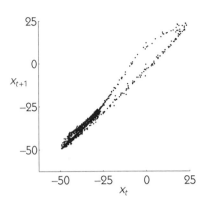

A return plot x_{t+1} versus x_t for the voltage across the membrane of the squid axon.

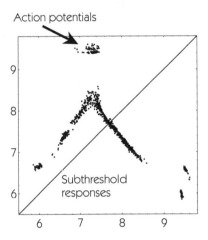

A_{i+1} versus A_i for the squid axon data, where A_i is the logarithm of the area under response i.

The bottom figure shows a return plot made by calculating the logarithm of the area under each stimulus response. The plot shows that the repetitive subthreshold responses seen in the time series result from an unstable fixed point; action potentials are generated only when the dynamics move away from this fixed point. The action potentials that appear to occur at random intervals in the top figure are really generated by a nonlinear dynamical system that can be largely characterized by the return plot.

For other systems, it may not be obvious how frequently to make measurements for the purpose of drawing a return plot. For example, the sunspot data shown in the preface were collected once per month. Nothing about a one-month interval relates to the dynamics of the sun—if we want to extract information about the dynamics, another measurement interval might be more appropriate.

In many cases, data have been collected from a continuous-time dynamical system properly described by differential equations rather than by finite-difference equations. In such cases, it may be appropriate to use the *phase-plane* or *embedding* reconstruction techniques described in the following sections. Sometimes, however, a return map does describe effectively the dynamics behind continuous-time data. In drawing such a return map, take care to select a time interval that reflects some important aspect of the dynamics.

RECONSTRUCTING THE PHASE PLANE

Consider data generated from the second-order differential equation describing a harmonic oscillator:

$$\frac{d^2x}{dt^2} = -bx. \tag{6.25}$$

As shown in Section 5.4, this equation can be rewritten in terms of two first-order differential equations,

$$\frac{dx}{dt} = y$$

$$\frac{dy}{dt} = -bx. \tag{6.26}$$

The variables x and y form the **phase plane**, and Eq. 6.26 describes the flow of the dynamics on this plane.

Suppose that we measure a time series $D(t) = x(t)$ from Eq. 6.25 (see Figure 6.15). How can we reconstruct the phase plane and the flow on it from the measured data? At any instant, the position of the system on the phase plane is given by the coordinates (x, y). The time series itself gives us D at every instant.

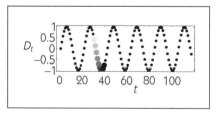

Figure 6.15
The quantity D_t measured from Eq. 6.25.

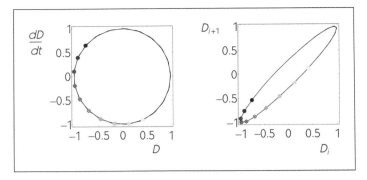

Figure 6.16 Two versions of the reconstructed phase plane for the data generated from Eq. 6.25. The gray dots indicate the position in the phase plane at the corresponding times in Figure 6.15.

We can measure $y(t)$ from $D(t)$ by noticing in Eq. 6.26 that $y = \frac{dD}{dt}$. If we plot out $\frac{dD}{dt}$ versus D, we get the **trajectory** of the system in the phase plane—this describes the flow based on the measured data (see Figure 6.16).

Given a time series $x(t)$, how do we calculate $\frac{dx}{dt}$? There are simple electronic circuits that act as differentiators, and in the past such a circuit might have been used to sketch out the trajectory on an oscilloscope screen. Today data typically are collected by computer, and so the measurement $D(t)$ actually consists of a sequence of measurements made at discrete times D_0, D_1, D_2, ... Using the textbook definition of the derivative of x at time t,

$$\frac{dx(t)}{dt} = \lim_{h \to 0} \frac{x(t + h) - x(t)}{h},$$

we are motivated to approximate the derivative at time t as

$$\frac{dD_t}{dt} = \frac{D_{t+h} - D_t}{h}.$$

For the discrete-time measurements, h can only take on the values 0, 1, 2, 3, ...—it cannot have a fractional value. The smallest useful value is $h = 1$, but sometimes, as we will see below, it is appropriate to select larger h.

Reconstructing the phase plane is thus a matter of plotting $\frac{D_{t+h} - D_t}{h}$ versus D_t. Notice that only two quantities are involved: D_{t+h} and D_t. They contain all the information in the plot, and it is effective simply to plot D_{t+h} versus D_t.

Equation 6.26 is a special case because $\frac{dx}{dt}$ gives us y. In general, dynamics on the phase plane are given by the pair of coupled differential equations (see Eq. 5.18)

$$\frac{dx}{dt} = f(x, y), \qquad \frac{dy}{dt} = g(x, y). \qquad (6.27)$$

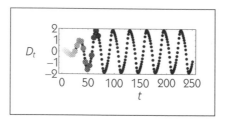

Figure 6.17
The quantity D_t measured from the van der Pol system, Eq. 5.25

If we measure only $x(t)$, how can we calculate the value of y? The answer is that often we cannot, but we do not need to in order to display relevant information about the dynamics in the phase plane. Notice that if we measure $x(t)$ and calculate $\frac{dx}{dt}$, we have both a direct measurement of x and a calculated value of $f(x, y)$. Some information about y is contained in the value of $f(x, y)$, and often this information is enough to allow us to get a good idea of the dynamics. Figures 6.17 through 6.19 give an example that shows how the reconstructed (D_t, D_{t+1}) phase plane compares to the original (x, y) phase plane.

To summarize, by making a series of measurements D_t and plotting D_{t+h} versus D_t, we can often reconstruct the phase-plane dynamics of a system, even though we never make direct measurements of the dynamical variable y.

EMBEDDING A TIME SERIES

As we saw in Chapter 4, a continuous-time system of ordinary differential equations that generates chaos must involve at least three equations. This means that the two-dimensional dynamics in a phase plane cannot represent chaotic be-

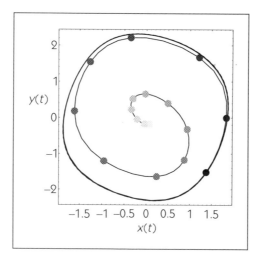

Figure 6.18
Dynamics in the original x, y phase plane for the van der Pol equation.

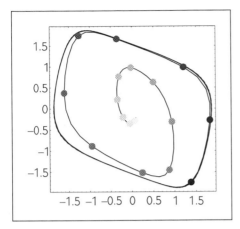

Figure 6.19
Dynamics of the van der Pol
equation in the reconstructed
D_{t+10} versus D_t phase plane.

havior. In order to reconstruct the geometry of a continuous-time chaotic system
from a time series, we can extend the technique developed for reconstructing the
phase plane. The phase-plane reconstruction involved plotting successive points
in a two-dimensional space. To reconstruct the dynamics in a three-dimensional
space, we plot the points as a three-dimensional coordinate:

$$(D_t, D_{t-h}, D_{t-2h}).$$

More generally, we can **embed** the time series in a p-dimensional space by taking
p-coordinates,

$$\mathbf{D}_t = (D_t, D_{t-h}, D_{t-2h}, \ldots, D_{t-(p-1)h}). \tag{6.28}$$

We use the boldface $\mathbf{D}_t$ to denote the embedded measurements, to differentiate
from D_t, which denotes a single measurement at time t. $\mathbf{D}_t$ incorporates measurements made at different times, ranging from t to $t - (p - 1)h$, but the index
t is used for notational convenience.

This technique of representing a measured time series as a sequence of
points in a p-dimensional space is called **time-lag embedding**. There is an important theorem (Taken's embedding theorem) that says the reconstructed dynamics
are geometrically similar to the original for both continuous-time and discrete-
time systems. The sequence of points created by embedding a time series is called
the trajectory of the time series. p is called the **embedding dimension**, and h is
the **embedding lag**.

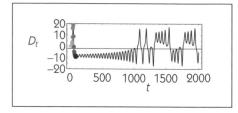

Figure 6.20
A measured signal D_t from the Lorenz system (Eq. 6.29).

As an example, consider the Lorenz system of three ordinary nonlinear differential equations that produce chaos:

$$\frac{dx}{dt} = 10(y - x),$$

$$\frac{dy}{dt} = 28x - y - xz, \qquad (6.29)$$

$$\frac{dz}{dt} = 28xy - \frac{8z}{3}.$$

If one could measure $x(t)$, $y(t)$, and $z(t)$ simultaneously, in a physical system, then by plotting out the three-dimensional coordinate $(x(t), y(t), z(t))$, we can reconstruct the dynamics in the three-dimensional **phase space**. But if we measure only one of the variables, so that $D(t) = x(t)$, we can create a reconstruction that is faithful to the geometry of the original, as shown in Figures 6.20 through 6.22.

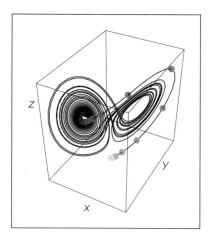

Figure 6.21
The trajectory of Eq. 6.29 in the original x, y, z phase space.

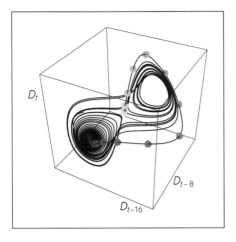

Figure 6.22
The reconstructed trajectory
of Eq. 6.29 using D_t, D_{t-8}, D_{t-16}.

✈ MODEL FIVE

The chaotic dynamics of Model Four were generated by a single equation involving a single state variable. Chaotic dynamics can also be generated by systems with more state variables, for instance the Lorenz equations (Eq. 6.29) have three state variables producing a chaotic attractor with a fractal dimension of approximately 2.06.

Although the dimension of a chaotic attractor may be less than the number of state variables, it can never exceed the number of state variables. In order to illustrate some of the properties of high-dimensional chaotic systems, we introduce a new model that produces chaotic dynamics, the Ikeda map:

$$x_{t+1} = 1 + \mu(x_t \cos m_t - y_t \sin m_t),$$

$$y_{t+1} = \mu(x_t \sin m_t + y_t \cos m_t), \tag{6.30}$$

where $m_t = 0.4 - \frac{6.0}{(1+x_t^2+y_t^2)}$ and $\mu = 0.7$. The Ikeda map has two dynamical variables, x_t and y_t. (m_t is just a convenience variable and can easily be eliminated from the equations by substitution.)

Since Eq. 6.30 has just two dynamical variables, any attractor it has can be at most two-dimensional. This is not very high, so let us consider another chaotic dynamical system, the Henon map:

$$z_{t+1} = 1.4 + 0.3v_t - z_t^2, \tag{6.31}$$

$$v_{t+1} = z_t.$$

This equation also has two variables, so its attractor can also be at most two-dimensional.

Taken together, however, the Ikeda map and the Henon map have four dynamical variables, v_t, w_t, x_t, y_t, so the attractor for the combined system can be at most four-dimensional. Suppose we measure

$$D_t = x_t + \beta z_t + W_t, \tag{6.32}$$

where W_t is random Gaussian white measurement noise. Our measured data will reflect the dynamics of both the Henon and Ikeda maps, and also the random noise W_t. Similarly, a natural or experimental time series may reflect the dynamics of several subsystems. Here, we will somewhat arbitrarily pick $\beta = 0.3$ and set the level of measurement noise to a standard deviation of 0.05 (see Figure 6.23).

This trick of adding signals from unrelated chaotic systems allows us to make a chaotic system of a higher dimension than any of the individual systems. We could add any number of such systems. Surprisingly, we could even add two or more copies of the same chaotic system, as long as the initial conditions were different in each copy.

Sometimes the dynamics of subsystems are coupled together so that one subsystem affects another. All of the sets of equations examined previously in this book have been this way. For Model Five, we will linearly couple the x variable of the Ikeda map to the z variable in the Henon map,

$$x_{t+1} = 1 + \mu(x_t \cos m_t - y_t \sin m_t) + 0.2z_t, \tag{6.33}$$

and leave the dynamical equations for the other variables as they are in Eq. 6.31.

Using a model of this sort in interpreting a measured time series, we might ask the following questions:

- How many variables are involved in the dynamics?

- Is there an attractor, and what is its dimension?

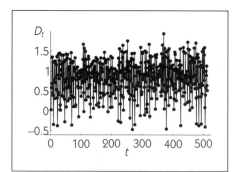

Figure 6.23
A simulated time series from Model Five, $D_t = x_t + \beta z_t + W_t$. The measurement noise W_t has standard deviation 0.05.

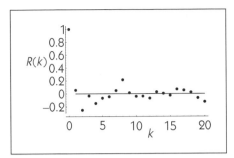

Figure 6.24
The autocorrelation function of the Model-Five data shown in Figure 6.23.

- Can we distinguish between the measurement noise and the deterministic dynamics?

- If the system is very high dimensional, is it even possible to detect the deterministic dynamics?

Again, we start our analysis of the data with the tools we have already introduced. The mean of the Model Five data is $M_{est} = 0.828$, and the standard deviation is $\sigma = 0.455$. The fluctuations about the mean are $V_t = D_t - M_{est}$. The autocorrelation function $R(k)$, shown in Figure 6.24, is consistent with white noise.

Although there is no dynamical noise in the equations, a scatter plot of V_{t+1} versus V_t for the Model Five data (Figure 6.25) does not show the simple geometry that was evident in the Model Four data (Figure 6.13). For Model Five, V_{t+1} is clearly not a function of V_t, even though we know that deterministic dynamics are at work. As we shall see, by using a two- or higher-dimensional embedding,

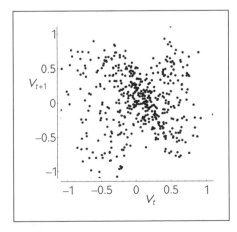

Figure 6.25
A return plot of fluctuations about the mean: V_{t+1} versus V_t for the Model Five data.

the deterministic relationship between V_{t+1} and previous values $(V_t, V_{t-1}, \ldots)$ becomes clearer.

                          □

6.7   CHARACTERIZING CHAOS

In Chapter 1, chaos was defined to be bounded, deterministic dynamics that are aperiodic and display sensitive dependence on initial conditions. In this section we will study time-series analysis techniques that allow us to investigate each of these characteristics in data.

BOUNDEDNESS

According to Chapter 1, dynamics are bounded if they stay in a finite range and do not approach ∞ or $-\infty$ as time increases. In practice, things are more subtle than this. An example is given by the simple linear system $x_{t+1} = Rx_t$. The solution is $x_t = R^t x_0$, that is, x_t grows or decays exponentially. Suppose that we measure $D_t = \frac{1}{x_t}$. For $|R| > 1$, the dynamics of x are unbounded, but D_t will go to zero as $t \to \infty$. For $|R| < 1$, the dynamics are bounded but $D_t \to \pm\infty$. This example shows that when dealing with measured data it is not sufficient to say that dynamics are bounded if a measured time series stays in a finite range, or unbounded if the time series blows up. In fact, if for no other reason than not having the opportunity to wait until $t \to \infty$, we can never definitively know from measurements whether the "true," unmeasured state variables stay bounded.

The definition of bounded as "staying in a finite range" is not very useful when dealing with data; any measured data will be in a finite range, since the mass and energy of the universe are finite. Infinity is a mathematical concept, not a physical one.

A different, but related concept for assessing boundedness in data is **stationarity**. We say that a time series is stationary when it shows similar behavior throughout its duration. One useful definition of "similar behavior" is that the mean and standard deviation remain the same throughout the time series. An operational definition might be that the mean and standard deviation in one third of the signal are not significantly different from those in the other two thirds—or one might prefer to use quarters or tenths, and so on.

If a time series is nonstationary, then it is questionable whether the techniques described in the following sections can be applied meaningfully. In this case we can attempt to generate stationarity by altering the time series. A simple and often effective technique is to **first-difference** the time series. That is, if the measurements are . . . , $x_i, x_{i+1}, x_{i+2}, \ldots$, then define $y_i = x_i - x_{i-1}$ and use y_i for further analysis.

Another technique for attempting to create stationarity is motivated by exponential growth. If $x_{t+1} = Rx_t$ for $|R| > 1$, then x_t will be nonstationary as will the first difference $y_t = x_t - x_{t-1}$. However, $\frac{x_t}{x_{t-1}}$ will be stationary.

APERIODICITY

Chaotic behavior is aperiodic. It might seem that the question of aperiodicity is one with a yes-or-no answer: Either a time series is periodic or it is not. However, in the presence of measurement noise, a measured time series from a truly periodic system can appear aperiodic. Because aperiodic systems can differ in their aperiodicity, it can be meaningful to quantify "how aperiodic" a time series is. Recall that aperiodicity means that the state variables never return to their exact previous values. However, in an aperiodic system, variables may return quite close to previous values. We can characterize aperiodicity by asking "How close?" and "How often?"

Since we often do not directly measure all of the state variables of a system, we need to use the embedding technique to represent all of our measured data's state variables. Recall that D_t is the measurement made at time t. By *embedding* the time series, we create a sequence

$$\mathbf{D}_t = (D_t, D_{t-h}, \ldots, D_{t-(p-1)h}),$$

where p is the embedding dimension and h is the embedding lag. Each $\mathbf{D}_t$ is a point in the p-dimensional embedding space, and the embedded time series can be regarded as a sequence of points, one point at each time t. Each point represents the state of the system at that time.

We can calculate the distance between the two points at times i and j:

$$\delta_{i,j} = |\mathbf{D}_i - \mathbf{D}_j|.$$

If the time series were periodic with period T, then $\delta_{i,j} = 0$ when $|i - j| = nT$, for $n = 0, 1, 2, 3, \ldots$. In contrast, for an aperiodic time series, $\delta_{i,j}$ will not show this pattern. Suppose we pick some distance r, and ask when $|\mathbf{D}_i - \mathbf{D}_j| < r$. One way to do this is to make a plot where i is on the horizontal axis, j is on the vertical axis, and a dot is placed at coordinate (i, j) if $|\mathbf{D}_i - \mathbf{D}_j| < r$. Such plots are called **recurrence plots** because they depict how the reconstructed trajectory recurs or repeats itself (see Figures 6.26 and 6.27).

For a periodic signal of period T, the plot looks like Figure 6.26 for very small r. This is a series of stripes at 45 degrees, with the stripes separated by a

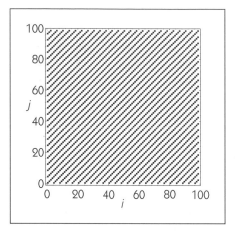

Figure 6.26

A recurrence plot for the quadratic map $x_{t+1} = 3.52x_t(1 - x_t)$. A black dot appears whenever $|\mathbf{D}_i - \mathbf{D}_j| < r$. The trajectory has a period of 4, so the recurrence plot consists of diagonal stripes separated by 4. The embedding dimension $p = 2$, and $r = 0.001$.

distance of T in the vertical and horizontal directions. (In all recurrence plots, there is a stripe along the diagonal corresponding to $i = j$.)

For a chaotic time series, the recurrence plot has a more complicated structure, sometimes with hints of almost periodic trajectories—one can see brief episodes where there are parallel stripes at 45 degrees (see Figures 6.28 and 6.29). For randomly generated numbers, such a structure is not evident (see Figures 6.30 and 6.31).

One thing to keep in mind is that the number of dots in a recurrence plot tells how many times the trajectory came within distance r of a previous value. The **correlation integral** $C(r)$ is defined to be the fraction of pairs of times i and

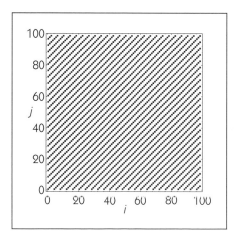

Figure 6.27

The same as Figure 6.26, but r is ten times bigger: $r = 0.01$. The plot is identical to Figure 6.26.

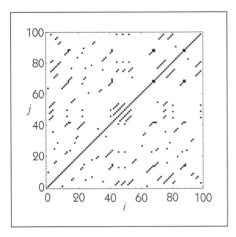

Figure 6.28
Recurrence plot for the chaotic
time series generated by
$x_{t+1} = 4x_t(1 - x_t)$; $p = 2$,
$r = 0.001$.

j where $\mathbf{D}_i$ and $\mathbf{D}_j$ are closer than r for $i \neq j$:

$$C(r) = \frac{\text{number of times } |\mathbf{D}_i - \mathbf{D}_j| < r}{N(N - 1)} . \qquad (6.34)$$

You can think of $C(r)$ as the density of ink in a recurrence plot. The numerator
is the actual number of dots in the plot, and the $N(N - 1)$ in the denominator is
the maximum possible number of dots. (Remember, we exclude the cases where
$i = j$. Otherwise, the denominator would be N^2.)

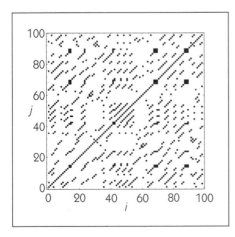

Figure 6.29
Same as Figure 6.28, but r is ten
times bigger.

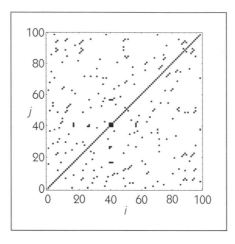

Figure 6.30
Recurrence plot for random white noise; $p = 2, r = 0.1$.

THE CORRELATION DIMENSION

The correlation integral is one of the most fundamental quantities in chaotic time-series analysis. What is important is not the value of $C(r)$ at any particular single value of r, but how $C(r)$ changes with r. As r is increased, more dots appear in the recurrence plots and so $C(r)$ increases. Figures 6.32, 6.33, and 6.34 show the correlation integral for the periodic data, the chaotic data, and the random white noise. For a perfectly periodic system, increasing r a little does not change the number of dots very much—compare Figures 6.26 and 6.27. For the chaotic data of Model Four, increasing r by the same amount causes more dots to appear (Figures 6.28 and 6.29), but the most dramatic increase occurs in the random white noise (Figures 6.30 and 6.31). $C(r)$ is flat for the periodic system

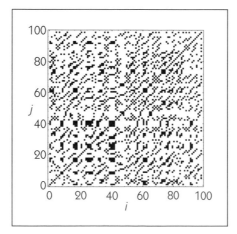

Figure 6.31
Same as Figure 6.30, but r is ten times bigger.

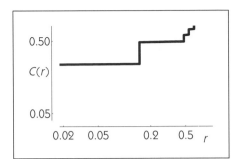

Figure 6.32
The correlation integral $C(r)$ of a periodic time series with period 4 generated from $x_{t+1} = 3.52x_t(1 - x_t)$. $N = 100$ data points were used, in an embedding dimension of $p = 2$. Note that $C(r)$ is plotted on a log-log scale.

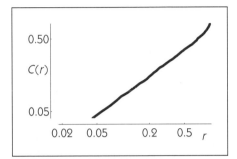

Figure 6.33
The correlation integral $C(r)$ from a chaotic time series generated from Model Four $(x_{t+1} = 4x_t(1 - x_t))$; $N = 100$, $p = 2$.

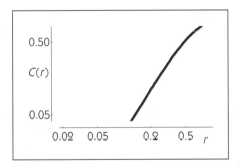

Figure 6.34
The correlation integral $C(r)$ from a time series produced by a computer random-number generator, $N - 100$, $p - 2$.

(Figure 6.32), has a gentle slope for the chaotic system (Figure 6.33), and has a steeper slope for the random system (Figure 6.34).

There is a close relationship between the correlation integral $C(r)$ and the concept of fractal dimension introduced in Section 3.3. Imagine for a moment that you have a set of points scattered more or less uniformly on a one-dimensional curve, as in Figure 6.35. Pick one of the points as a reference, and count how many of the other points are within distance r of the reference. As r is increased, the number of points within distance r will increase directly as the length r. Now imagine that the points are scattered more or less uniformly on a two-dimensional surface (Figure 6.36). Choosing one of the points as a reference, we can see that

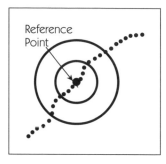

Figure 6.35
When points are scattered along a one-dimensional curve, the number of points closer than distance r to a reference point increases linearly with r.

the number of points within distance r of the reference will be related to the area of a circle of distance r, that is, πr^2. Similarly, if the points were scattered throughout a three-dimensional volume, the number of points within distance r of a reference point would be related to the volume of a sphere of radius r, that is, $\frac{4}{3}\pi r^3$. In general, for points scattered throughout a ν-dimensional object, the number of points closer than distance r to a reference point is proportional to r^ν.

In calculating the correlation integral of a set of points, one uses each of the points as a reference and counts how many of the other points are within distance r. This suggests that the correlation integral of a scattering of points throughout a ν-dimensional volume will be proportional to r^ν, that is,

$$C(r) = Ar^\nu, \tag{6.35}$$

where A is a constant of proportionality. Taking the logarithm of both sides of Eq. 6.35 gives

$$\log C(r) = \nu \log r + \log A. \tag{6.36}$$

In order to find ν, we simply need to plot $\log C(r)$ versus $\log r$ and find the slope of the resulting line. This procedure can also be applied to estimate the

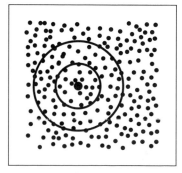

Figure 6.36
When points are scattered on a two-dimensional surface, the number of points closer than distance r to a reference point increases as the area of a circle of radius r.

fractal dimension of an object, in place of the box-counting technique described in *Dynamics in Action* 5.

One way that the correlation dimension has been used in time-series analysis is to look for attractors in time series. The initial idea, proposed by Grassberger and Procaccia (1983), was based on the observation that the attractors of chaotic systems are often self-similar and can be described by a fractal dimension. If a time series comes from a dynamical system that is on an attractor, then the trajectory made from the time series by embedding will have the same topological properties as the original attractor—as long as the embedding dimension is large enough. In particular, the reconstructed trajectory will have the same dimension as the original one. Takens (1981) proved that if the original attractor has dimension v, then an embedding dimension of $p = 2v + 1$ will be adequate for reconstructing the attractor. In practice, $p \geq v$ will often be adequate, but the only guarantee comes when $p \geq 2v + 1$.

Since the objective of the Grassberger-Procaccia analysis is to find the dimension v, one does not know at the outset what embedding dimension p to use. The solution to this problem is to calculate v from the correlation integral at many different values of p, as shown in Figure 6.37.

For a time series from a system that is on a v-dimensional attractor, the correlation dimension of the time series offers a means to estimate the dimension of the attractor. However, for systems that are not on an attractor, the interpretation of v can be much more difficult.

One relatively simple case for interpreting v is random white noise. Consider a sequence of random white noise measurements, such as those from Model One. From Figure 6.6, you can see that when the data from Model One are embedded with $p = 2$, they create a solid-looking blob. Since this blob covers the whole plot with ink (or at least it would if there were many more data points), it is two-dimensional (i.e., $v = 2$ when $p = 2$). Similarly, an embedding with $p = 3$ would create a three-dimensional blob that would completely fill a three-dimensional volume, and so $v = 3$ when $p = 3$. In the ideal case for random

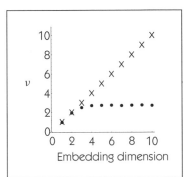

Figure 6.37
An idealized case of correlation dimension v versus embedding dimension. The dots display v for a time series with attractor dimension 2.7, while the x symbol gives v for random white noise.

white noise, $\nu = p$. Here, "ideal" means "we have an infinite amount of data." Of course, it is impossible to have an infinite amount of data, but even for small data sets the relationship $\nu \approx p$ may hold. One theoretical rule of thumb is that 10^p data points are needed to show that $\nu \approx p$ is true up to any given p; thus 1000 (or 10^3) points are needed to show that $\nu = p$ for $p = 3$. In practice, this rule is quite conservative, and ν can be shown to increase with p even for much shorter time series.

When introduced in the early 1980s, the correlation dimension was greeted with incredible enthusiasm and optimism. Now it has fallen into some disrepute. As shown in Figure 6.37, for a time series from a system on an attractor, ν levels out with increasing p once p is large enough, while for random white noise, ν increases with p. There has been a strong temptation for people to invert this logic and to believe that if ν levels out with increasing p, then the time series reflects an attractor. Sometimes this is the case, but sometimes it is not. There are cases where ν levels out but there is no attractor. A particularly important case is that of $\frac{1}{f}$ noise (see *Dynamics in Action* 6). To guard against the incorrect interpretation of the correlation integral, it is important to use surrogate data, as described in Section 6.8.

❏ EXAMPLE 6.4

Estimate the dimension of the chaotic attractor underlying the Model Five data.

Solution: The first step is to embed the time series. This requires the choice of an embedding dimension p and an embedding lag h. One way to choose an embedding lag is to take the smallest value of h at which the autocorrelation function $R(h) \approx 0$. In this case, Figure 6.24 shows that $R(1) \approx 0$, so we will use $h = 1$.

Rather than picking a single embedding dimension, we will repeat the calculations for $p = 1, 2, \ldots, 10$. At each of these embedding dimensions, we repeat the same steps:

1. Calculate the correlation integral $C(r)$ using Eq. 6.34.
2. Using Eq. 6.36, use $C(r)$ to calculate the dimension ν. One way to do this is to plot $\log C$ versus $\log r$. ν is the slope of this graph:

$$\nu = \frac{d \log C}{d \log r}.$$

However, this slope generally depends on the value of r selected. To avoid this problem for the moment, we will plot out the slope ν as a function of r.

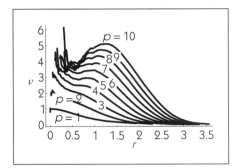

Figure 6.38
Slope ν versus r for embedding dimensions $p = 1$ through $p = 10$.

Figure 6.38 shows how the slope ν changes with r for different embedding dimensions. For the largest values of r found in the embedded time series, the slope approaches zero, regardless of the embedding dimension used. Estimating a dimension by using large r is somewhat like looking at the object from a great distance; no matter what the object, it will look like a single point—an object of dimension 0—just as a distant star looks like a single point of light.

For the smallest values of r, the slope ν depends on and increases with the embedding dimension. This is characteristic of noise and reflects the measurement noise in the Model Five data.

For $r \approx 0.5$ the slope is roughly the same for many different embedding dimensions. Figure 6.39 shows ν (at $r = 0.5$) for $p = 1, 2, \ldots, 10$. The pattern is similar to that seen in Figure 6.37, and we conclude that the attractor of the Model Five data has a dimension of approximately 3.9. A range of values of r at which ν is fairly constant is often called a **scaling region**.

The need to pick a specific range for r is one of the difficulties, and a great weakness, of estimating dimensions. In this case, we chose a range near $r = 0.5$ because that value of r gives us the results closest to the ideal form shown in Figure 6.37. Here we have the advantage of knowing that there is an attractor, and therefore we have good reason to believe we are justified in our choice of r. Without this information, interpreting the meaning of the dimension calculation

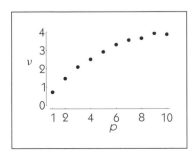

Figure 6.39
The correlation dimension versus embedding dimension p for $r = 0.5$.

could be quite challenging and problematic, and the results should be treated with skepticism.

⬜

DETERMINISM

We say that a system is deterministic when future events are causally set by past events. A finite-difference equation like $x_{t+1} = f(x_t)$ is deterministic as long as $f(x_t)$ has only one value for each possible value of x_t; given the past value x_t, the function $f()$ determines the future value x_{t+1}. For Model Four, which is a finite-difference equation that produces chaos, if we knew x_0 then by iteration we could calculate all future values of x_t using Eq. 6.23.

But, of course, we do not know x_0 exactly, since our measurements are made with noise: $D_t = x_t + W_t$. If we take D_0 as our estimate of the initial condition x_0, and iterate from this using Eq. 6.23, then sensitive dependence on initial conditions will cause our predictions to become faulty. For instance, suppose the true initial condition is $x_0 = 0.37$ but that our measurement of

Table 6.2 x_t and y_t from two identical finite-difference equations, $x_{t+1} = 4x_t(1 - x_t)$ and $y_{t+1} = 4y_t(1 - y_t)$. Although $x_0 \approx y_0$, by time $t = 5$ the values of x and y have moved far apart.

x_t	y_t	t
0.370	0.380	0
0.932	0.942	1
0.252	0.217	2
0.754	0.680	3
0.741	0.870	4
0.767	0.451	5
0.715	0.990	6
0.814	0.038	7
0.605	0.147	8
0.956	0.501	9
0.167	0.999	10

the initial condition is $D_0 = 0.38$. As shown in Table 6.2, our predictions based on Eq. 6.23 will diverge from the true values. At first the predictions will be quite good, but after five or so time steps, they become completely wrong. Even when the predictions are good, they are not perfect because of the measurement noise.

We can decide from data whether an underlying deterministic system is present: Use the data to construct a model of the dynamics, and then see whether the predictions made from this model are accurate. If the predictions are perfect, then the system is *completely* deterministic. If the predictions are good, but not perfect, then the system has a deterministic *component*. If the predictions are terrible, then the system is *not* deterministic at all.

We can construct dynamical models from data in a number of different ways. One of the simplest methods works as follows. Suppose that we make our measurements up to time T and that we want to make a prediction of the value at time $T + 1$.

1. Embed the time series to produce $\mathbf{D}_t$.

2. Take the embedded point at time T,

$$\mathbf{D}_T = (D_T, D_{T-h}, \ldots, D_{T-(p-1)h}),$$

   and look through the rest of the embedded time series to find the point that is closest to $\mathbf{D}_T$. Let's say that this closest point has time index a. This means that $\mathbf{D}_a$ is closer to $\mathbf{D}_T$ than any other $\mathbf{D}_t$.

3. The definition of determinism is that future events are set causally by past events. $\mathbf{D}_T$ describes the past events to D_{T+1}. Similarly $\mathbf{D}_a$ describes the past events to the measurement D_{a+1}. If $\mathbf{D}_T$ is close to $\mathbf{D}_a$, and if the system is deterministic, then we expect that D_{a+1} will be close to D_{T+1}. So we take as our prediction of D_{T+1} the measured value D_{a+1}. We will call this prediction $\mathcal{P}_{T+1}$.

This is a funny kind of model. Our previous models have consisted of sets of explicit equations. This model, which is used for prediction, consists of a data set (the measured time series) and a set of instructions (e.g., "find the nearest point $\mathbf{D}_a$"). The set of instructions is called an **algorithm**, and the model exists implicitly in the set of data and the algorithm. Such data-implicit models were uncommon before the advent of computers, but now they are commonplace and of increasing importance.

There are many variations on this simple model of dynamics. One elaboration is to take not just the time a where $\mathbf{D}_a$ is closest to $\mathbf{D}_T$, but to take K different times $a_1, a_2, \ldots, a_K$ where $\mathbf{D}_{a_1}, \mathbf{D}_{a_2}, \ldots, \mathbf{D}_{a_K}$ are all close to $\mathbf{D}_T$. Then the prediction of D_{T+1} is taken as the average of $D_{a_1+1}, D_{a_2+1}, \ldots, D_{a_K+1}$:

$$\mathcal{P}_{T+1} = \frac{1}{K} \sum_{i=1}^{K} D_{a_i+1}. \qquad (6.37)$$

Given a method for making a prediction $\mathcal{P}_{T+1}$, we need to make an actual measurement of D_{T+1} in order to decide if the prediction is good or bad. The difference between $\mathcal{P}_{T+1}$ and D_{T+1} is the **prediction error**, which tells us about the quality of the prediction. Of course, a single prediction might be good or bad just by chance. To give a more meaningful indication of the determinism in the data, we can take the average of many prediction errors. Suppose we make $2T$ measurements of a time series. We take the first half of the time series to construct a data-implicit model of the dynamics. Then we use the model to predict the values of the second half of the time series.

There are two ways to do this. One is to use the model to predict the value at time $T + 1$. Then, we construct a new embedded point using this predicted value $\mathcal{P}_{T+1}$:

$$\mathbf{D}_{T+1} = (\mathcal{P}_{T+1}, D_{T+1-h}, \ldots, D_{T+1-(p-1)h}).$$

We then find the nearest points to $\mathbf{D}_{T+1}$ to make a prediction of the value at time $T + 2$, which we call $\mathcal{P}_{T+2}$. This process can be iterated—we use past predictions to make future predictions. This method can in fact be used to extrapolate a time series beyond its measured values.

Although such extrapolation is useful to make predictions far in the future, for the purposes of assessing determinism in data it is better to use the measured data directly. In this second way of making predictions, in order to predict the value at time $T + 2$, we make the embedded point

$$\mathbf{D}_{T+1} = (D_{T+1}, D_{T+1-h}, \ldots, D_{T+1+(p-1)h}).$$

Note that here the measurement at time $T + 1$ is used, and not the prediction $\mathcal{P}_{T+1}$; we are not using the past predictions to make future predictions.

Once we have made predictions for the second half of the time series, we can calculate a mean prediction error, $\mathcal{E}$:

$$\mathcal{E} = \frac{1}{T} \sum_{k=1}^{T} (D_{T+k} - \mathcal{P}_{T+k})^2. \qquad (6.38)$$

Very large $\mathcal{E}$ means the predictions are bad and the system is not deterministic. Conversely, small $\mathcal{E}$ suggests that the system is deterministic.

How do we decide if $\mathcal{E}$ is large or small? What do we compare it to as a standard? Suppose that we are very lazy and that instead of calculating a new prediction for each time $T + k$, we made the same prediction for all times. Presumably this would be a bad method of prediction, since it completely ignores the dynamics of the data. What is the best value to use for this bad method of prediction? We want to choose a value $\mathcal{P}_{\text{lazy}}$ that minimizes the mean prediction error,

$$\mathcal{E}_{\text{lazy}} = \frac{1}{T} \sum_{k=1}^{T} (D_{T+k} - \mathcal{P}_{\text{lazy}})^2. \tag{6.39}$$

Compare Eq. 6.39 to Eq. 6.5. They are very similar; the minimization we are doing here is almost identical to the minimization we performed to find the sample mean M_{est}. In fact, a good value for $\mathcal{P}_{\text{lazy}}$ is the sample mean of the time series. Given that we set $\mathcal{P}_{\text{lazy}} = M_{\text{est}}$, the mean prediction error $\mathcal{E}_{\text{lazy}}$ in Eq. 6.39 is very similar to the variance of the time series, σ^2, as can be seen by comparison to Eq. 6.8.

A convenient way to decide if $\mathcal{E}$ is large or small is to compare it to $\mathcal{E}_{\text{lazy}}$, or rather to the variance of the time series σ^2. We can do this by taking the ratio

$$\frac{\mathcal{E}}{\sigma^2}.$$

If this ratio is close to one, then the mean prediction error is large. If the ratio is close to zero, then the mean prediction error is small.

❏ EXAMPLE 6.5

We can examine the data sets from Models One through Four to look for determinism. Rather than using just the closest neighboring point in the embedded time series to make the prediction, we will use K nearby points, as in Eq. 6.37.

Solution: For the example here, we will use an embedding dimension $p = 1$ so that $\mathbf{D}_t = D_t$. As discussed in Section 6.6, it often makes sense to pick $p > 1$.

For the Model-One data, Figure 6.40 shows the ratio of the prediction error to the variance, $\frac{\mathcal{E}}{\sigma^2}$, as a function of the number of neighbors K used to make the prediction. When K is small, the ratio is greater than 1. This says that the model makes worse predictions than the lazy method of simply predicting the mean. As K becomes large, the ratio goes to unity.

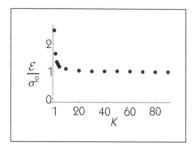

Figure 6.40
Prediction error $\frac{\mathcal{E}}{\sigma^2}$ versus number of neighbors K used in the prediction for the data from Model One.

Recall that there are no active dynamics in Model One. The system is at a fixed point and all of the variability in the measurements is due to the random measurement noise W_t. There are no deterministic dynamics to predict, so it is not surprising that prediction is ineffective. Since there are 100 points in the time series, when K is near 100 virtually all of the points in the time series are being averaged together to produce the prediction, and Eq. 6.37 yields a prediction that is basically the mean, M_{est}. This is therefore the same as the lazy prediction method of using M_{est}, and so $\mathcal{E} = \sigma^2$. In fact, since there are no dynamics to the data, we cannot do better than using M_{est} to predict the time series, since M_{est} is the quantity that minimizes the prediction error, as in Eq. 6.5. When K is small, the number the prediction algorithm generates will vary around the mean since only a few of the points are used in the averaging. As described in Section 6.3, the fewer points used, the more the prediction will vary around the mean. Since the mean gives the best possible prediction for this data, any deviation from the mean will give worse predictions.

For the Model-One data, the prediction error is large (i.e., $\frac{\mathcal{E}}{\sigma^2} \geq 1$) and we are justified in concluding that the data are random, consistent with the known mechanism of the model.

Model Two, in contrast, shows definite predictability. The ratio $\frac{\mathcal{E}}{\sigma^2}$ is shown in Figure 6.41. Here the ratio is less than unity for small K, and approaches unity as K approaches 100, the number of points in the time series. At very small K, the predictions are worse than at intermediate K—averaging the five to ten nearest

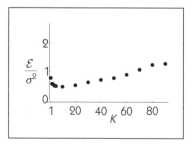

Figure 6.41
$\frac{\mathcal{E}}{\sigma^2}$ versus K for the data from Model Two.

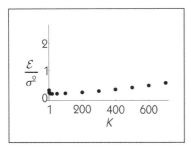

Figure 6.42
$\frac{\mathcal{E}}{\sigma^2}$ versus K for the data from Model Three.

points produces a better prediction than simply using the single nearest point. This prediction is substantially better than using M_{est}. Therefore, we conclude that the data from Model Two contain some determinism but are not completely deterministic. This is consistent with Eq. 6.11, which has a deterministic component to its dynamics (ρx_t) in addition to the random dynamical noise (v_t) and measurement noise (W_t). The 1000 data points from Model Three produce quite similar results, as shown in Figure 6.42.

Model Four is completely deterministic. The data analysis using prediction error confirms this; the prediction error is virtually zero for small K and, as expected, the ratio $\frac{\mathcal{E}}{\sigma^2}$ approaches unity as K approaches the number of points in the time series (see Figure 6.43).

The prediction results for Models One, Two, and Three could have been anticipated from the the autocorrelation function. The autocorrelation function $R(k)$ for Model One shows no correlation between measured values D_T and D_{T+1} (Figure 6.9). The autocorrelation functions for the data from Models Two and Three show quite strong correlations between D_T and D_{T+1} (Figures 6.10 and 6.11). This is not the whole story, however. Note that although the autocorrelation function for Model Four (Figure 6.14) is much the same as that for Model One, the prediction results are completely different. The prediction method is sensitive to the nonlinearity in Model Four, whereas the autocorrelation function is not.

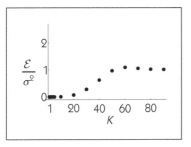

Figure 6.43
$\frac{\mathcal{E}}{\sigma^2}$ versus K for the data from Model Four.

[Technical note: In this example we have made a slight modification to the calculation of $\mathcal{E}$ described in the body of the text. There we divided the time series into two halves and used the first half to construct the data-implicit model, while using the second half to evaluate the predictive abilities of the model. Here we do not divide the time series. We use all of the data in constructing the model, and we evaluate the predictions based on the same data. However, when making a prediction $\mathcal{P}_{T+1}$, we exclude the point $\mathbf{D}_T$ from the data used to generate the model. If we did not do this, then the closest point to $\mathbf{D}_T$ would obviously be itself, which would give $\mathcal{P}_{T+1} = D_{T+1}$ (for $K = 1$). This would a perfect prediction, but completely worthless since we would be predicting what we already knew. By excluding $\mathbf{D}_T$, we avoid this problem and can use all of the data at once.] ☐

DYNAMICS IN ACTION

19 PREDICTING THE NEXT ICE AGE

Over the past millions of years, glaciers have repeatedly built up in the northern hemisphere, covering land that is now in temperate climates. The last ice age ended roughly 10,000 years ago.

When will the next ice age come? This is a question for climate prediction, as opposed to the short-term weather prediction with which we are all familiar from the nightly news. Unlike the day-to-day weather, the fundamental principles underlying climate are largely unknown. This means that data-implicit models may have an important role to play. The following application of data-implicit modeling to ice-age prediction is drawn from Hunter (1992).

An indirect record of global ice volume is contained in the ratio of two oxygen isotopes, O^{16} and O^{18}, found in the shells of Formanifera that are found at the bottom of the ocean. Cores taken at the ocean bottom indicate this $\frac{O^{16}}{O^{18}}$ ratio over the past 800,000 years, a period that includes roughly eight ice ages.

The mechanism that causes ice ages is not known. The Milankovich theory is based on the idea that the amount of summer sunlight in the Northern hemisphere is a dominant factor. If summer sunlight is too low, snow that fell during the winter cannot all melt in the summer, and so ice gradually accumulates.

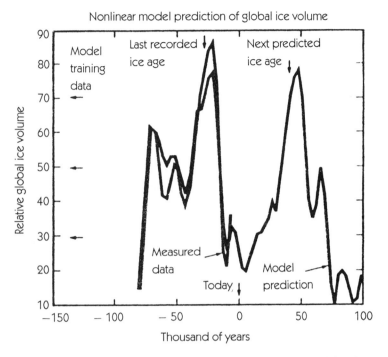

Nonlinear model prediction of global ice volume

Measured global ice volume and predictions from a data-implicit model. Redrawn from Hunter (1992).

The amount of summer sunlight depends on the luminosity of the Sun, but also on parameters of the Earth's orbit. The closer the Earth is to the Sun, the more light falls on the Earth. The Sun-Earth distance varies over the course of the year and is governed by the **eccentricity** of the Earth's orbit. The axis of the Earth's rotation is slightly inclined with respect to its orbital plane; this **obliquity** is what causes the yearly seasonal cycle. The angle of inclination changes over time, just as a spinning top wobbles. This is called *precession*. Scientists have a good understanding of these orbital parameters and are able to calculate their past and future values.

What is not known, however, is how the accumulation of snow depends on these parameters. What seems to be important is the eccentricity, which modulates the amplitude of precession. The eccentricity is therefore related to the variability in the angle of inclination. When there is much variability, past accumulations of snow have an occasional chance to melt; when there is little variability, snow accumulations may not have the opportunity to melt completely.

Other factors also make modeling difficult. When there is snow on the ground over large fractions of the Earth's surface, more sunlight is reflected back into space, increasing the propensity for snow to accumulate. However, changes in ocean level and cloud cover may have countervailing effects.

Hunter used past records of global ice volume, as inferred from measured $\frac{O^{16}}{O^{18}}$ ratios in ocean cores, and constructed a data-implicit model of global ice volume (see the figure on the previous page). Since future orbital parameters are well known, he used them as well.

The indirectly measured global ice volume and the calculated orbital parameters for 800,000 years ago until 60,000 years ago were used to construct a data-implicit model. This model was iterated until the present, in order to confirm that the model could have predicted the last ice age, which occurred 10,000 years ago. Starting at the present, and using calculated future values of orbital parameters, the model is iterated to predict future ice volume. According to the model's predictions, the next ice age will start in 30,000 years and will peak in 50,000 years.

❏ EXAMPLE 6.6

From the data from Model Five, use nonlinear predictability to estimate how many variables are involved in the dynamics.

Solution: Nonlinear prediction allows us to look for a functional relationship between V_{t+1} and previous values of V. If the predictability is good—if $\mathcal{E}$ is small—then V_{t+1} is determined by previous values of V. Figure 6.44 shows $\mathcal{E}$ for embedding dimensions $p = 1, 2, 3,$ and 4. The best predictions are made when roughly ten nearest neighbors are used, and these predictions appear to be improving as p is increased. Figure 6.45 shows $\mathcal{E}$ for $k = 10$ nearest neighbors for embedding dimensions $p = 1$ through $p = 10$: The predictions are best for $p = 3$ or $p = 4$, suggesting that three or four previous values of V do the best job of determining V_{t+1}. This is consistent with the fact that four coupled dynamical equations were used to generate the data.

Perhaps it is surprising that using more than four previous values of V does not lead to a better prediction. After all, using more information can't hurt, can it? Due to the sensitive dependence on initial conditions in chaotic systems, values

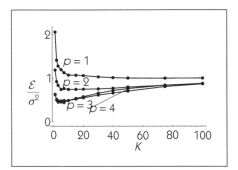

Figure 6.44
Nonlinear predictability $\frac{\mathcal{E}}{\sigma^2}$ versus the number of nearest neighbors K used to make the prediction. Results are shown for embedding dimensions $p = 1$ through $p = 4$.

of V from far in the past do not contain much information about the value of V_{t+1}. If we use these irrelevant values in finding nearest neighbors, predictions will be poor. This irrelevance of the distant past limits our ability to investigate high-dimensional chaotic systems using time-lag embedding.   ◘

SENSITIVE DEPENDENCE ON INITIAL CONDITIONS: LYAPUNOV EXPONENTS

Suppose that we have two copies of Model Four—one using the variable x, the other using y—that are identical except that their initial condition can be made to differ. We start with x_0 and y_0 very close together. As we iterate the system from the two initial times, x_i and y_i start to move apart, slowly at first and then more rapidly. Eventually, x_i and y_i show no correlation with one another, yet the dynamics of both arise from the same equation (see Table 6.2 on page 326).

This "stretching apart" of the distance between initially nearby points is called **sensitive dependence on initial conditions.** One way to characterize a chaotic dynamical system is to measure the strength of this sensitive dependence.

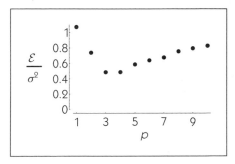

Figure 6.45
Nonlinear predictability $\frac{\mathcal{E}}{\sigma^2}$ versus embedding dimension. $K = 10$ nearest neighbors were used to make the prediction.

In order to develop some ideas about how to measure sensitive dependence on initial conditions, let's assume that we have perfectly deterministic dynamics

$$x_{t+1} = f(x_t). \tag{6.40}$$

If we have two initial conditions x_0 and y_0 whose initial separation $|x_0 - y_0|$ is very small, the separation after one time step is

$$|x_1 - y_1| = |f(x_0) - f(y_0)| = \frac{|f(x_0) - f(y_0)|}{|x_0 - y_0|} |x_0 - y_0| \approx \left| \frac{df}{dx} \right|_{x_0} |x_0 - y_0|,$$

where we make use of the definition of the derivative

$$\left. \frac{df}{dx} \right|_{x_0} = \lim_{y_0 \to x_0} \frac{f(x_0) - f(y_0)}{x_0 - y_0}.$$

The strength of the sensitive dependence on initial conditions is therefore $\left| \frac{df}{dx} \right|_{x_0}$. Clearly, this depends on the initial condition x_0. What we want, though, is a number that describes sensitive dependence for the map as a whole, and not just at one initial condition; we want to "average" all initial conditions. We can motivate the proper form of averaging by noting that

$$|x_2 - y_2| \approx \left| \frac{df}{dx} \right|_{x_1} |x_1 - y_1| \approx \left| \frac{df}{dx} \right|_{x_1} \frac{df}{dx} \bigg|_{x_0} |x_0 - y_0|$$

and, by iteration,

$$|x_n - y_n| \approx \left| \prod_{t=0}^{n-1} \frac{df}{dx} \right|_{x_t} |x_0 - y_0|$$

(where $\prod$ means multiplication in the same way that $\sum$ means summation). Recalling from Chapter 1 that the solution to the linear finite-difference equation $x_{t+1} = ax_t$ is $x_n = a^n x_0$, we see that the average separation per iteration (which is a for the linear system) is

$$\left(\left| \prod_{t=0}^{n-1} \frac{df}{dx} \right|_{x_t} \right)^{\frac{1}{n}}.$$

This is the **geometric mean** of the quantities $\left| \frac{df}{dx} \right|_{x_t}$. The term **Lyapunov exponent** is used for the logarithm of this average separation per iteration.

A procedure, then, for quantifying the sensitive dependence on initial conditions from a one-dimensional finite-difference map is as follows:

1. Iterate the map to generate a sequence of values $x_0, x_1, x_2, \ldots, x_{n-1}$.

2. Calculate the slope of the map at each of the points $x_0, \ldots, x_{n-1}$.

3. Calculate the absolute value of the geometric mean of the values in step (2). (If you are doing this on a computer, beware of round-off errors.) This value represents the sensitive dependence on initial conditions of the map as a whole.

❏ **EXAMPLE 6.7**

Estimate a Lyapunov exponent for the Model Four data.

Solution: The first step is to use the data to construct a prediction model as described earlier in this section. We can then use this prediction model as the function $f(x)$ in Eq. 6.40.

A prediction model of the form of Eq. 6.37 is not adequate for the purpose of finding Lyapunov exponents from data. Although the data-implicit model of Eq. 6.37 provides us with a value of $f(\ )$ at each data point, it does not tell us what $\frac{df}{dx}$ is, and this information is needed to find the Lyapunov exponent.

Instead, we need to fit a prediction model that does specify the slope $\frac{df}{dx}$ at each data point. Many different models could do this job. Possibly the simplest is to fit short line segments to the data—a **locally linear model**. The slope of these line segments then gives $\frac{df}{dx}$.

Figures 6.46 and 6.47 show a locally constant model (Eq. 6.37) and a locally linear model fit to some of the Model Four data in a return plot (a one-dimensional embedding). For these plots, $K = 3$ points were used. In a two-dimensional

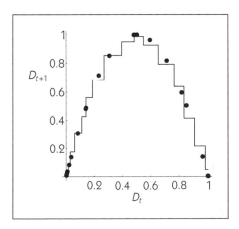

Figure 6.46
A model of the form Eq. 6.37 fits the data to short, level line segments—a locally constant model.

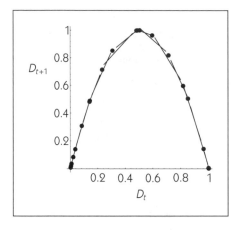

Figure 6.47
A locally linear model fits the data to short line segments. The slope of the line segment at each point gives $\frac{df}{dx}$ at that point.

embedding, small portions of planes would be used instead of line segments; in a higher-dimensional embedding, hyperplanes would be used.

⊓

✈ MODEL SIX

Models One, Two, and Three are linear models. A general form of a multi-dimensional, linear, finite-difference equation is the **autoregressive** model,

$$x_{t+1} = a_0 x_t + a_1 x_{t-1} + a_2 x_{t-2} + \cdots + a_{p-1} x_{t-(p-1)} + v_t. \tag{6.41}$$

In this equation, x_{t+1} depends on the p previous values: $x_t, \ldots, x_{t-(p-1)}$. The parameters $a_0, \ldots, a_{p-1}$ are fixed in time and play the same role as ρ in Eq. 6.3 or Eq. 6.11. The dynamical noise at time t is v_t and is almost always assumed to be Gaussian white noise. Here we will assume that there is no measurement noise, that is, $D_t = x_t$.

Equation 6.41 is capable of producing many different types of output, depending on the values of the parameters $a_0, \ldots, a_{p-1}$. Three different examples are shown in Figures 6.48, 6.49, and 6.50.

The analysis of Eq. 6.41 is central to a number of fields in science and technology, and, correspondingly, there are a number of different names that can be found in the technical literature: Statisticians tend to use the term "autoregressive (AR) model," control engineers use "all-pole model," signal processing engineers use "infinite impulse-response filter," while physicists prefer "maximum entropy model."

Whatever the name, the dynamics displayed by the model are those we have already seen in linear models: exponential growth and decay, and oscillations whose amplitudes either grow or decay exponentially. However, in contrast to

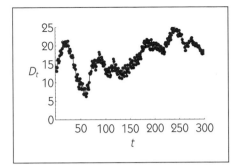

Figure 6.48
An output of Model Six for
$a_0 = 1.39, a_1 = -0.703,$
$a_2 = 0.038, a_3 = 0.735,$
$a_4 = -0.46.$

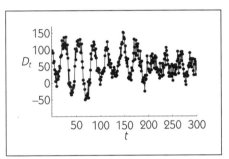

Figure 6.49
An output of Model Six for
$a_0 = 0.677, a_1 = 0.175,$
$a_2 = 0.297, a_3 = 0.006,$
$a_4 = -0.114, a_5 = -0.083,$
$a_6 = -0.025.$

the linear models we have already studied, Eq. 6.41 can produce several different frequencies of oscillation at the same time, with the amplitudes of the different frequencies growing or decaying exponentially at different rates. The result is that Eq. 6.41 is quite general, suitable for modeling many diverse types of data.

For any given time series, the question of how to find the best $a_0, a_1, \ldots, a_{p-1}$ can be addressed in the spirit of the prediction models we have already studied. We use Eq. 6.41 to make a **linear prediction** at time $T + 1$ using the measurements D_t made prior to that time:

$$\mathcal{P}_{T+1} = a_0 D_T + a_1 D_{T-1} + \cdots + a_{p-1} D_{T-(p-1)}.$$

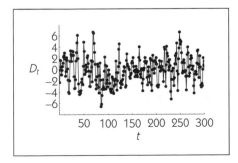

Figure 6.50
An output of Model Six for
$a_0 = 1.05, a_1 = -0.5.$

We want to select the parameters $a_0, a_1, \ldots, a_{p-1}$ to minimize the prediction error using a least-squares criterion:

$$\mathcal{E} = \sum_{i=p}^{N-1} (\mathcal{P}_i - D_i)^2$$

$$= \sum_{i=p}^{N-1} (v_i)^2. \tag{6.42}$$

Finding the parameters $a_0, a_1, \ldots, a_{p-1}$ that minimize $\mathcal{E}$ is somewhat technical, but the upshot is that there is a formula that specifies the parameters in terms of the autocorrelation function $R(k)$ of the data. This means that the autocorrelation function uniquely specifies a linear model of the data in the form of Eq. 6.41. This model is sometimes called an **optimal linear model** because it uses the parameters $a_0, a_1, \ldots, a_{p-1}$ that minimize $\mathcal{E}$, but it should be understood that the model is "optimal" only relative to other linear models and that nonlinear models might produce a smaller prediction error.

The question of how to select p, called the **model order**, is more subtle. Ultimately, this is a philosophical question, and the technical issues surrounding it are well beyond the scope of this text.

Fortunately, we will see that the model order p is not important for our purposes in this chapter. The only facts about the autoregressive model that we need to keep in mind are

1. It is a model with linear dynamics.
2. Optimal model parameters $a_0, a_1, \ldots, a_{p-1}$ can be selected that minimize the prediction error $\mathcal{E}$ for any given time series.
3. The optimal parameters can be calculated from the autocorrelation function $R(k)$.

In particular, this last point means that if two time series have the same autocorrelation function, then they have the same optimal linear model.

The main question we will attempt to answer using Model Six is, are the data well described by a linear model, or is there evidence in the data for nonlinear dynamics?

6.8   DETECTING CHAOS AND NONLINEARITY

We have a time series and we want to know whether the system that produced it is chaotic. How can we tell?

The answer is easy: We cannot. Any finite amount of data might come from a chaotic system, or might come from a random system. The situation is similar to the famous scene of monkeys at typewriters: If we put enough monkeys at enough typewriters for long enough, all the works of Shakespeare will eventually be produced. So, given a Shakespearean tragedy, how can we know for sure whether it was produced by the Immortal Bard, or by a monkey pecking randomly at a typewriter?

> O heavy lightness, serious vanity,
> Misshapen chaos of well-seeming forms,
> Feather of lead, bright smoke, cold fire, sick health,
> Still-waking sleep, that is not what it is!
> *William Shakespeare (1564–1616), Romeo and Juliet, Act 1, Scene 1*

> ,Fs a teetsdl,ss t cfrihohpincusfs l e
> od egt acgl,tm gtkiwitv waolakate ihoe-s to mheii eeia mslsy
>   sihnofsyStena ovs
> ilwi,rrb elehilOg h ! i,Mhskohr ,pnf rlana hset-eea n
> *A typing monkey (simulated)*

Of course, only a fool would claim that the works of Shakespeare were generated by a typing monkey. We can look at even a small fragment of Shakespeare's works, and see structure such as words and syntax, and divine more abstract structure such as meaning. The chances of seeing such structure in randomly generated letters are so small that we discount the very possibility as absurd.

We can look at time series in a similar way. Suppose that we look for chaotic structure in a time series. If we see it, then we can argue that the time series is unlikely to have been generated by random noise.

But what is "chaotic structure"? We have already seen that the definition of chaos includes three elements:

- determinism,
- aperiodicity, and
- sensitive dependence on initial conditions.

In Section 6.7 we introduced several ways to quantify these elements in a time series.

The fourth element in the definition of chaos, "boundedness," is not of much use to us here. It is easy to generate random numbers that are bounded. For instance, if we write each number from a time series on a deck of cards, and then shuffle the cards, the deck will serve as a random-number generator that is bounded. So, whatever structure there is in "boundedness" cannot distinguish between chaos and randomness.

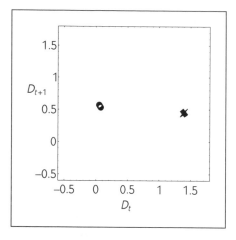

Figure 6.51
The Model-Five dynamics started at several nearby initial condition. Each o marks an initial condition plotted as D_{t+1} versus D_t; there are 30 of them. The x's mark the state after iterating the Model-Five dynamics for 5 time steps, from each of the 30 initial conditions.

Actually, we have to be careful even in using the other three elements in the definition of chaos. Consider the use of determinism in detecting chaos. Models Two and Three show deterministic structure (see Figures 6.41 and 6.42) even though they have only linear dynamics and are therefore incapable of producing chaos.

A similar problem arises when looking at sensitive dependence on initial conditions. Figures 6.51 and 6.52 show what happens to two small clouds of initial conditions in the dynamics of Model Five. The sensitive dependence on initial conditions in the chaotic dynamics causes the clouds to broaden over time. Very similar behavior can be observed in Figures 6.53 and 6.54, which show the linear dynamics of Model Three. In this case, the cloud broadening is due to dynamical noise, not chaos.

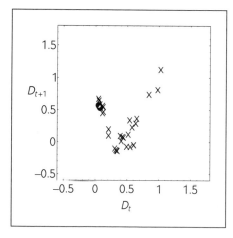

Figure 6.52
After 200 time steps of the chaotic Model Five dynamics, the cloud of initial conditions spread outs, showing the sensitive dependence on initial conditions.

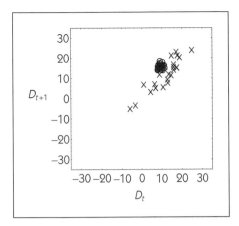

Figure 6.53   The Model-Three dynamics, started at several nearby initial conditions. Each of the o's marks one initial condition, plotted as D_{t+1} versus D_t. The x's mark the position that the Model-Three dynamics take each initial condition after 5 time steps. The cloud of initial conditions has spread out, reflecting the influence of the noise in the Model-Three dynamics, but visually, it is hard to distinguish this from sensitive dependence on initial conditions.

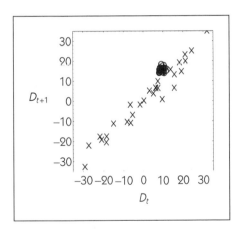

Figure 6.54
After 200 time steps of the linear Model Three dynamics

TOWARD AN APPROPRIATE NULL HYPOTHESIS

Scientists often work by putting forward a hypothesis and then trying to find an example to refute it, to show that the hypothesis is incorrect. As applied to chaos and time series, following this procedure means that one does not try to prove that a time series is chaotic, but rather to refute or reject some other hypothesis. The hypothesis that one is trying to reject is called the **null hypothesis.**

What is an appropriate null hypothesis, when thinking about the possibility of chaos in a time series? Up until now, we have pointed to the dichotomy between chaos and randomness, suggesting that we should use randomness as the null hypothesis. But what do we mean by randomness?

One possibility is white noise: Each measurement D_t is independent of every other measurement. This is a convenient hypothesis because it readily suggests a test; if we can find any dependence between measurements, then we can reject the null hypothesis. Unfortunately, we have already seen cases where we can reject the white noise null hypothesis even when there is no chaos. For example, in the case of Models Two and Three, the autocorrelation function shows that there is dependence between successive measurements, even though these models involve only linear dynamics and therefore cannot produce chaos.

The white noise null hypothesis is somewhat like the hypothesis of typing monkeys. It is not too often that we have to decide whether a sentence was written by Shakespeare or by a typing monkey. More likely, the problem is one of deciding whether a work was written by Shakespeare or, say, by Alexander Pope—typing monkeys can be ruled out from the very beginning, and doing so tells us nothing useful about the true author. White noise is simply too restrictive to be a good null hypothesis when testing for chaos.

> Lo! thy dread Empire CHAOS! is restor'd;
> Light dies before thy uncreating word;
> Thy hand, great Anarch! lets the curtain fall;
> And Universal Darkness buries All.
>
> *Alexander Pope (1688–1744), The Dunciad*

A better null hypothesis is provided by Model Six, which gives an optimal linear model of any data set. The hypothesis here is that the dynamics are linear, with Gaussian white noise random inputs. We will therefore call this the **linear-dynamics null hypothesis**. This null hypothesis is inconsistent with the possibility of chaos, since linear dynamics cannot produce chaos. This means that if a time series is chaotic, we should in principle be able to reject the null hypothesis.

TESTING THE NULL HYPOTHESIS WITH SURROGATE DATA

We have a measured time series and a null hypothesis. How do we test whether the time series is inconsistent with the null hypothesis? We use what is called a **discriminating statistic**, some quantity that can be computed both from the measured time series and also from a time series that is consistent with the null hypothesis. Three discriminating statistics that are relevant to chaos are the nonlinear predictability $\mathcal{E}$, the Lyapunov exponent, and the correlation dimension, but other discriminating statistics can potentially be used.

We test whether the time series is consistent with the null hypothesis in the following way: First, calculate the value of the discriminating statistic on the measured time series. We will call this value $\mathcal{D}$. Then find the range of values for the discriminating statistic for time series that are consistent with the null hypothesis. If $\mathcal{D}$ falls within this range, then the discriminating statistic cannot distinguish between the null hypothesis and the measured time series. On the other hand, if $\mathcal{D}$ falls outside the range, then the time series is inconsistent with the null hypothesis.

One way of finding the range of values of the discriminating statistic for a time series consistent with the null hypothesis is this: Generate many different time series that are consistent with the null hypothesis, and then calculate the value of the discriminating statistic for each of these time series. We will call this value S_i for each of the null hypothesis time series. Data generated to be consistent with the null hypothesis are called **surrogate data**. This process of using surrogate data to find the range of values for data consistent with the null hypothesis is called **bootstrapping**.

There is a particularly simple method for generating surrogate data consistent with the null hypothesis of linear dynamics with Gaussian white noise inputs. In Section 6.5, we saw that a linear dynamical system can be characterized by a transfer function, which consists of two parts: the transfer gain $G(\omega)$ and the transfer phase $\Phi(\omega)$. The transfer function describes the relationship between any input and the output of the linear dynamical system. In order to calculate the transfer function, we need to measure both the input and the output. However, if the input is Gaussian white noise, then even if we do not measure the input we can calculate the transfer gain $G(\omega)$. The transfer phase $\Phi(\omega)$ will be random numbers between 0 and 2π at each ω. Or, to be more precise, since we don't measure the input, the phases $\Phi(\omega)$ look random to us, even though they are determined by the input.

If we took the same linear dynamical system and gave as input a new sequence of Gaussian white noise random inputs, then the transfer gain would be the same as before, but the transfer phase would be a new set of random numbers. In order to simulate this, we can take the following steps:

1. Compute the Fourier transform of the original time series. This will consist of an amplitude $A_{\text{output}}(\omega)$ and a phase $\phi_{\text{output}}(\omega)$ at each frequency ω.

2. Replace the phases $\phi_{\text{output}}(\omega)$ with random numbers ranging between 0 and 2π. Note that this has no effect on the amplitude $A_{\text{output}}(\omega)$. (Technical note: In the original time series, $\phi_{\text{output}}(\omega) = -\phi_{\text{output}}(-\omega)$, and this symmetry should be maintained when assigning random phases.)

3. Compute the inverse Fourier transform of $A_{\text{output}}(\omega)$ and the randomized $\phi_{\text{output}}(\omega)$. This produces a new time series, the surrogate data.

The surrogate data has the same $A_{\text{output}}(\omega)$ as the original time series. Since the power spectrum is proportional to $A_{\text{output}}^2(\omega)$, the surrogate data time series has exactly the same power spectrum as the original. Since the autocorrelation function is the Fourier transform of the power spectrum, the surrogate data also have exactly the same autocorrelation function as the original time series. This means that it is impossible to discriminate between the surrogate and the original based on the autocorrelation function or anything that is derived from the autocorrelation function.

Recall from Model Six that the parameters in the optimal linear model of a time series are derived from the autocorrelation function. Since the surrogate data and the original data have exactly the same autocorrelation function, both the surrogate data and the original have identical optimal linear models. In generating surrogate data in this manner, we do not need to specify the model order p of the linear model: The surrogate data and the original time series have the same optimal linear model for any model order.

Because we want to find the range of values for the discriminating statistic for data consistent with the null hypothesis, we will want to make many different surrogate data time series. Each one is called a **realization** of the null hypothesis. If we want to make many different realizations of the null hypothesis, then we follow the same process, using different random numbers for the phases $\phi_{\text{output}}(\omega)$ in step 2. Typically, 10 to 100 different realizations are used.

Now the procedure is easy: Calculate the value of the discriminating statistic for the original time series and for each of the surrogate data time series. If the value for the original time series is outside the range of values found for the surrogates, then the original time series is inconsistent with the null hypothesis.

We have considerable latitude in choosing a discriminating statistic. If one is interested in chaos, then an appropriate discriminating statistic is the nonlinear predictability $\mathcal{E}$, or the Lyapunov exponent, or the correlation dimension. However, in principle, any discriminating statistic could be used, even if it has nothing whatsoever to do with chaos. Whatever discriminating statistic is being used, the result indicates whether the original time series is consistent with the null hypothesis of linear dynamics with Gaussian white noise inputs.

❑ EXAMPLE 6.8

Use surrogate data to indicate whether the data from Model Three and the data from Model Five reflect linear or nonlinear dynamics.

Solution: We follow this sequence of steps:

- Generate many different realizations of surrogate data for each of the data sets. In this case, we will use ten realizations for each data set. Some examples are shown in Figures 6.9 through 6.14.

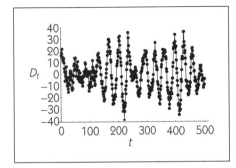

Figure 6.55
A realization of surrogate data for Model Three.

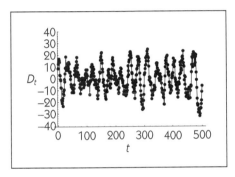

Figure 6.56
A second realization of surrogate data for Model Three.

- Calculate a discriminating statistic on the original data and on the corresponding surrogates. For this example, we will use nonlinear predictability $\frac{\mathcal{E}}{\sigma^2}$ as a discriminating statistic. We will use an embedding dimension of $p = 4$ for both the Model Three and Model Four data.

- See whether the value of the discriminating statistic for the original data lies outside the range for the many realizations of the surrogate data.

Figure 6.59 shows the nonlinear predictability $\frac{\mathcal{E}}{\sigma^2}$ for the Model Three data and for ten surrogates generated from this data. The Model Three data's predictability lies within the range of the surrogates. This means that nonlinear

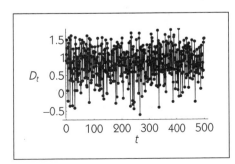

Figure 6.57
A realization of surrogate data for Model Five.

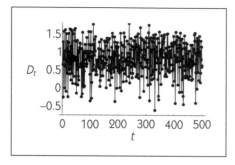

Figure 6.58
A second Model Five surrogate.

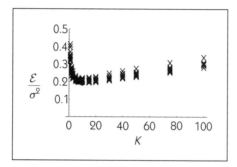

Figure 6.59
Nonlinear predictability $\frac{\mathcal{E}}{\sigma^2}$ versus K for the Model Three data (dots) and ten surrogate data sets (x). An embedding dimension of $p = 4$ was used.

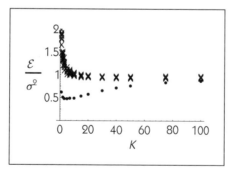

Figure 6.60
Nonlinear predictability $\frac{\mathcal{E}}{\sigma^2}$ versus K for the Model Five data (dots) and ten surrogate data sets (x).

predictability does not refute the null hypothesis that the data arise from a linear model. Note that $\frac{\mathcal{E}}{\sigma^2} \ll 1$ for the Model Three data. This means that there is some determinism in Model Three. However, the surrogate data analysis tells us that this determinism is consistent with linear dynamics.

The results for the Model Five data are different. (See Figure 6.60). For small values of K, the Model Five data's predictability lies well outside the range of values found for the surrogate data. This allows us to reject the linear dynamics null hypothesis.

6.9 ALGORITHMS AND ANSWERS

Suppose you have a time series from some field measurement, for example the Standard & Poor's stock price index measured each day. Suppose also that you have two computer programs, one to calculate a Lyapunov exponent and one to calculate a correlation dimension. You run the programs on your time-series data, setting parameters such as the number of nearest neighbors to use or the scaling region. The computer prints a message saying that the Lyapunov exponent is 0.2 and the correlation dimension is 3.1.

Does this mean that stock prices have a self-similar attractor with a dimension of 3.1 and that there is sensitive dependence on initial conditions? Not at all! Most computer programs are written to provide an output for any input. In designing the algorithm, the programmer makes certain assumptions. For example, the algorithm for quantifying sensitive dependence on initial conditions, described in Section 6.7, assumes that data are well described by a deterministic finite-difference equation. The algorithm for calculating the correlation dimension assumes that the trajectory lies on an attractor. If the data do not satisfy these assumptions, then the output of the algorithms should not be interpreted as answers to questions such as "Is there sensitive dependence on initial conditions?" or "Is there an attractor with a fractal dimension?"

The advantage of using surrogate data and testing the null hypothesis is that the assumptions behind the algorithms become unimportant. This is because we are no longer answering questions such as "Is there an attractor with a fractal dimension?" Instead, we are asking whether or not the time series is consistent with the null hypothesis.

It is tempting to believe that if we use a discriminating statistic that is motivated by chaos—for instance, the nonlinear predictability $\mathcal{E}$—then finding that the original time series is inconsistent with the linear dynamics null hypothesis means that the time series is chaotic. This is incorrect. All we can conclude, no matter which discriminating statistic is used, is that the time series is inconsistent with the null hypothesis. Some nonchaos phenomena that can lead to rejection of the null hypothesis are

- nonstationarity of the data;

- non-Gaussian white noise random inputs;

- nonlinearities in the measurement process;

- nonlinearities in the dynamics that do not involve chaos, such as the nonlinearity seen in the Lotka-Volterra equations, Section 5.5.

If the linear dynamics null hypothesis is rejected, then we have still not proved that the dynamics are chaotic. As of this writing, there is no general and standard test for any of the above nonchaos phenomena in time series that involve measurement noise or dynamical noise.

Conversely, if we cannot reject the null hypothesis, then all we can say is that "the measured data are consistent with the null hypothesis." This does not mean that the null hypothesis is correct—it means that we don't have any evidence that the hypothesis is incorrect. There might be too much measurement noise to reject the linear dynamics null hypothesis, or the dynamics might be chaotic but of such high dimension or high Lyapunov exponent that we do not have enough data to see the chaotic structure.

SOURCES AND NOTES

There are many branches in the literature surrounding time series analysis, but the root of time series analysis emerges from statistics. A knowledge of basic statistics is indispensable to the study of time series, and there are many introductory statistics textbooks such as Snedecor and Cochran (1989). The "standard toolbox" of techniques for analysis of time series from linear systems is based in spectral analysis and the auto- and cross-correlation functions. The principles are laid out in Box and Jenkins (1976) and Jenkins and Watts (1968). Somewhat less comprehensive introductions that provide an introduction to probability theory are Bendat and Piersol (1971) and Peebles (1987).

Time series analysis is particularly important in the closely-related engineering fields of signal processing and control. There are a large number of textbooks in this area, including Oppenheim and Schafer (1989) and Rabiner and Gold (1975) for signal processing, and Kailath (1980) for linear systems control theory. An important subject is estimation—how one deduces the values of unmeasured variables from measured ones—and also has a large literature. An overview is provided by Gelb et al. (1974). There is also a large engineering literature dealing with nonlinear control systems; Isidori (1989) provides an introduction.

The subject of time series analysis of chaotic systems is quite new, and there are no standard texts on the subject. Instead, one must resort to the technical literature, which can be quite intimidating. A good place to start is with review articles; two excellent ones are Grassberger et al. (1991) and Abarbanel et al. (1993). An intermediate-level introduction to chaos and randomness is given in Eubank and Farmer (1990).

The review articles mentioned above contain many references to the research literature. Here, we mention some articles that are particularly germane to the presentation of this chapter. The basis for almost all nonlinear dynamics time series analysis methods is time-lag-embedding of data. The first application of this technique to chaotic time series was by Glass and Mackey (1979) in the context of delay-differential equations, and the technique was introduced more generally in Packard et al. (1980) based on a suggestion by Ruelle. An important theorem was proved by Takens (1981) and extended and elaborated upon by Sauer et al. (1991). The influence of noise is considered in Casdagli et al. (1991).

Recurrence plots were introduced by Eckmann et al. (1987). Somewhat earlier, Grassberger and Procaccia (1983) had shown that the correlation dimension was a practical means of characterizing chaotic attractors. This technique has been widely used in applications, despite difficulties in interpreting results in data that may not be chaotic. Nonlinear prediction techniques were introduced by Farmer and Sidorowich (1987) in part to overcome this difficulty in interpretation. A paper written for non-specialists is Sugihara and May (1990). The presentation given in Chapter 6 is strongly influenced by Casdagli (1989), and the ice-age example is drawn from Hunter (1992). Methods for detecting determinism without constructing prediction models are described in Kaplan and Glass (1992, 1993) and Kennel et al. (1992). Of course, prediction techniques may be of ultimate use in forecasting the future. Many of the scientists involved in developing these methods have left academia for Wall Street. A popular review of the possible connections between chaos and finance is given in *The Economist* (Oct. 9, 1993).

The use of surrogate data is essential for deciding whether an irregular time series arises from nonlinear deterministic chaos or linear stochastic dynamics. The method was introduced by Theiler et al. (1992). An early application of phase-randomization to biological data is found in Kaplan and Cohen (1990).

The nonlinear techniques described in Chapter 6 are still part of the ongoing research enterprise. We do not know which methods will grow in use and which will wither as useless historical diversions. We also do not know what new techniques will emerge as important to using nonlinear dynamics to understand time series, but given that the field had its inception as recently as the late 1970s, it is likely that changes will be dramatic.

✐ EXERCISES

✐ **6.1** Time Series A (see Table 6.3) was produced by a computer random number generator. The mean of the entire time series is $M_{est} = 0.178$, and the standard deviation is $\sigma^2 = 1.045$. Is M_{est} significantly different than zero?

Calculate the mean of the first ten points of Time Series A, and the last ten points. Are the two means statistically different from zero? (If we want to know

Table 6.3 Time Series A

1	0.372	2	−0.161	3	0.526	4	2.06
5	−1.04	6	0.206	7	1.23	8	−2.83
9	0.452	10	−0.4	11	0.323	12	1.83
13	1.9	14	−0.353	15	−0.596	16	0.66
17	1.54	18	0.283	19	−2.21	20	−0.565
21	−0.812	22	2.39	23	−0.383	24	−0.449
25	−1.59	26	−2.24	27	0.534	28	−0.226
29	−1.15	30	0.464	31	−0.0285	32	−0.6
33	0.947	34	0.696	35	0.0939	36	0.615
37	−0.134	38	−0.162	39	0.812	40	−0.0927
41	−0.266	42	−0.987	43	0.451	44	−0.623
45	0.31	46	0.426	47	0.963	48	−1.02
49	0.259	50	0.649	51	−1.72	52	−2.14
53	0.642	54	0.415	55	−1.45	56	1.58
57	1.46	58	−0.105	59	1.03	60	1.93
61	0.0236	62	0.573	63	−0.263	64	0.129
65	−0.617	66	1.31	67	−0.446	68	1.08
69	−0.116	70	−1.17	71	2.47	72	1.15
73	0.984	74	1.44	75	0.447	76	−0.311
77	0.515	78	−0.193	79	−0.915	80	−0.486
81	0.43	82	0.225	83	−0.496	84	−0.98
85	−0.0647	86	1.92	87	1.79	88	−0.179
89	−0.539	90	1.24	91	0.0622	92	2.13
93	−0.224	94	0.266	95	−0.491	96	0.296
97	2.21	98	0.181	99	0.77	100	−0.0416

whether the two means are statistically different from each other, Student's t-test can be used, and is described in almost any introductory statistics textbook.)

6.2 In Section 6.3 the estimated mean M_{est} was found as the value that minimizes the squared difference between itself and the values in the time series:

$$E = \sum_{t=1}^{N}(D_t - M_{est})^2. \tag{6.43}$$

Another familiar quantity is the **median**, which is the value that half of the points are above and half below. Show that the median $\mathcal{M}$ is the result of minimizing

$$E = \sum_{t=1}^{N} |D_t - \mathcal{M}|. \tag{6.44}$$

(HINT: The derivative of $|D_t - \mathcal{M}|$ with respect to $\mathcal{M}$ is equal to ± 1, depending on whether D_t is greater than or less than $\mathcal{M}$.)

6.3 Each year the Happy Valley School District administers standardized tests to its students. The tests consist of 100 questions, each of which has a yes or no answer. A student gets one point for each question answered correctly, and zero points for each incorrect answer. The results of the testing are shown to parents in the form of a histogram, for all the students, as shown in Figure 6.61. The data fit the famous "bell-shaped curve," which we have been calling a Gaussian distribution.

1. Given that the mean score is 60.2, is there any reason to think that the students do better than they would if they answered questions randomly? (HINT: If all 100 questions were answered at random, the mean score would be 50 and the standard deviation would be 5.)

2. Your daughter, otherwise an A student, has done badly, scoring 40 on the test. Normally she scores a 90 on such tests. The school claims that she has tried intentionally to give the wrong answer on every question, but your daughter claims she was sick on the day of the test and couldn't read the exam questions. Is your daughter's answer plausible?

3. An angry parent complains that the school isn't doing its job, and that the students haven't learned anything except how to mark the exam sheet

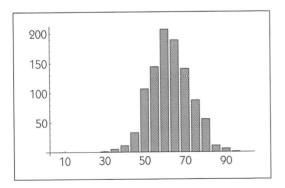

Figure 6.61 A histogram of the number of the scores received by students on a standardized test. The mean score is 60.2, and the standard deviation is 10.1. There are 1000 students' scores recorded here.

at random. The parent has read *Dynamics in Action* 7 of this book, and knows that a random walk produces a Gaussian-shaped distribution. The parent claims that the scores show that 30 of the questions were so easy that anyone could answer them, and the remaining 70 questions were answered at random. Do the data support the parent's claims? (HINT: Use the fact that the standard deviation of the distances moved by random walkers goes as the square root of the number of steps, to calculate what the standard deviation would be for 70 questions.)

6.4 Use the return plot given in *Dynamics in Action* 18 to construct functions $A_{t+1} = f(A_t)$ that fit the data.

1. Construct a piecewise constant model.

2. Construct a piecewise linear model.

Can either model produce an irregular series of action potentials? Can either model produce chaos?

6.5 In studying the Model 1 and Model 4 data, it was claimed that the respective autocorrelation functions were consistent with white noise. (See Figure 6.9 and 6.14.) The autocorrelation function for ideal white noise is $R(0) = 1$ and $R(k > 0) = 0$. In the two figures, it is apparent that while $R(k > 0)$ is close to zero, it is not exactly zero. How close is good enough?

Like the sample mean, the calculated value of $R(k)$ will vary from the "true" value because of sampling fluctuations. Given that the signal is really white noise, the calculated $R(k > 0)$ from any particular dataset of length N is a random number picked from a distribution with a mean of zero and a standard deviation of $1/\sqrt{N}$.

Are the graphs of $R(k)$ given in Figures 6.9 and 6.14 consistent with white noise? (100 data points were used to construct the graphs).

6.6 One test for the stationarity of a time series is whether the variance in the first half of a time series is the same as the variance in the second half. Of course, the two calculations are unlikely to produce exactly the same values, so we need to have some way to decide whether the variances are similar enough to justify saying that they are the same statistically.

The standard statistical test for comparing two variances is the F-test, which is based on the ratio of the two variances. If the variances were the same, then the ratio would be 1. Figure 6.62 gives 95 percent confidence levels for the ratio, as a function of the length of the time series. (We assume that the two time series have the same length.) If the ratio is within the two lines, then there is no statistically significant difference between the two variances.

Calculate the variance of the first 10 points in Time Series A, and of the last 10 points. Are they statistically different?

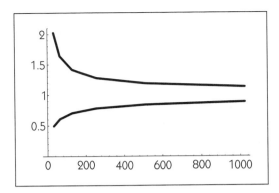

Figure 6.62 The 95 percent confidence levels for the ratio of the variances of two time series, as a function of the time series' length N.

COMPUTER PROJECTS

Project 1 Write a computer program to perform nonlinear prediction on a time series, as described in Section 6.7.

Project 2 Write a computer program to calculate the correlation integral $C(r)$ of a time series. Your program should read in the time series, and also an embedding dimension and an embedding lag. (A good choice for the embedding lag is the value k at which the autocorrelation function first falls to $1/e$.)

At any given r, the correlation integral is easily calculated: calculate the distance from each embedded point to every other embedded embedded point, and count how many of those distances are smaller than r. The value of $C(r)$ is then

$$C(r) = \frac{\text{Number of distances} < r}{\text{Total number of distances}}.$$

Given a time series of N points, and using an embedding dimension of p and embedding lag of h, then there are $N - (p - 1)h$ embedded points. The total number of distances is $(N - (p - 1)h)(N - (p - 1)h - 1)/2 \approx N^2/2$.

One is often interested in calculating $C(r)$ at many different values of r. Considerable efficiency can be gained by calculating all of the distances between points $|\mathbf{D_i} - \mathbf{D_j}|$ for $j = i + 1$ to N and $i = 1 - (p - 1)h$ to N and making a histogram of the result. The correlation integral is then the number of counts in the histogram to the left of the desired value of r, divided by the total number of counts. In order to facilitate looking at small values of r, it is useful to make the histogram based on the logarithm of the distances between points, rather than the distances themselves.

Project 3 Write a program to calculate the correlation dimension of a time series. One way to do this is to follow the procedure outlined in Example 6.4, which requires selecting a scaling region. This can be a subjective procedure, and difficult to apply to surrogate data.

A simple method for estimating the correlation dimension is to select two length scales r_1 and $r_2 < r_1$, and calculate

$$v = \frac{\log C(r_1) - \log C(r_2)}{\log r_1 - \log r_2}.$$

Theiler and Lookman (1993) point out that it is highly effective to select r_2 so that $C(r_1)/C(r_2) \approx 5$, which reduces the problem to selecting a single length scale r_1. It is convenient to set r_1 to be roughly $\sigma/4$, where σ is the standard deviation of the time series.

Project 4 Write a computer program to create surrogate data.

You will need the following ingredients, each of which is described in Press (1992), or is available from many commercial packages such as MATLAB® or MATHEMATICA®.

- A Fourier transform subroutine such as an FFT. Some FFT subroutines will only work with data that is a power of two in length, for example, 256, or 512. To understand this exercise, you will have to understand how the results of the FFT are stored in your computer, and you can only get this information by reading the manual that comes with your Fourier transform software.

- A random number generator. The random generator should have a **seed** that can be set to initialize the generator.

Your program should follow these steps:

1. Read in the time series. If you have an FFT subroutine that requires that your data be a power of two in length, you will need to truncate your data to the nearest power of two before proceeding.

2. Take the Fourier transform of your data. You now have an array of complex numbers. In principle, each of these complex numbers has a form $x + iy$, but different computers and software packages will store complex numbers differently.

3. Set the seed of the random number generator to a value you specify.

4. For each of the complex numbers in (2), except the first and the last one, do the following:
   - Calculate $r = \sqrt{x^2 + y^2}$.
   - Generate a random number θ uniformly distributed between zero and 2π. Most computer random number generators create a number

that is uniformly distributed between zero and one, so all you need to do is multiply the output of the random number generator by 2π.

■ Replace x by $r\cos\theta$ and replace y by $r\sin\theta$. Many Fourier transform routines perform calculations for both positive and negative frequencies. If this is the case for you, then at any given frequency you will generate only one θ at each frequency, using θ for the positive frequency and $-\theta$ for the negative frequency. (When taking the Fourier transform of a real time series, the result at frequency $-\omega$ is the complex conjugate of the result at ω.)

Leave the first and last—often termed DC and Nyquist frequency—alone.

5. Take the inverse Fourier transform of the phase-randomized data you generated in (4). The inverse Fourier transform is often calculated using the same subroutine as the Fourier transform; your manual can explain how to perform the inverse.

6. Print out the real part of the result of (5). If you have done things correctly, the numbers should all be real, except perhaps for a tiny imaginary component due to computer round-off error. In order to produce a different realization of the surrogate data, change the random seed that was set in step (3).

In practice, a number of mistakes can be made. The most common is to forget to use the same θ for corresponding positive and negative frequencies. If you find that, after taking the inverse Fourier transform, the imaginary part of the answer is not negligible, then you have probably made this mistake. Another common error arises from the complicated manner that some FFT subroutines store their output. Often, the DC component is stored as the first element of an array, and the Nyquist is stored next.

To test your program, generate a sine wave that has an integer number of cycles. For example, if you have N points in your time series, then $\sin(2\pi t\,\frac{10}{N})$ for $t = 1,\ldots,N$ will have 10 cycles. The surrogate data generated from this sine wave should have exactly the same number of cycles, and be shifted only in phase. If you make a sine wave with a non-integer number of cycles (say, 10.5), then you will notice that the surrogate data looks like a sine wave whose amplitude slowly changes.

Make a long random time series that consists of zeros and ones. The surrogate data generated from this time series will have the same autocorrelation function, but will not be zeros and ones. The amplitudes in the surrogate data will have a Gaussian distribution.

Project 5 As pointed out in Exercise 4, the method of generating surrogate data using phase-randomization of the Fourier transform produces data with a

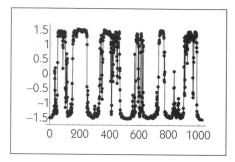

Figure 6.63
A time series from a linear dynamical system, subjected to a nonlinear measurement, $D_i = \arctan(x_i)$.

Gaussian distribution of values. Often, the original data does not have a Gaussian distribution, and so it is easy to distinguish the original data from the surrogates by using a discriminating statistic that looks for non-Gaussian distributions. This can be misleading when using surrogate data to look for nonlinear dynamics, because a non-Gaussian distribution can be created by a measurement function that is nonlinear, even if the underlying dynamics are linear and Gaussian. For instance, the time series shown in Figure 6.63 was produced by a linear dynamical system, but subjected to a nonlinear measurement—the arctangent of the data was taken, producing values that tend to be near ±1.5. The phase-randomized surrogate data looks qualitatively different from the original data, because its values do not cluster near ±1.5 but instead form a Gaussian distribution.

There is a technique that helps to avoid being mislead by nonlinear measurement functions: apply nonlinear measurement transformations to the phase-randomized surrogate data to give it a distribution identical to the original data. This is called **amplitude-adjusted surrogate data**, and often looks much more like the original data (see Figure 6.65). The Null Hypothesis behind amplitude-adjusted surrogate data is "linear dynamics with a possibly nonlinear, monotonically increasing measurement function." This Null Hypothesis is somewhat more general than the "linear dynamics, linear measurement" hypothesis behind the phase-randomized surrogate data.

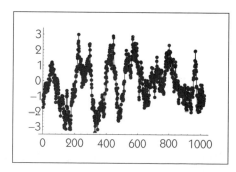

Figure 6.64
Surrogate data of the signal in Figure 6.63 generated by phase randomization of the Fourier transform.

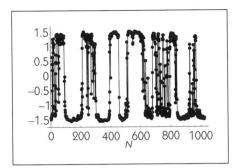

Figure 6.65
Surrogate data of the signal in Figure 6.63 generated using amplitude adjustment before and after phase randomization of the Fourier transform.

Amplitude-adjusted surrogate data can be created by shuffling the original time series in a very careful manner. Each point in a time series can be thought of as having two indices, which we will call the *time index* and the *amplitude index*. The time index refers to the temporal order of the points. The first point has time index 1, the second has time index 2, and so on. The amplitude index refers to the actual values, irrespective of their order in time. From this perspective, the *smallest* value has amplitude index 1, the next smallest has amplitude index 2, and the *largest* has amplitude index N. In order to apply a nonlinear measurement transformation, we first generate a target time series that has the desired distribution. Then, we take the source time series, and replace each point by the value of the point in the target time series that has the same amplitude index. This can be accomplished by sorting the target and source time series in the following sequence:

1. Sort the source time series according to amplitude index, keeping track of the time index. After the sorting, the values will be in increasing amplitude order, but the time index associated with each value will be out of order.

2. Sort the target time series in the same way.

3. Replace the amplitude values in the sorted source time series, with the corresponding amplitude values in the sorted target time series. Make sure to leave the time indices as they were in the sorted time series. Call this the "mixed" time series.

4. Sort the mixed time series in ascending time index order.

The result will be that the amplitude values in the target time series replace those of the source time series, but the time order remains that of the source time series.

Write a program that applies this sorting algorithm to transform a source time series to the amplitude distribution of a target time series. You can test this program by using a sine wave as a source, and uniformly distributed numbers (e.g., 1, 2, 3, . . .) as a target. The result should be a triangle wave that increases and decreases in phase with the original sine wave.

Overall, the process for making amplitude-adjusted surrogate data is as follows:

1. Amplitude transform the original data to a Gaussian distribution. Use the original data as the source time series, and Gaussian white noise as the target time series.

2. Make the phase-randomized surrogate of the transformed data.

3. Amplitude transform the surrogate data to the original data. Now, the original data is the target time series, and the surrogate data is the source time series.

Surrogate data produced in this way will have exactly the same distribution as the original time series. In fact, the surrogate data is the original time series, but shuffled in order. The shuffling has been carefully done so that the result is not necessarily white noise—which is the result if you randomly shuffle the order of a time series—but has an autocorrelation function that is quite similar to the original time series' autocorrelation function.

A Multi-Functional Appendix

In dynamics, one sees many equations of the form

$$y = f(x), \tag{A.1}$$

$\frac{dx}{dt} = f(x)$, or $x_{t+1} = f(x_t)$. In these equations, a dependent variable (y or $\frac{dx}{dt}$ or x_{t+1}) is expressed as a **function** of an independent variable (x or x_t). Saying that y is a function of x is just another way of saying that for a given value of x, we can calculate the unique corresponding value of y. Exactly how this calculation is done, of course, depends on the "form of the function." For example, the function

$$f(x) = 2x - 7x^2$$

can be easily evaluated; when $x = 3$ this function has the value $2 \times 3 - 7 \times 3^2 = -57$. When $x = 3.1$, the value is -61.07. Other forms of functions are not always simple to evaluate in one's head or using just paper and pencil. For example, the function $\cos(x)$ evaluated at $x = 3$ has the value -0.9899925, although almost everyone would need a calculator to find this out.

Just a few different forms of functions cover most of the territory in dynamics. After becoming familiar with the shape of the graphs of these functions, one can often use intuition to understand important aspects of an equation. If you know what context different functions arise in, you can often quickly see in an equation the underlying physical or biological mechanism.

To determine the geometrical features of a graph of a function, $y = f(x)$ you have to carry out only a small number of computations. You are probably already familiar with these from calculus, but here is a quick summary.

- The x-intercept or zeroes. Set the dependent variable y equal to 0 and solve for x. This is the problem people are solving when they factor an equation or use numerical techniques such as Newton's method.

- The y-intercept. Set x equal to 0 and solve for y.

- The behavior at $x = \pm\infty$ and 0. Substitute these values for x in the equation and determine the value of y. If y is indeterminate (e.g., 0/0 or $0 \times \infty$) you will have to determine which term grows the fastest in the neighborhood of the point under consideration. This is often easy to see geometrically, but if you have a problem you will have to apply l'Hôpital's rule (see your calculus book).

- The maxima and minima. Compute the first derivative, $\frac{dy}{dx}$, of Eq. A.1 and set it equal to 0. The values of x that satisfy the resulting equation are usually maxima or minima. For the maxima the second derivative $\frac{d^2y}{dx^2}$ is negative, whereas for minima it is positive. Caveat: This does not work all the time, so be aware of tricky functions that will confuse you if you do things mechanically without thinking. For example, the functions $y = x^3$ and $y = x^4$ are simple to graph, but you must be careful applying this rule.

- The inflection points. These are values of x for which the sign of the first derivative changes sign. They can usually be found by computing the value of x for which $\frac{d^2y}{dx^2}$ is zero. The caveat above concerning tricky functions applies here as well, so be careful.

- Singular values. For some values of x, y approaches $\pm\infty$. For example, in the function $f(x) = \frac{1}{(x-7)}$, the denominator is zero when $x = 7$.

We now discuss several functions that are found in applications. Although most of the functions can be written in more general fashion by translation of the origin and rotations of the axes, we present the functions in the most usual and useful representations. Lowercase Roman and Greek letters (with the exception of x, y, and t) refer to real constants. The same symbol, such as b, will have different meanings in the different functions in which it appears as a parameter, but this should not cause any confusion. The dependent variable is y and the independent variable is x or t (t will be used for those functions that in practice usually have time as the independent variable).

A.1   THE STRAIGHT LINE

The straight line

$$y = mx + b$$

is of great importance. The graph of this function is a straight line of slope m. The y-intercept is b (see Figure A.1). Many physical relations are well described by a straight line (sometimes with $b = 0$), at least as a good first approximation. Thus Boyle's law states that the pressure of a fixed volume of gas is proportional to the absolute temperature, and Ohm's law states that the current through a resistor is proportional to the voltage.

In analyzing dynamical equations, nonlinear functions are often approximated by a straight line. In addition, there are many examples in which nonlinear functions can be transformed to a linear function. This leads to a powerful technique to plot data and determine parameters.

❑ **EXAMPLE A.1**

Exponential decay (see Chapter 4) is described by the function $y = ke^{-\alpha t}$. Interpret the graph of ln y as a function of t.

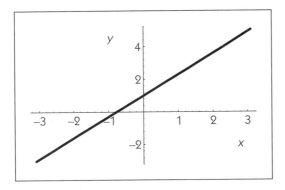

Figure A.1   The straight line $y = mx + b$ with $m = 1.3$ and $b = 1$.

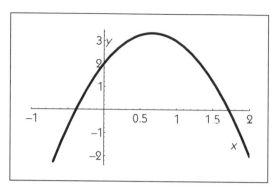

Figure A.2 The quadratic function $y = ax^2 + bx + c$ with $a = -3, b = 4$, and $c = 2$.

Solution: Take the natural logarithm of both sides of the exponential decay function to obtain $\ln y = \ln k - \alpha t$. The plot of $\ln y$ as a function of t is thus a straight line with slope $-\alpha$ and y-intercept $\ln k$.

A.2 THE QUADRATIC FUNCTION

By adding a term proportional to x^2 to the right-hand side of the equation of a straight line we obtain a quadratic function, generally written as

$$y = ax^2 + bx + c.$$

This equation—which is the equation of a curve called a **parabola** (see Figure A.2)—has a single maximum or minimum that is easily found by setting the first derivative equal to zero. The extremal point falls at $x = \frac{-b}{2a}$ and it is a maximum if a is negative and a minimum if a is positive. Nonlinear finite-difference equations where the right-hand side is a quadratic function are considered in detail in Chapter 1.

A.3 THE CUBIC AND HIGHER-ORDER POLYNOMIALS

A polynomial function is a function of the form

$$y = \sum_{n=0}^{p} a_n x^n = a_0 + a_1 x + a_2 x^2 + \cdots + a_p x^p,$$

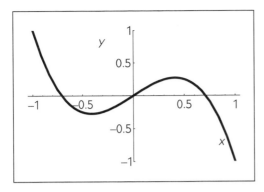

Figure A.3
The cubic function
$y = -2x^3 + x$. Note
the 2 extremal points at
$x = \pm 0.408$ and the three
roots at $x = 0, \pm 0.707$.

where the sum is taken over non negative integers, the a_n are constants, and p is the **order** of the polynomial. Thus the quadratic function considered above is a second-order polynomial, and the third-order polynomial is also called the **cubic function** (see Figure A.3). Generally, your life will not be much disturbed by polynomials of order higher than 3. However, there are two things you should know about the higher-order polynomials:

- The number of values of x where $y = 0$ is less than or equal to the order of the polynomial.
- The number of extremal points of an nth-order polynomial is less than or equal to $n - 1$.

Three main places where cubic functions appear in applications are the finite-difference equations where the right-hand side is a cubic function, see Chapter 1; the van der Pol equation, a second-order nonlinear equation that generates limit cycle oscillations, see Chapter 5; and the Fitzhugh-Nagumo equation, a second-order nonlinear equation for excitable systems, which is also described in Chapter 5.

A.4   THE EXPONENTIAL FUNCTION

The exponential function,

$$f(x) = e^{mx},$$

is probably the most important nonlinear function that arises in applications (see Figure A.4). The derivative of the exponential function is proportional to itself:

$$\frac{df(x)}{dx} = \frac{de^{mx}}{dx} = me^{mx} = mf(x).$$

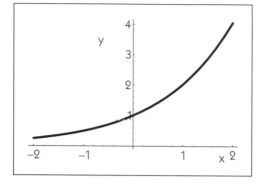

Figure A.4
The exponential function $y = e^{mx}$ with $m = 0.7$.

This leads to the appearance of the exponential function in problems involving growth and decay, where the rate of change of a substance x is proportional to the amount of x present.

❏ **EXAMPLE A.2**

Consider the differential equation $\frac{dy}{dt} = \alpha y$, where α is a constant. Show that the solution of this equation is $y(t) = ke^{\alpha t}$, where k is a constant.

Solution: The solution of a differential equation is an expression that when substituted into both sides leads to an identity. The derivative of $y(t)$ is $\frac{dy}{dt} = k\alpha e^{\alpha t} = \alpha y(t)$.

❏

Exponential functions arise, along with the sine and cosine functions (see Section A.6), as solutions of linear ordinary differential equations. Thus, whenever an applied mathematician finds that data can be described by an exponential function, or a sum of exponential functions, a theoretical model posed as a system of linear ordinary differential equations is immediately suggested. Such sorts of models have been particularly popular in compartmental analysis and in studies of kinetics of ionic channels.

A.5 SIGMOIDAL FUNCTIONS

Sigmoidal functions have a characteristic shape that starts at one value and rises smoothly to another value as $x \rightarrow \infty$, with a single inflection point. One can imagine many algebraic expressions to represent such curves, but in applications, only a small number of different functions are encountered frequently. Here we discuss four different functions; the Hill function, the hyperbolic tangent, the logistic function, and the Heaviside function. Which of these functions is selected for a given application may depend on the system under consideration, or on the personality and training of the investigator. We do not know of good theorems concerning the substitution of one function for another—but if you see a dynamical equation containing one sigmoidal function, then substitution of another sigmoidal function with the same steepness and upper and lower asymptotes often will give equivalent dynamics.

THE HILL FUNCTION

This function looks like the English name of its originator, A.V. Hill (see Figure A.5). The function

$$f(x) = \frac{x^n}{\theta^n + x^n}$$

is often used to describe the cooperative binding of molecules to proteins, for example, the binding of oxygen to hemoglobin. Consequently, the Hill function is the sigmoidal function of choice for dynamics in biochemical networks.

THE HYPERBOLIC TANGENT

Anyone who really wants a fancy sigmoidal function will choose the hyperbolic tangent

$$f(x) = \tanh \beta x = \frac{e^{\beta x} - e^{-\beta x}}{e^{\beta x} + e^{-\beta x}}.$$

Since hyperbolic functions are omitted from most elementary calculus courses these days ("We ran out of time, and no one really uses these functions anyway!"),

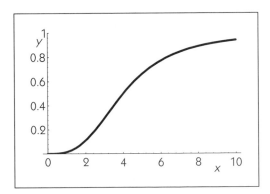

Figure A.5
The Hill function
$y = \frac{x^n}{\theta^n + x^n}$ with $n = 3$, $\theta = 4$.

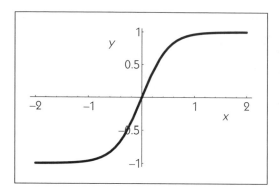

Figure A.6 The hyperbolic tangent function $y = \tanh \beta x$ with $\beta = 2$.

only those with pretensions of higher mathematical knowledge (mathematicians or physicists) will ever use these functions. The symmetry of the *tanh* function $f(x) = -f(-x)$ distinguishes it from the Hill and logistic functions, but this feature is not often exploited in applications (see Figure A.6).

THE LOGISTIC FUNCTION

The function

$$y = \frac{1}{1 + be^{-kx}}$$

arises as the solution of the logistic differential equation (Chapter 4). This function, which is depicted in Figure A.7, is favored by physicists and engineering sorts, and as such it often appears in theoretical models of neural networks.

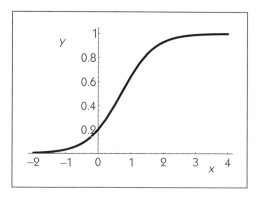

Figure A.7
The logistic function
$y = \frac{1}{1+be^{-kx}}$ with $b = 4$,
$k = 2$.

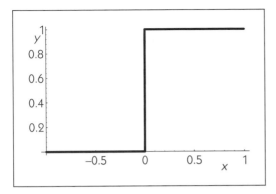

Figure A.8 The Heaviside function.

THE HEAVISIDE FUNCTION

The Heaviside function,

$$f(x) = \begin{cases} 0 & \text{if } x < 0, \\ 1 & \text{if } x \geq 0, \end{cases}$$

sometimes called the step function, is exploited in physics and engineering applications. The function is discontinuous at 0. The Heaviside function is the limiting function that arises when the slope of sigmoidal functions becomes infinitely steep (see Figure A.8). In models, the dynamics are often pretty much the same when one uses a very steep sigmoid function, or a Heaviside function. Using a Heaviside function instead of one of the other sigmoidal functions will sometimes turn an intractable nonlinear equation, whose properties can only be determined using numerical integration, into a piecewise linear equation that can be analytically studied.

A.6   THE SINE AND COSINE FUNCTIONS

In a right triangle, the *sine* of an angle is the ratio of the length of the opposite side divided by the length of the hypotenuse; the *cosine* is the ratio of the length of the adjacent side to the length of the hypotenuse. In dynamics, these trigonometric functions arise in a different context since variables may show fluctuations over time that are well described by sine or cosine functions. The equation describing a simple harmonic oscillator (e.g., a mass on a spring—see

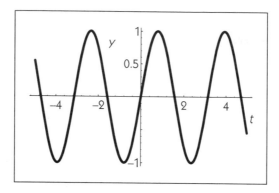

Figure A.9   The sine function $f(x) = \sin(\omega x)$ with $\omega = 2$.

Chapter 5)

$$\frac{d^2x}{dt^2} = -\omega^2 x$$

has a sine or cosine as a solution.

The graph of the sine function, $y(t) = \sin \omega t$ is shown in Figure A.9. There is a regular oscillation that repeats with a period, $T = \frac{2\pi}{\omega}$, and the amplitude of the oscillation is k. The connection between exponential, sine, and cosine functions is expressed as

$$e^{i\omega t} = \cos \omega t + i \sin \omega t,$$

where $i = \sqrt{-1}$. This relationship can be derived directly from the power series expansions of the exponential, sine, and cosine functions.

A.7   THE GAUSSIAN (OR "NORMAL") DISTRIBUTION

If one takes measurements of a single characteristic in a population of individuals, it often happens that the measured values cluster around some central value. The function that gives a commonly observed distribution of measurements is called the **Gaussian** or "**normal**" **distribution**, and is given by

$$y = G(x) = \frac{1}{\sqrt{2\pi}\sigma} \exp\left(-\frac{(x-\mu)^2}{2\sigma^2}\right),$$

where μ is the average (mean) value and σ is a constant called the standard deviation. The graph of the Gaussian distribution is the familiar but nevertheless mystical bell-shaped curve (see Figure A.10); the standard deviation σ is proportional to the width of the bell. To interpret the normal distribution in the statistical sense described above, we say that the probability that a measured value lies in a range between x and $x + \delta x$ is $G(x)\delta x$.

A large fraction of conventional statistical methods is based on the assumption that what is being measured is Gaussian-distributed. But why is this rather bizarre function so ubiquitous? The often-quoted reason is the "central limit theorem" that says, roughly, that the sum of many independent quantities will have a Gaussian distribution.

One way to derive the Gaussian distribution is from a dynamical process called a **random walk**. A random walk can take place in any number of dimensions, but for the moment just imagine a one-dimensional random walk along a line. Start at the origin and randomly take one step to the right or left. Then take a second step, but once again choose randomly whether to go to the left or right. Repeat this process N times, each time choosing a random direction. The exact probability that the random walker will be any given distance from the origin can be derived using the binomial distribution, and in the case when N is large, the resulting binomial distribution can be approximated by the Gaussian distribution. This is consistent with the central limit theorem because the position after N steps in a random walk is the sum of N random numbers.

An important application of the Gaussian distribution is in the study of **diffusion**. The thermal motion of molecules leads individual particles to undergo erratic paths, first observed by Robert Brown when he examined tiny particles floating in water under a microscope. The irregular motion, sometimes called **Brownian motion** is a physical example of a random walk leads to a Gaussian distribution, see *Dynamics in Action 7*. A wonderful way to review your knowledge of some basic mechanical operations of calculus is to carry out computations

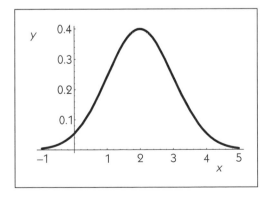

Figure A.10
The Gaussian function
$$y = \frac{1}{\sqrt{2\pi}\sigma} \exp{-\frac{(x-\mu)^2}{2\sigma^2}}$$
with $\mu = 2$ and $\sigma = 1$.

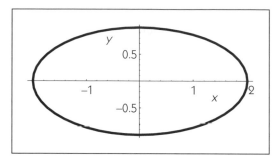

Figure A.11 The ellipse $\frac{x^2}{a^2} + \frac{y^2}{b^2} = 1$ with $a = 2, b = 1$.

involving the Gaussian distribution and diffusion. The problems at the end of this appendix offer many chances to do this.

A.8 THE ELLIPSE

The ellipse, shown in Figure A.11, is a friendly oval fellow satisfying the equation

$$\frac{x^2}{a^2} + \frac{y^2}{b^2} = 1.$$

The special case when $a = b$ is a circle. Note that in the above equation, we have not used the format $y = f(x)$. This is because y is not a function of x; for values of x in the range $-a < x < a$, there are two possible values for y corresponding to the positive and negative square roots.

One way the ellipse enters into dynamics is in phase-plane plots of differential equations (see Chapter 5). This is illustrated in the following example.

❏ EXAMPLE A.3

Consider a system in which the position as a function of time is $y(t) = k \sin \omega t$. Show that the curve in which the velocity is plotted as a function of the position is an ellipse.

Solution: Taking the derivative of $y(t)$ we find $v - \frac{dy}{dt} = k\omega \cos \omega t$. From this we immediately find that $y^2 + \frac{v^2}{k^2\omega^2} = 1$, which is the equation of the ellipse.

❏

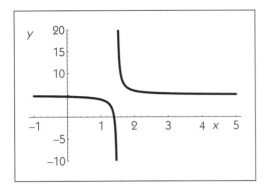

Figure A.12
The hyperbola
$y = a + \frac{c}{x-b}$. In this case,
the singularity occurs at
$x = 1.5$, where $a = 5$,
$b = 1.5$, and $c = 0.5$.

A.9 THE HYPERBOLA

The hyperbola

$$y = a + \frac{c}{x - b}$$

is an important function, but it has singular behavior (i.e., $y \to \infty$) as x approaches b. In many cases, though, constraints on x prevent the appearance of the singularity (see Figure A.12). A good example is in the study of enzyme kinetics, where the Michaelis-Menten expression for the initial rate of transformation of a substrate, S, by an enzyme, E, is $v = \frac{V_{max}[S]}{K_m+[S]}$, where $[S]$ is the concentration of S, V_{max} is the maximum rate, and K_m is constant called the Michaelis-Menten constant. Since V_{max} and K_m are positive, and concentrations are positive, the annoying singularity is never encountered. Hikers might recognize hyperbolae as marking the appearance of mountain passes on contour maps. This geometric signature of mountain passes is likewise important in studies of dynamics in two-dimensional flows; see Chapter 5.

✏ **EXERCISES**

The following integrals may be useful in the solution of the Exercise in Appendix A.

$$\int_0^\infty x^n e^{-ax}dx = \frac{n!}{a^{n+1}} \qquad \int_0^m xe^{-ax^2}dx = \frac{1}{2a}(1 - e^{-am^2})$$

$$\int_0^\infty xe^{-ax^2}dx = \frac{1}{2a} \qquad \int_0^\infty x^2 e^{-ax^2}dx = \frac{1}{4a}\sqrt{\frac{\pi}{a}}$$

✏   **A.1** Draw graphs of the following piecewise linear functions $y = f(x)$ where $0 \le x \le 1$.

a. $f(x) = 2x, \quad 0 \le x \le 0.5, \ f(x) = 2 - 2x, \quad 0.5 < x \le 1$;

b. $f(x) = 0.25 + 1.5x; \quad 0 \le x \le 0.5, \ f(x) = -0.25 + 0.5x, \quad 0.5 < x \le 1$;

c. $f(x) = 2x(\text{mod } 1)$.

The dynamics that are found when these piecewise linear functions are used as the right-hand side of one-dimensional finite-difference equations can be surprisingly complicated.

A.2 Consider the two curves $y = x$ and $y = \lambda x(1 - x)$. There is always a point of intersection of both curves at $y = x = 0$. For what values of λ is there a second point of intersection that lies in the range

a. $x < 0$;

b. $0 < x < 0.5$;

c. $0.5 < x < 1$?

For each of the above cases sketch the graph.

A.3 Consider the function $y = -x^3 + \lambda x$, for all real values of λ. Sketch this function for

a. $\lambda < 0$;

b. $\lambda = 0$;

c. $\lambda > 0$. Be sure to identify all intercepts, maxima, minima, and inflection points.

A.4 Consider the function

$$f(x) = Cx^2(2 - x),$$

where C is a positive constant.

a. What are the maxima, minima, and inflection points for this function?

b. Sketch the function for $C = \frac{25}{16}$ for both positive and negative values of x.

A.5 Consider the functions

$$y_1(t) = e^{-t} + e^{-3t},$$

$$y_2(t) = e^{-t} - e^{-3t},$$

Consider $t \ge 0$. For each function,

a. Sketch the function;

b. Plot $\ln y_1$ and $\ln y_2$ as a function of time. Are any regions of the graph approximately linear?

A.6 Consider the Hill function,

$$f(x) = \frac{Ax^n}{\theta^n + x^n}, \qquad x \geq 0,$$

where n is a real number greater than 2.

a. Sketch this function. Be sure to determine the extremal and inflection points, if any, and indicate the behavior as $x \to \infty$.

b. Determine the slope of the Hill function at the inflection point.

c. The plot of

$$\ln \frac{\frac{f(x)}{A}}{1 - \frac{f(x)}{A}}$$

as a function of $\ln x$ is often called a *Hill plot*. Assuming that $f(x)$ is given by the Hill function, interpret the Hill plot, and show how it can be used to determine the Hill coefficient, n.

A.7 Figure A.13 shows the binding of oxygen to hemoglobin. The fraction of hemoglobin saturated with oxygen is shown as a function of the percentage of

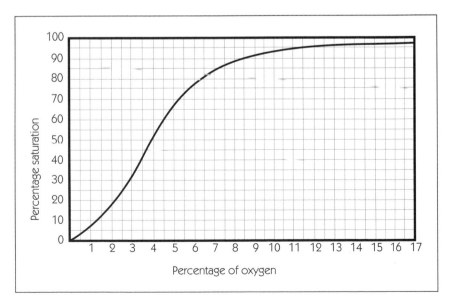

Figure A.13

oxygen in the air being breathed. Fit this data to the Hill function to determine the values of the parameters giving the best fit to the data.

✎ **A.8** Consider the function

$$f(x) = a \frac{\theta^2}{\theta^2 + x^2} + b, \qquad x \geq 0, \tag{A.2}$$

where a, b, and θ are positive real numbers. Sketch this function. Be sure to show any maxima, minima, and inflection points (these should be determined algebraically).

✎ **A.9** In inducible enzyme synthesis in bacteria, the synthesis of a given enzyme depends on binding of repressor molecules to a region of the chromosome called the operator. The repressor molecules can bind either to the operator or to a molecule called the effector (or inducer). The enzyme synthetic rate is proportional to the fraction of free operators, α. Yagil and Yagil (1971) propose that the fraction of free operators can be written as

$$\alpha = \frac{\alpha_b + \frac{\alpha_b E^n}{K_1}}{1 + \alpha_b + \frac{\alpha_b E^n}{K_1}},$$

where E is the effector concentration, K_1 is a rate constant, and $\alpha_b (0 < \alpha_b \ll 1)$ is approximately the fraction of free operators at zero effector concentration (n, α_b, K_1, and E are positive).

a. Show that $\frac{d\alpha}{dE} \geq 0$.

b. Sketch α as a function of E. Be sure to show the behavior when $E = 0$ amd when $E \to \infty$.

c. Show that $\log\left(\frac{\alpha}{1-\alpha} - \alpha_b\right) = n \log E + \log \frac{\alpha_b}{K_1}$.

d. If $\log\left(\frac{\alpha}{1-\alpha} - \alpha_b\right)$ is plotted as a function of $\log E$, sketch the resulting graph. Indicate any relevant features such as slopes and intercepts.

✎ **A.10** In respiration in man, the ventilation response function is given by

$$V = \frac{V_m y^n}{\theta^n + y^n},$$

where V is the ventilation, y is the partial pressure of CO_2, V_m is the maximal ventilation, and θ and n are parameters to be determined. When the partial pressure of CO_2 is y_0, the slope of the ventilation response function is S_0, and the ventilation is V_0.

a. Demonstrate that

$$n = \frac{V_m S_0 y_0}{V_0(V_m - V_0)}$$

$$\theta = y_0 \left(\frac{V_m - V_0}{V_0} \right)^{1/n}$$

b. Compute n and θ, assuming $V_m = 48$ L/min, $y_0 = 40$ mmHg, $V_0 = 8$ L/min, and $S_0 = 1$ L/min mmHg.

A.11 Show that the logistic function

$$N(t) = \frac{N(0)k}{[k - \alpha N(0)]e^{-kt} + \alpha N(0)},$$

where k, α, and $N(0)$ are positive constants, is a solution of the differential equation

$$\frac{dN}{dt} = kN - \alpha N^2.$$

A.12 Show that

$$y(t) = k \cos \omega t,$$

where k and ω are constants, is a solution of the differential equation

$$\frac{d^2 y}{dt^2} = -\omega^2 y.$$

A.13 Sketch $f(x) = 0.6 \sin(\pi x)$ and $f(x) = 0.6(\sin(\pi x))^2$ for $0 \le x \le 1$. Determine all maxima, minima, and inflection points.

A.14 Consider a variable x that is described by a Gaussian distribution,

$$G(x) = \frac{1}{\sigma \sqrt{2\pi}} \exp \left(\frac{-(x - \mu)^2}{2\sigma^2} \right).$$

The mean value of x, called $\bar{x}$, is given by the integral

$$\int_{-\infty}^{\infty} x G(x) dx.$$

The variance of x is given by the integral

$$\int_{-\infty}^{\infty} (x - \bar{x})^2 G(x)dx.$$

Evaluate the integrals to find the mean and the variance of x.

✐   **A.15** If I place A molecules at the origin $x = 0$ at time $t = 0$ in a one-dimensional system, the molecules will diffuse so that at time t, the average density of molecules at position x is

$$P(x, t) = \frac{A}{2\sqrt{\pi Dt}} \exp\left(\frac{-x^2}{4Dt}\right).$$

a. Sketch $P(x, t)$ for $D = 10^{-5}$ cm^2/sec and $t = 1$ sec. Use linear scales.

b. Compute $\frac{\partial P(x,t)}{\partial t}$.

c. Compute $D \frac{\partial^2 P(x,t)}{\partial x^2}$. This should be equal to $\frac{\partial P(x,t)}{\partial t}$.

d. Compute $\int_{-\infty}^{\infty} P(x, t)dx$.

✐   **A.16** The number density $P(r, t)$ for molecules diffusing from a point source introduced at $t = 0$ in n dimensions is

$$P(r, t) = \frac{A}{(2\sqrt{\pi Dt})^n} \exp\left(\frac{-r^2}{4Dt}\right),$$

where A is the total number of molecules, D is the diffusion coefficient, t is the time, and r is the distance from the source.

a. For $n = 1, 2, 3$, compute the time when the number density is a maximum.

b. If neurotransmitters are introduced to a neural preparation using iontophoresis (passing an electrical current through a microelectrode containing ionic solution), the maximum response of a neuron occurs when the number density of the neurotransmitter at the receptor is a maximum. Assume diffusion in three dimensions with a diffusion coefficient of 10^{-5} cm^2/sec. What is the distance from the microelectrode to the neuron if the maximal response occurs at $t = 1.5 \times 10^{-3}$ sec?

✐   **A.17** In a study of the time course of acetylcholine release, Katz and Miledi (1965) analyze time delays resulting from diffusion of acetylcholine to its receptor. Diffusion from an instantaneous point source is characterized by the curve shown in Figure A.14.

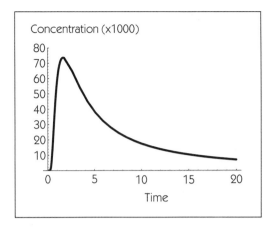

Figure A.14
$D = 10^{-5}$ cm^2 sec^{-1},
$r = 0.01$ cm.

This curve can be calculated from the equation

$$\text{Concentration} = \frac{Q}{8(\pi Dt)^{\frac{3}{2}}} \exp\left(\frac{-r^2}{4Dt}\right),$$

where r is the distance from the point source to the point at which the concentration is measured (i.e., the receptor), Q is the quantity released, and D is the diffusion coefficient.

a. Determine the time that the concentration is a maximum at the receptor (in terms of the parameters in the equation).

b. What is the concentration at that time?

c. Katz and Miledi state that the time until the concentration reaches one half of its maximum value is about 44 percent of the time needed to reach maximum value. Show that this is true algebraically.

A.18 This problem is based on an article by Fatt and Katz (1951) that concerns neuromuscular transmission in frogs. If a charge q_0 is placed at time $t = 0$ at a point $x = 0$ on a nerve fiber, the membrane voltage V at time t at a point a distance x away from the charge is

$$V(x, t) = \frac{q_0}{2C_m\lambda\sqrt{\frac{\pi t}{\tau_m}}} \exp\left(-\frac{x^2\tau_m}{4\lambda^2 t} - \frac{t}{\tau_m}\right)$$

where τ_m is the time constant of the membrane, λ is the space constant of the membrane, and C_m is the capacitance of the membrane per unit length of the fiber.

a. Show that the time T when V is a maximum at a particular point $x = R$ satisfies the equation

$$\frac{R^2}{\lambda^2} = \frac{4T^2}{\tau_m^2} + \frac{2T}{\tau_m}.$$

b. Sketch the graph for $\frac{R^2}{\lambda^2}$ as a function of $\frac{T}{\tau_m}$.

A.19 This question deals with the distribution of molecules along the length of a linear blue-green algae following release of molecules from either one source or two sources. A pulse of N_0 molecules is released from a source at time $t = 0$. The concentration $N(r, t)$ of molecules at a distance r from the cell is

$$N(r, t) = \frac{N_0}{2\sqrt{\pi Dt}} \exp\left(\frac{-r^2}{4Dt}\right).$$

a. At what time is the concentration of molecules at a distance L away from the source a maximum (express the time in terms of L and D)? Compute the time for $L=2$ cm and $D = 2 \times 10^{-5}$ cm^2 / sec. What is the concentration at this time (within 10 percent)?

b. If two cells act as sources, the concentration of molecules can be found by adding up the contribution from each source. If a cell is at a distance L_1 from one source and L_2 from a second source, write down the formula for the total contribution from both sources.

c. Consider a cell equidistant from two sources 4 cm apart so that $L_1 = L_2 = 2$ cm. Each source releases N_0 molecules at $t = 0$. At what time is the concentration at the cell a maximum ($D = 2 \times 10^{-5}$ cm^2/sec)? What is the concentration at this time (within 10 percent)?

d. Consider a cell 2 cm from one source and 4 cm from a second source. Both sources release N_0 molecules at $t = 0$ ($D = 2 \times 10^{-5}$ cm/sec. The time when the concentration at this cell is a maximum is called t_{max}. Is t_{max} greater than, less than, or equal to the time computed in part c? Justify your answer (lengthy additional computations are not needed).

A.20 Let $f_1(x)$ be a Gaussian distribution with mean value 0 and standard deviation σ_1, and let $f_2(x)$ be a Gaussian distribution with mean value 0 and standard deviation σ_2. Compute

$$P(x) = \int_{-\infty}^{\infty} dx' f_1(x - x') f_2(x').$$

This integral is called the **convolution integral**. $P(x)$ describes the probability distribution of the sum of two independent random variables, one chosen from distibution $f_1(\cdot)$ and the other from distribution $f_2(\cdot)$. The results of this problem are used in many places, for example in the computation of the standard deviation of the distribution of synaptic potentials generated from the summation of several quanta (del Castillo and Katz, 1954).

✏️ **A.21** A cell at the left-hand border of a filamentous blue-green algae produces a pulse of 10^4 molecules at $t = 0$. The molecules diffuse with a diffusion coefficient of D $(cm^2 sec^{-1})$ and decay at a rate γ (sec^{-1}). The average number of molecules at time t in a cell of length Δx whose center is a distance x away from the left-hand border is $\Delta x P(x, t)$, where

$$P(x, t) = \frac{10^4}{\sqrt{\pi D t}} \exp \left(-\frac{x^2}{4Dt} - \gamma t \right).$$

a. Show that the time when the average number of molecules in a cell whose center is a distance x away from the left-hand border is a maximum is given by

$$t_{max} = -\frac{1}{4\gamma} + \frac{1}{4\gamma} \left(1 + \frac{4\gamma x^2}{D} \right)^{\frac{1}{2}}.$$

b. Consider a cell 10-μ long whose center is 50 μ from the left-hand border. Assume $D = 10^{-5}$ cm^2 sec^{-1}, $\gamma = 10^{-4}$ sec^{-1} $(1\mu = 10^{-4}$ cm). For this cell compute t_{max} and the average number of molecules in the cell at t_{max}.

✏️ **A.22** Consider a system in which the position as a function of time is $y(t) = k \sin \omega t$. Show that the curve in which $y(t + \tau)$ is plotted as a function of $y(t - \tau)$ is an ellipse.

✏️ **A.23** A series of action potentials in a nerve cell is described by the Poisson process. According to this, the probability that the time interval between an event and the second following event lies between t and $t + \Delta t$ is $p(t)\Delta t$, where

$$p(t) = R^2 t e^{-Rt}, \qquad t \geq 0,$$

where R is a positive constant.

a. Sketch $p(t)$ as a function of t. Show all maxima, minima, and inflection points.

b. Evaluate $\int_0^\infty p(t)dt$. What is the interpretation of this integral?

c. Evaluate $\int_0^\infty tp(t)dt$. What is the interpretation of this integral?

✎   **A.24** This question deals with random walks in 2 dimensions. A drunk man takes n steps. Each step is exactly 1 foot long and each step is in a randomly chosen direction. The probability that he will be at a distance lying between R and dR, where R is in feet is given by

$$P(R) = \frac{2R\ e^{-\frac{R^2}{n}}}{n}.$$

a. Evaluate the integral

$$\int_0^\infty P(R)\ dR.$$

b. Evaluate the integral

$$\int_0^\infty R\ P(R)\ dR.$$

What is your interpretation of this integral in terms of the random walk?

c. Consider the situation after the man has taken 20000 steps. Sketch $P(R)$. Be sure to indicate the value of the function and the slope of the function at $R = 0$, the value of the function at any maxima or minima, and the asymptotic behavior as $R \rightarrow \infty$. You do not need to calculate the inflection points.

d. After 20000 steps, the man has almost walked a total of almost 4 miles. However, do you expect to find him in a radius of 300 feet centered around his starting point? Explain and if possible justify with calculations.

APPENDIX B

A Note on Computer Notation

There is a very familiar notation for routine mathematical operations. For example, everyone knows that $u + b$ means "the sum of a and b," or that c^d means "raise c to the d power," or that e/f means "divide f into e." This notation is so common that it seems natural. It has in fact developed over hundreds of years.

The notation that has developed for algorithms and computer programs has not had such a long time to develop and become standardized. There are many different approaches to writing down an algorithm. One approach is to use pseudocode, wherein each step in an algorithm is described by English-language terms mixed with mathematics notation.

Another approach is to use a computer language such as FORTRAN or Pascal. The advantage of this approach over pseudocode is that the written form of the algorithm can easily be put on a computer. The disadvantage is that each computer language has its own quirks of syntax and notation that can be unfamiliar.

The approach we are taking here is to use a standard computer language, C, to describe the algorithms for drawing fractals. However, we are only using those parts of the language that are more or less self-explanatory so that there is no need to read a C-language manual in order to understand the examples given here. For the most part, the algorithms will be written in a `typewriter` font. Those parts of the algorithm that are of interest only to C programmers will be written in a different *italic* font: readers who are not interested in using C can safely ignore these *italized* parts of the algorithm.

Here is the small amount of knowledge of the C language that you will need to have to understand the algorithms in this chapter.

Variable assignment   In order to give a variable, say a, a value, say 7, we write a statement

```
a = 7;
```

The semicolon (;) simply indicates the end of the statement, just as a period indicates the end of an English-language sentence. The statement `a = b + c*d;` says to give the variable a the value b plus c times d.

Function evaluation   The mathematical notation for a function is something like $f(x)$ or $f(x, y)$. In C, the notation is almost exactly the same, `f(x);` or `f(x,y);`, a difference being that C-language functions often have a large number of arguments, like `f(a,b,c,d,e,f,g,h,i);`.

If we have a mathematical function $f(x) = \cos x$, then $f(\pi)$ is -1. A C-language function can work in just the same way: a statement like `a = cos(3.14159);` puts the value -1 into the variable a. In addition, C-language functions can do things other than calculations, like drawing shapes on a computer display or printer. For example, we can have a statement

```
drawLine(x1,y1,x2,y2);
```

which draws a line on a display from the point (x_1, y_1) to the point (x_2, y_2).

Function definition   Suppose we wanted to define a function, called `drawSquare(x1,y1,x2,y2)` that draws a square whose diagonal corners are the points (x_1, y_1) and (x_2, y_2). In the C language, this function would be defined as follows:

```
drawSquare(x1,y1,x2,y2)
  double x1,y1,x2,y2; (Ignore this line.)
{
    drawLine(x1,y1,x1,y2);
    drawLine(x1,y2,x2,y2);
    drawLine(x2,y2,x2,y1);
    drawLine(x2,y1,x1,y1);
}
```

This function uses the function `drawLine()` four times to draw the four lines that make up the square. The sequence of statements that makes up the function is enclosed in a pair of curly braces { }.

Conditionals   The statement

```
if( x >= 7 ) {
    a = b;
}
```

means: if the value of x is greater than or equal to 7, then give the variable a the value of the variable b, otherwise, don't do anything. Similarly, the series of statements

```
if( x >= 7 ) {
    a = b;
}
else {
    a = c;
}
```

means: if the value of x is greater than or equal to 7, set a to the value of b, otherwise set a to the value of c.

One quirk of C notation is that the test for equality involves a double equal sign, e.g.,

```
if( a == 4 ) {
/* do something when a equals 4 */
}
```

Contrast this to the single equal sign (=) used for assignment.

Recursion   Functions can contain themselves as one of their statements. For example, suppose we have a function defined as

```
silly(x)
  double x;
{
    print_out(x);
    if( x <= 10)
        silly(x+1);
}
```

prints out the value of the variable x, and then executes itself with the value $x + 1$. If the statement `silly(5);` were part of a program, the result would be a printout that looks like 5 6 7 8 9 10.

Recursion is closely related to self-similarity. This is used extensively in Chapter 3 where the fractal-drawing programs are recursive and reflect directly the self-similarity of the objects the programs draw.

Stuff you don't really need to know   Just in case you are curious, the italized statements like *double a;* are instructions to the computer that say what type of variable a is—in this case a double-precision floating point number. So far as non-computer-programmers are concerned, all the variables used here are just numbers, and follow all the familiar rules for addition, multiplication, etc.

Solutions to Selected Exercises

CHAPTER 1

✐ **1.4**

a. See Figure S.1.

b. There is a single fixed point at $x_t = 10$. The slope evaluated at the fixed point is -0.2. Therefore, the fixed point is stable and is approached in an oscillatory fashion.

c. This fixed point is approached as $t \to \infty$.

✐ **1.7**

a. There is a fixed point at $x_t = 0$. The slope evaluated at this fixed point is α. Therefore, this fixed point is stable for $\alpha < 1$ and unstable for $\alpha > 1$. The dynamics in the neighborhood of this fixed point are monotonic. There is a second fixed point at $x_t = \frac{\alpha-1}{\beta}$. However, since $x_t \geq 0$, this fixed point is found only for $\alpha > 1$. The slope evaluated at this fixed point is $\frac{1}{\alpha}$. Therefore, this fixed point is always stable and is approached in a monotonic fashion.

b. In this case you cannot determine stability for $\alpha = 1, \beta = 1$ by only determining the slope evaluated at $x_t = 0$. However, by drawing a graph and using the cobweb method you can determine that $x_t = 0$ is monotonically approached in the limit $t \to \infty$, and therefore $x_t = 0$ is a stable fixed point.

c. By algebraic iteration and induction, you can demonstrate that $x_{t+n} = \frac{x_t}{1+nx_t}$. Therefore, as $n \to \infty$, we find that $x_{t+n} \to 0$, in accord with part (b).

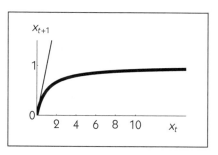

Figure S.1
Graph for Exercise 1.4.

Figure S.2
Graph for Exercise 1.7, part b.

 1.9

a. This is the graph of a hyperbola. There are no maxima, minima, or inflection points.
b. There is a single fixed point at $x_t = 115$ msec.
c. The slope evaluated at this fixed point is -0.6. Therefore, this fixed point is stable and is approached in an oscillatory fashion.
d. There is an oscillatory approach to the fixed point that is similar to "alternans" in cardiac electrophysiology.

 1.11 This problem looks a lot harder than it really is.

a. Since $\frac{pN_t^2}{1+N_t^2} \approx 0$, we have $N_{t+1} = N_t e^r$. Since $r > 0$, for $0 < N_0 \ll 1$ we have $N_1 > N_0$.

b. Now we find that $\frac{pN_t^2}{1+N_t^2} \approx p$, so that $N_{t+1} = N_t e^{r(1-p)}$. Since $p > 1$ and $r > 0$, $N_1 < N_0$ for $N_0 \gg 1$.

c. There are fixed points at $N_t = 0$ and $N_t = \frac{1}{\sqrt{p-1}}$.

d. Courage in carrying through the algebra is all that is needed.

$$\frac{dg(N_t)}{dN_t} - \left\{\left[\frac{-2prN_t^2}{(1+N_t^2)^2}\right] + 1\right\} \times \exp\left[r\left(1 - \frac{pN_t^2}{1+N_t^2}\right)\right].$$

e. There is a minimum at $N_t \approx 1.54$ and a maximum at $N_t \approx 0.65$.

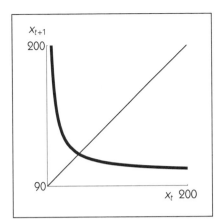

Figure S.3
Graph for Exercise 1.9.

f. The slope evaluated at $N_t = 0$ is e^r. Since this is greater than 1, this fixed point is always unstable. For $p = 2$, the second fixed point is at $N_t = 1$. The slope evaluated at this fixed point is ≈ -0.2 so that this fixed point is stable and is approached in an oscillatory fashion.

g. See Figure S.4.

1.12

a. See Figure S.5. There is a minimum at $x_t = 0$, a maximum at $x_t = \frac{4}{3}$, and an inflection point at $x_t = \frac{2}{3}$. The value of x_{t+1} at the maximum is $\frac{50}{27}$.

b. There are fixed points at $x_t = 0$, $x_t = \frac{2}{5}$, and $x_t = \frac{8}{5}$.

c. The slope evaluated at $x_t = 0$ is 0; this is a stable fixed point with a monotonic approach. The slope evaluated at $x_t = \frac{2}{5}$ is $\frac{7}{4}$; this is an unstable fixed point with a monotonic departure from the neighborhood of the fixed point. The slope evaluated at $x_t = \frac{8}{5}$ is -2; this is an unstable fixed point with an oscillatory departure from the neighborhood of the fixed point.

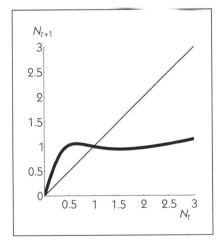

Figure S.4
Graph for Exercise 1.11.

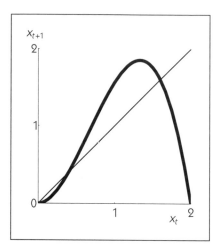

Figure S.5
Graph for Exercise 1.12.

d. Starting at $x_t = \frac{1}{3}$, the dynamics approach the fixed point at $x_t = 0$, since $\frac{1}{3} < \frac{2}{5}$. Starting at $x_t = 1$, you are in a different attractor (all points stay in the interval between about 0.79 and $\frac{50}{27}$). Therefore, you know that with the initial condition of $x_t = 1$ the system will not go to extinction. It takes further analysis to determine if the dyanamics are periodic or chaotic. This is an example of multistability, since there are 2 attractors.

   1.17

a. These are equations of parabolas. At the maximum $\phi_t = \frac{1}{4}$, and $\phi_{t+1} = \frac{3}{4}$. At the minimum, $\phi_t = \frac{3}{4}$ and $\phi_{t+1} = \frac{1}{4}$. (b) There are four fixed points. At the fixed points $\phi_t = 0$ and $\phi_t = 1$, the slope is 6; these fixed points are unstable with a monotonic departure from the neighborhood of the fixed point. At the fixed points $\phi_t = \frac{5}{12}$ and $\phi_t = \frac{7}{12}$, the slope is -4; these fixed points are unstable with oscillatory departure from the neighborhood of the fixed points. (c) The cycle of period 2 is between the two extremal points, $\phi_t = \frac{1}{4}$ and $\phi_t = \frac{3}{4}$. Since the cycle goes through extremal values it is guaranteed to be stable. (Actually, it is "superstable" since the slope is zero).

   1.19

a. See Figure S.7.

b. There are no fixed points.

c. Starting at $\phi_0 = 0.65$, there is a period 4 cycle $0.65 \rightarrow 0.45 \rightarrow 0.85 \rightarrow 0.25 \rightarrow 0.65 \rightarrow \ldots$. Starting at $\phi_0 = 0.95$, there is a period 5 cycle $0.95 \rightarrow 0.35 \rightarrow 0.75 \rightarrow 0.15 \rightarrow 0.55 \rightarrow 0.95 \rightarrow \ldots$.

d. Neither of these cycles is stable since starting at an initial condition close to a point on either cycle will lead to a different cycle. In the theoretical model this behavior would only occur if the ratio between the two frequencies of the cardiac oscillators is a rational number and if there is no interaction between the oscillators. These conditions would never be realized in practice.

   1.21 The dynamics are not chaotic but are quasiperiodic.

   1.22

d. At all points, the slope of the graph is greater than 1. Consequently, neighboring initial conditions will always diverge. Thus, there is sensitive dependence on initial conditions. Any graph of x_{t+n} versus x_t will also have a slope greater than 1, so all periodic cycles are unstable. (Remember, the slope of x_{t+n} versus x_t at any cycle $x_1, x_2, \ldots, x_n$ is given

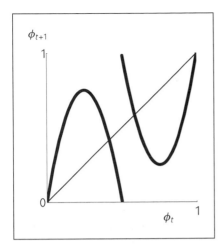

Figure S.6
Graph for Exercise 1.17.

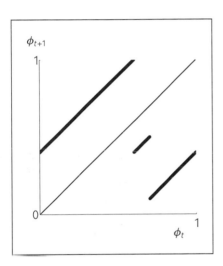

Figure S.7
Graph for Exercise 1.19.

by $\frac{df}{dx}\big|_{x_1}$, $\frac{df}{dx}\big|_{x_2}$, ..., $\frac{df}{dx}\big|_{x_n}$, which will be $m^n > 1$. The dynamics are also bounded and deterministic, so all four elements of the definition of chaos are satisfied.

CHAPTER 2

✏ **2.3**

a. $10 \rightarrow 11 \rightarrow 01 \rightarrow 00 \rightarrow 10 \rightarrow \ldots$

b. $100 \rightarrow 110 \rightarrow 111 \rightarrow 011 \rightarrow 001 \rightarrow 000 \rightarrow 100 \rightarrow \ldots$

c. For any value of n, there is a cycle of length $2n$. The cycle passes through the following states: $100\ldots00 \rightarrow 110\ldots00 \rightarrow \ldots \rightarrow 111\ldots10 \rightarrow 111\ldots11 \rightarrow 011\ldots11 \rightarrow 001\ldots11 \rightarrow \ldots \rightarrow 000\ldots01 \rightarrow 000\ldots00 \rightarrow 100\ldots00 \rightarrow \ldots$

2.5

b. The state in which all cells are 0 is a steady state. There are many different cycles in the network. For example, the state in which cells 1,3,5,6,7,8 are 1 is on a cycle of period 6. There cannot be chaos since this is a system with a finite number of states, and the dynamics must eventually repeat.

c. Without any work, we can say that the maximum cycle length must $< 2^{10}$. This is because there are 2^{10} different states of the system, and we already know from above that there is a steady state and a short cycle.

2.7

b. Any initial conditions in which at least one cell is 1 leads to a final state in which all the cells are 1.

c. The number of ways you can choose 3 cells out of 25 is $\frac{25 \times 24 \times 23}{3 \times 2 \times 1}$. The denominator is necessary because the order in which you pick the different cells does not matter. In this situation, if you take into consideration configurations that are the same under the symmetry of the square, the number of different configurations is much smaller. This computation is practically useful since it shows the way to compute the odds of winning lotteries in which you have to select several integers in a given range.

d. For an initial condition in which the three cells that are 1 are not adjacent to each other or the boundary, there is a transient of three iterations until the final state in which all cells are 1. Many other initial conditions also have a transient of length three, but some initial conditions have a longer transient.

2.9

a. We make the left side of Table S.1 just by writing down all the possible states in some convenient order. Then we use the transition information in the problem to match each entry with the succeeding state.

b. $x_{t+1} = \text{IDENTITY}(y_t)$. $y_{t+1} = \text{IDENTITY}(z_t)$. $z_{t+1} = \text{INVERSE}(x_t)$.

c. All the networks are frustrated networks with $n = 3$. For example, see Exercise 2.4, part (c) for another example. There are eight different networks of this sort and all have qualitatively similar dynamics. We can think about his by identifying each state with the corner of cube, as shown in Figure S.8. The truth table tells us the order in

Table S.1

xyz_t	xyz_{t+1}
000	001
001	011
010	101
011	111
100	000
101	010
110	100
111	110

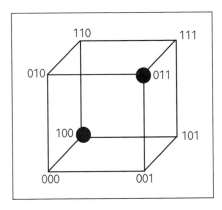

Figure S.8
Graph for Exercise 2.9.

which the corners are visited. To flip all three states in a cycle of length two, the order must connect two diagonally opposed corners. In a cube, there are 4 such pairs. The remaining 6 corners (i.e., states) must be visited in an order that involves walking down an edge of the cube, without backtracking. Each edge connects corners that differ by one state. There are two such paths that avoid the two corners already consumed by the cycle of period two. Altogether, we can find $4 \cdot 2 = 8$ such networks.

CHAPTER 4

4.3
a. $x(t) = x(0)e^{Ct}$.
b. $C = \frac{\ln 2}{20}$ hr$^{-1} \approx 0.0345$ hr^{-1}.
c. The density will increase to 8 times its initial size after 3 doublings. This takes 60 hr. The time to increase to 10 times the initial density is given by $\frac{\ln 10}{C} \approx 66.74$ hr.

4.4
a. Calling y the ratio $\frac{C^{14}}{C^{12}}$, we find that $y(t) = 1.6 \times 10^{-12}e^{-\alpha t}$, where the time is expressed in years and $\alpha = \frac{\ln 2}{5720}$ yr^{-1}.
b. The preserved sample has $\frac{1}{4}$ the amount of C^{14} as the original sample. Therefore it was formed approximately 11440 (5720 × 2) years ago.

4.5
a. Direct integration of the equation gives $p(t) = p(0)e^{\frac{-t}{\tau}}$.
b. Since $\int_0^\infty p(0)e^{\frac{-t}{\tau}} dt = \tau p(0)$, we find $p(0) = \frac{1}{\tau}$.
c. The fraction of channels that open at $s = 0$ and close by time t is given by $\int_0^t p(0)e^{\frac{-s}{\tau}} ds = \tau p(0) = 1 - e^{\frac{-t}{\tau}}$. Therefore, the theoretical expression for the percentage shown in the graph is $100(1 - e^{\frac{-t}{\tau}})$.
d. By examining the graph, we find that about 50% of the channels have closed by 15 msec so that $\tau \approx \frac{15}{\ln 2}$ msec ≈ 22 msec. Neurophysiologists carry out this sort of computation routinely.

4.7 This computation from a classical paper is based on the linear first order differential equation.
a. Taking the natural logarithm of both sides of the expression for β_n we find that $\ln \beta_n = \ln C_1 + \frac{V}{C_2}$. Therefore, in the graph of $\ln \beta_n$ versus V the y-intercept is $\ln C_1$ and the slope is $\frac{1}{C_2}$. We find that C_1 is approximately 0.11 msec^{-1} and C_2 is approximately 111

mv. The data in the original article, is based on data from several axons, whereas the data in this problem is based on data from only one axon.

b. This is the equation for exponential decay with a shift in the origin. The solution is

$$n(t) = n_0 e^{-(\alpha_n + \beta_n)t} + \frac{\alpha_n}{\alpha_n + \beta_n} \left[1 - e^{-(\alpha_n + \beta_n)t} \right].$$

c. Substituting the solution above into Eq. 4.26, and equating coefficients of corresponding terms leads to the following results. $g_{k\infty} = \left(\frac{\alpha_n}{\alpha_n + \beta_n} \right)^4 g_k$, $g_{k0} = n_0^4 \bar{g}_k$, and $\tau_n = \frac{1}{\alpha_n + \beta_n}$.

4.8 Although this problem uses partial derivatives, at each point in space there is an exponential approach to a homogeneneous solution, and the problem can be done using concepts in Chapter 4.

   b. At $t = 0$, we have $C(x, 0) = C_0 \left[1 - \frac{2}{\pi} \cos \left(\frac{\pi x}{L} \right) \right]$, and at $t \to \infty$, we have $C(x, \infty) = C_0$.

   d. Calling $t_{\frac{1}{2}}$ the time needed to go one-half way from the initial to the final concentration at each point, we find

$$C(x, t_{\frac{1}{2}}) = \frac{1}{2} [C(x, \infty) - C(x, 0)] + C(x, 0).$$

   Substituting the expressions found above, we determine $t_{\frac{1}{2}} = \frac{L^2 \ln 2}{\pi^2 D}$. Substituting the values in the text, we have $t_{\frac{1}{2}} = 7.0 \times 10^5$ sec. This gives a good idea for the time constant for homogenization from an initial nonuniform distribution of an electrolyte in an aqueous solution in a 10 cm tube.

4.12

a. This is the equation for exponential growth, $\frac{dV}{dt} = kV$, where V is the tumor volume and k is a constant.

b. The solution of this equation is $V(t) = V(0)e^{kt}$, where $k = \frac{\ln 2}{138}$ days$^{-1} \approx 5 \times 10^{-3}$ days^{-1}. Since $V = \frac{4}{3} \pi r^3$ where r is the tumor radius, we find $r(t) = r(0)e^{\frac{kt}{3}}$.

c. From the above if $\ln r(t)$ is plotted as a function of t, the y-intercept is $\ln r(0)$ and the slope is $\frac{5}{3} \times 10^{-3}$ days^{-1}.

4.17

a. There are fixed points at $x = 0$, $x = 1$, and $x = \frac{-1+\sqrt{5}}{2} \approx 0.618$. The last fixed point must exist from the graph, but can also be computed algebraically, once the other 2 fixed points are known by factoring the original fourth order equation and using the quadratic formula.

b. The slope evaluated at the fixed at $x = 0$ is -1. Since this is negative, the fixed point is stable. Similarly, the slope evaluated at the fixed point $x = 1$ is $-\frac{1}{2}$, so this fixed point is also stable. The slope evaluated at the fixed point at $x \approx 0.618$ is ≈ 0.42 which is greater than 0, so this fixed point is unstable. Notice that there is alternation of stability of the fixed points in this problem.

c. All initial conditions between $x = 0$ and the fixed point at $x \approx 0.618$ approach the origin as $t \to \infty$, whereas all other initial conditions approach the fixed point at $x = 1$ as $t \to \infty$.

4.20

a. The amount of drug in the body following the last dose is given by $(D_0 + 100)e^{-\alpha t}$ mg, where $\alpha = \frac{\ln 2}{4}$ hr^{-1}.

b. As an approximation, we can assume that after 10 days of the drug administration, the level of drug is the same just before each new dose is given: $(D_0 + 100)e^{-4\alpha} = D_0$. Since $e^{-4\alpha} = \frac{1}{2}$, we find that $D_0 = 100$ mg. In choosing timing for drug administration, the half-life must be taken into account.

4.21

c. $c_1 = \ln A - \ln \omega_0; c_2 = \omega_0; c_3 = -1$.

CHAPTER 5

5.5

a. See Figure S.9.

b. See Figure S.10.

c. From the sketch you should see that starting from an initial condition of $r(0) = r_0$ and $\mu(0) = 0$, μ first increases and then decreases, whereas r monotonically decreases. In the limit $t \to \infty$ both approach 0. Call t_{max} the time when μ is a maximum. From the graph, we have $\mu(t_{max}) = \frac{k_1}{k_2} r(t_{max})$.

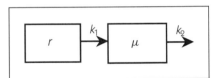

Figure S.9
Graph for Exercise 5.5.

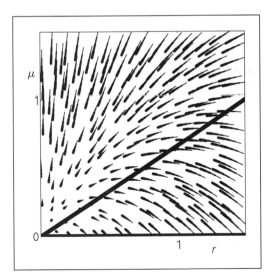

Figure S.10   Diagram for Exercise 5.5, part b. The thin line shows the r-isocline, and the thick line shows the μ-isocline.

d. $\frac{d^2\mu}{dt^2} + (k_1 + k_2)\frac{d\mu}{dt} + k_1k_2\mu = 0.$

e. $r(t) = r_0e^{-k_1t}$; $\mu(t) = \frac{k_1r_0}{k_2-k_1}e^{-k_1t} - \frac{k_1r_0}{k_2-k_1}e^{-k_2t}$. From the above result, by taking the derivative of μ with respect to time, and setting equal to 0, we determine that $k_2e^{-k_2t_{max}} = k_1e^{-k_1t_{max}}$. Substituting the analytic expressions for $\mu(t)$ and $r(t)$ at t_{max}, we once again obtain $\mu(t_{max}) = \frac{k_1}{k_2}r(t_{max})$. This example shows how a graphical analysis of a linear second order differential equation can provide information about the dynamics. The same information can be obtained from the analytical solution, but only after a bit of a struggle.

5.7

a. $\frac{d^2y}{dt^2} + (2\alpha + \gamma)\frac{dy}{dt} + \alpha\gamma = 0.$

b. The characteristic equation is $\lambda^2 + (2\alpha + \gamma)\lambda + \alpha\gamma = 0$. Solving this quadratic equation we find

$$\lambda_1 = \frac{-(2\alpha + \gamma) + \sqrt{4\alpha^2 + \gamma^2}}{2}, \qquad \lambda_2 = \frac{-(2\alpha + \gamma) - \sqrt{4\alpha^2 + \gamma^2}}{2}.$$

When $\gamma \gg \alpha$, $\sqrt{4\alpha^2 + \gamma} \approx \gamma$ and taking the positive sign we compute $\lambda_1 \approx -\alpha$, and taking the negative sign, we find that $\lambda_2 \approx -\gamma$.

c. The solution is $y(t) = c_1e^{\lambda_1t} + c_2e^{\lambda_2t}$. Using the initial conditions $y(0) = 0$ and $dy/dt(0) = \alpha N$, we find $c_1 + c_2 = 0$ and $\lambda_1c_1 + \lambda_2c_2 = \alpha N$, giving $c_1 = \frac{\alpha N}{\lambda_1-\lambda_2}$ and $c_2 = -\frac{\alpha N}{\lambda_1-\lambda_2}$. For $\gamma \gg \alpha$, we have $\lambda_1 - \lambda_2 \approx \gamma$, so that $y(t) \approx \frac{\alpha N}{\gamma}e^{-\alpha t} - \frac{\alpha N}{\gamma}e^{-\gamma t}$.

d. Taking the derivative of y and setting it equal to 0, we find that y is a maximum at $t \approx -\ln 10^{-3}$ hr ≈ 6.9 hr. Substituting this value for the expression for $y(t)$, the maximum value of y is approximately $10^{-3}N$ — only $1/1000$ of the drug dose. Although this is a hypothetical example, an important problem in chemotherapy is to get a sufficient quantity of drug to the target organ.

e. Since $\gamma \gg \alpha$ most of the destruction of x for short times comes about by a process of exponential decay so that $x(t) \approx x(0)e^{-\gamma t}$. Therefore, the time when x has fallen to half its initial value is well approximated by $t_{\frac{1}{2}} \approx \frac{\ln 2}{\gamma} \approx 0.69$ hr.

5.11

a. See Figure S.11.

c. $\frac{d^2y}{dt^2} + (k_1 + k_2 + k_3)\frac{dy}{dt} + k_1(k_2 + k_3)y = 0.$

d. The eigenvalues are $\lambda_1 = \alpha + \beta$ and $\lambda_2 = \alpha - \beta$ where $\alpha = \frac{-(k_1+k_2+k_3)}{2}$ and $\beta = \frac{\sqrt{(k_1+k_2+k_3)^2-4k_1k_2}}{2}$. The solution of the differential equation is $y(t) = c_1e^{\lambda_1t} + c_2e^{\lambda_2t}$ where $c_1 = \frac{1}{2} + \frac{k_1-k_2-k_3}{4\beta}$ and $c_2 = \frac{1}{2} - \frac{k_1-k_2-k_3}{4\beta}$.

e. (i) If $k_1 = 0$, then there are no transitions from S_1 to S_2. For this case we find $y(t) = e^{-(k_1+k_3)t}$. (ii) If $k_3 = 0$, there will never be any population of S_1 and $y(t) = e^{-k_2t}$. The special cases here also follow from the general formulae in part (d). This provides a partial check on the computations.

5.13

a. Since the solution is a sum of three exponentials it can be generated from a third order ordinary differetial equation.

b. For $t > 180$ min, the solution of the equation is approximately $c(t) = x(180)e^{-\frac{t-180}{65.7}}$ since the other 2 terms are negligible by this time. The half-life for this exponential decay is approximately $\ln 2 \times 65.7$ min ≈ 45 min. Therefore, at 225 min the concentration will be approximately half of what it was at 180 min.

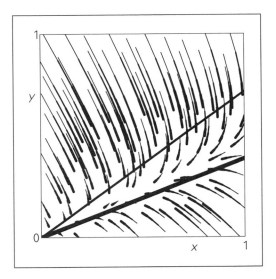

Figure S.11   Diagram for Exercise 5.11, part a. Flow in the x, y plane. The x-isocline is the thin line, and the y-isocline is the thick line.

c. The time constant of 65.7 min is associated with elimination of lidocaine from the plasma. This could be associated with several different physiological processes such as degradation in the liver or by circulating enzymes, or excretion in the kidneys.

5.16

a. There are three steady states: $s = 0, l = 0$; $s = 1, l = 0$; $s = \frac{3}{4}, l = \frac{1}{4}$.
b. The only steady state that does not have one of the variables equal to zero, at $s = \frac{3}{4}, l = \frac{1}{4}$, is a stable focus.
c. See Figure S.12.
d. Notice that from the equations, if the initial value of any variable is 0, then it is 0 for all future times. We therefore find: conditions (i) and (ii) approach the origin as $t \to \infty$; condition (iii) leads to a state in which $s = 1, l = 0$ at $t \to \infty$; condition (iv) leads to $s = \frac{3}{4}, l = \frac{1}{4}$ as $t \to \infty$.

5.19

a. There are three steady states: $(x^* = 0, y^* = 0)$, $(x^* = 1, y^* = 1)$ and $(x^* = 4, y^* = 4)$.
b. We start by linearizing the original equations:

$$\frac{dx}{dt} = f(x, y) = y - x$$

$$\frac{dy}{dt} = g(x, y) = \frac{5x^2}{4 + x^2} - y$$

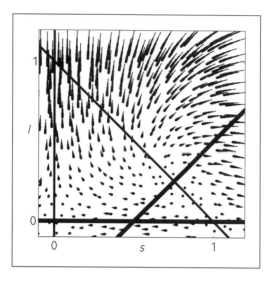

Figure S.12
Diagram for Exercise 5.16.
Flow in the s, l plane. The
s-isoclines are the thin
lines, the l-isoclines are
the thick lines

in order to find

$$A = \left.\frac{\partial f}{\partial x}\right|_{(x^*, y^*)} \qquad B = \left.\frac{\partial f}{\partial y}\right|_{(x^*, y^*)}$$

$$C = \left.\frac{\partial g}{\partial x}\right|_{(x^*, y^*)} \qquad D = \left.\frac{\partial g}{\partial y}\right|_{(x^*, y^*)}$$

At $x^* = 0$, $y^* = 0$, we find $A = -1$, $B = 1$, $C = 0$, and $D = -1$. The eigenvalues
are therefore -1, -1 so this is a stable node. (We can do the same analysis using linear
algebra. The characteristic equation is

$$\begin{vmatrix} -1 - \lambda & 1 \\ 0 & -1 - \lambda \end{vmatrix} = 0$$

This is equivalent to the quadratic equation $\lambda^2 + 2\lambda + 1 = 0$.)

At $x^* = 1$, $y^* = 1$, we linearize to find $A = -1$, $B = 1$, $C = \frac{8}{5}$, and
$D = -1$. The eigenvalues are therefore $\frac{-2 \pm \sqrt{\frac{32}{5}}}{2}$. One of these is positive and the
other is negative, so this is a saddle point.

At $x^* = 4$, $y^* = 4$, we find $A = -1$, $B = 1$, $C = \frac{2}{5}$, and $D = -1$. The
eigenvalues are therefore $\frac{-2 \pm \sqrt{\frac{8}{5}}}{2}$. Both of these are negative real numbers so this is a
stable node.

c. See Figure S.13.
d. Depending on the initial condition the state asymptotically approaches either the steady
state at the origin or the steady state at $x = 4$, $y = 4$. Since there are two stable steady
states in the same equation, this type of mechanism could be a model for differentiation.

5.21
a. There is a steady state at $x_1 = \frac{1}{\sqrt{2}}$, $x_2 = 1$.

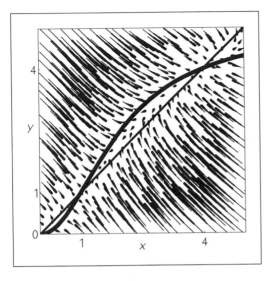

Figure S.13
Diagram for Exercise 5.19.
Flow in the x, y plane.
The x-isocline is the thin
line, the y-isocline is the
thick curve.

b. Linearizing, we find $A = -k$, $B = -\frac{n}{2}$, $C = 1$, and $D = -k$. The eigenvalues are therefore $-k \pm i\,\frac{n}{2}$. Independent of the value of n, the eigenvalues are imaginary with a negative real part. Therefore, the steady state is always a stable focus.

c. See Figure S.14.

5.23

a. There are three steady states: $y = 0$, $x = 0$; $y = 0$, $x = 1$; $y = 0$, $x = -1$.

b. The steady state at $x = 0$, $y = 0$ is a saddle point, whereas the other two steady states are stable foci.

c. See Figure S.15.

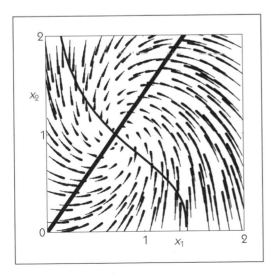

Figure S.14
Diagram for Exercise 5.21.
Flow in the x_1, x_2 plane
for $n = 3$, $K^2 = 1/2$.
The x_1-isocline is the thin
curve. The x_2-isocline is
the thick line.

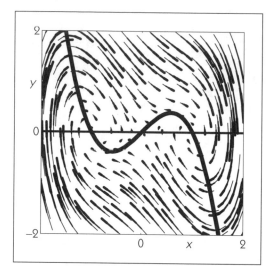

Figure S.15
Diagram for Exercise 5.15.
Flow in the x, y plane.
The x-isocline is the thin
line. The y-isocline is the
thick curve.

d. An initial condition $x(0) = 0$, $y(0) > 0$ approaches the stable focus at $y = 0$, $x = 1$
    in the limit $t \to \infty$.

✎   **5.25**

a. See Figure S.16.

b. There are three steady states: $x = -\sqrt{\frac{18}{5}}$, $y = 0$; $x = 0$, $y = 0$; and $x = 2$, $y = \frac{1}{2}$.

c. See Figure S.16.

d. Linearizing the equation at $x = 0$, $y = 0$, we find $A = \frac{9}{4}$, $B = 1$, $C = 0$, and
    $D = -1$. The eigenvalues are therefore $\frac{9}{4}$ and -1 so this is a saddle point.

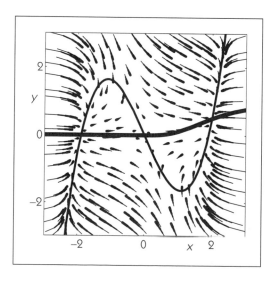

Figure S.16
Diagram for Exercise 5.16.
Flow in the x, y plane.
The x-isocline is the thin
curve. The y-isocline is
the thick curve.

At $x = -\sqrt{\frac{18}{5}}$, $y = 0$, we have $A = -\frac{18}{4}$, $B = 1$, $C = 0$, and $D = -1$. The eigenvalues are therefore $-\frac{18}{4}$ and -1, so this is a stable node.

At $x = 2$, $y = \frac{1}{2}$, $A = -\frac{21}{4}$, $B = 1$, $C = \frac{3}{8}$, and $D = -1$. The eigenvalues are therefore $\frac{-\frac{25}{4} \pm \sqrt{\left(\frac{25}{4}\right)^2 - \frac{39}{2}}}{2}$. Both of these are negative real numbers so the steady state is a stable node.

Depending on the initial condition the state asymptotically approaches either the steady state at $x = -\sqrt{\frac{18}{5}}$, $y = 0$, or the steady state at $x = 2$, $y = \frac{1}{2}$. Many models in neurobiology associate different stable steady states with different "memories", but this equation does not model a realistic situation.

APPENDIX A

A.6

c. If the function $f(x)$ is described by the Hill function, then the Hill plot is a straight line with slope n and with y-intercept $-n \ln \theta$.

A.16

a. For a point a distance r away from the point source, the number density is a maximum at time $t = \frac{r^2}{2nD}$, where n is the number of dimensions and D is the diffusion coefficient. This is an important result since it gives you an easy way to estimate the time scale for diffusion.

b. The distance from the microelectrode to the neuron is 3×10^{-4} cm.

A.24

a. This integral is equal to 1. It must be since it is the probability the man is somewhere.

b. This integral is the average displacement from the origin. It is equal to $\frac{\sqrt{\pi n}}{2}$.

c. From the formula in (b), the average displacement displacement is about 125 feet. Therefore, the man is likely to be in a circle of a radius of 300 feet centered around his starting point. For an exact computation, you know that the total probability that the man is in a circle of radius K after n steps is

$$\int_0^K P(R) dR = 1 - e^{-\frac{K^2}{n}} \approx 0.99$$

Notice that the dispacement increases as the square root of the number of steps.

Bibliography

Abarbanel, H. D. I. , Brown, R., Sidorowich, J. J., and Tsimring, L. S., (1993). The analysis of observed chaotic data in physical systems, *Rev. Mod. Phys.*, **65**, 1331–92.

Alberts, B., Bray, D., Lewis, J., Raff, M., Roberts, K., and Watson, J. D. (1983). *Molecular Biology of the Cell*. New York: Garland Publishing.

Ascioti, F. A., Beltrami, E., Carroll, T. O., and Wirick, C. (1993). Is there chaos in plankton dynamics? *J. Plankton Res.* **15**, 603–17.

Baker, G. L. and Gollub, J. P. (1990). *Chaotic Dynamics: An Introduction.* Cambridge: Cambridge University Press.

Barnsley, M. F. (1992). *Fractals Everywhere, 2nd edition.* New York: Academic Press.

Bass, T. A. (1985). *The Eudaemonic Pie: Or Why Would Anyone Play Roulette without a Computer in His Shoe?* Boston: Houghton Mifflin.

Bassingthwaighte, J. B., Liebovitch, L. S., and West, B. J. (1994). *Fractal Physiology.* New York: Oxford University Press.

Bélair, J., and Glass, L. (1983). Self similarity in periodically forced oscillators. *Phys. Lett.* **96A**, 113–16.

Bendat, J. S., and Piersol, A. G. (1971). *Random Data: Analysis and Measurement Procedures.* New York: John Wiley and Sons.

Berger R. D., Saul J. P., and Cohen R. J. (1989). Transfer function analysis of autonomic regulation. I. Canine atrial rate response. *Am. J. Physiol.* **256**, H142–H152.

Blaxter, K. L., Graham, N. M. and Wainman, F. W. (1956). Some observations on the digestibility of food by sheep, and on related problems. *Brit. J. Nut.* **10**, 69–91.

Bray, W. C. (1921). A periodic reaction in homogeneous solution and its relation to catalysis. *J. Am. Chem. Soc.* **43**, 1262–67.

Box, G. E. P. and Jenkins, G. M. (1976). Time series analysis forecasting and control. San Francisco: Holden-Day.

Bullough, W. S., and Laurence, E. B. (1968). Chalones and cancer. *Nature* **220**, 134–35.

Casdagli, M. (1989). Nonlinear prediction of chaotic time series. *Physica D* **35**, 335–56.

Casdagli, M., Eubank S., Farmer, J. D., and Gibson, J. (1991). State space reconstruction in the presence of noise. *Physica D* **51**, 52–98.

Chahinian, A. P., and Israel, L. (1976). Rates and patterns of growth of lung cancer. In: Israel, L. and Chahinian, A. P., eds. *Lung Cancer: Natural History, Prognosis, and Therapy.* New York: Academic Press, 63–79

Chen, C. T. (1984). *Linear System Theory and Design,* New York: Holt, Rinehart, and Winston.

Chess, G. F., and Caleresu, F. R. (1971). Frequency response model of vagal control of heart rate in the cat. *Am. J. Physiol.* **220**, 554–57.

Chou, T.-C. (1991). *Electrocardiology in Clinical Practice, 3rd Edition.* Philadelphia: W. B. Saunders Co.

Cooper, E., and Shrier, A. (1985). Single-channel analysis of fast transient potassium currents from rat nodose neurones. *J. Physiol.* **369**, 199–208.

Cotton, F. A., and Wilkinson, G. (1980). *Advanced Inorganic Chemistry: A Comprehensive Text, 4th edition.* New York: Wiley-Interscience.

Crutchfield, J. P., Farmer, J. D., Packard, N. H., and Shaw, R. S. (1986). Chaos. *Scientific American* **255** (Dec.), 46–57.

Crutchfield, J. P., and Young, K. (1990). Computation at the onset of chaos. In: Zurek, W., ed. *Entropy, Complexity, and the Physics of Information. SFI Stud. Sci. Complexity, Proc. Vol. VIII.* Reading, MA: Addison-Wesley, 223–69.

Crutchfield, J. P., and Mitchell, M. (1994). The evolution of emergent computation. *SFI Tech. Rep.* SFI-94-03-012. *Proc. Natl. Acad. Sci.* (USA) (submitted).

Cvitanovic, P., ed. (1989). *Universality in Chaos, 2nd edition.* Bristol: Adam Hilger.

Das, R. Mitchell, M., and Crutchfield, J. P. (1994). A genetic algorithm discovers particle-based computation in cellular automata. In: Davidov, Y., Schwefel, H.-P., and Männer, R., eds. *Lect. Notes Comp. Sci.* Berlin: Springer-Verlag, 344–53.

Davidenko, J. M., Pertsov, A. V., Salomonosz, R., Baxter, W., and Jalife, J. (1992). Stationary and drifting waves of excitation in isolated cardiac muscle. *Nature* **355**, 349–51.

del Castillo, J. and Katz, B. (1954). Quantal components of the end-plate potential. *J. Physiol.* **124**, 560–73.

de Silva, J. A. F., Bekersky, I., and Puglisis, C. V. (1974). Spectrofluorodensitometric determination of flurazepam and its major metabolites in blood. *J. Pharm. Sci.* **63**, 1837–41.

Devaney, R. L. (1992). *A First Course in Chaotic Dynamical Systems: Theory and Experiment.* Reading, MA: Addison-Wesley.

Eckmann, J.-P., Kamphorst, S. O. and Ruelle, D. (1987). Recurrence plots of dynamical systems. *Europhys. Lett.* **4**, 973–77.

Edelstein-Keshet, L. (1988). *Mathematical Models in Biology.* New York: Random House.

Eden, M. (1961). A two-dimensional growth process. In: Neyman, J., ed. *Proceedings of the Fourth Berkeley Symposium on Mathematical Statistics and Probablility, Volume IV: Biology and Problems of Health.* Berkeley: University of California Press, 223–82.

Edgar, G. A., ed. (1993). *Classics on Fractals.* Reading, MA: Addison-Wesley.

Ermentrout, G. B., and Edelstein-Keshet, L. (1993). Cellular automata approaches to biological modeling. *J. Theor. Biol.* **160**, 97–133.

Eubank, S. and Farmer, D. (1990). An introduction to chaos and randomness. In: Jen, E., ed. *1989 Lectures in Complex Systems. SFI Stud. Sci. Complexity, Lect. Vol. II,* Reading, MA: Addison-Wesley.

Family, F., and Vicsek, T., eds. (1991). *Dynamics of Fractal Surfaces.* Singapore: World Scientific.

Farmer, J. D., and Sidorowich, J. S. (1987). Predicting chaotic time series. *Phys. Rev. Lett.,* **62**, 845–48.

Fatt, P., and Katz, B. (1951). An analysis of the end-plate potential recorded with an intra-cellular electrode. *J. Physiol.* **115**, 320–70.

Feigenbaum, M. J. (1980). Universal behavior in nonlinear systems. *Los Alamos Sci.* **1**, 4–27. This paper is reprinted in Cvitanovic (1989).

Folkman, J., and Hochberg, M. (1973). Self-regulation of growth in three dimensions. *J. Exp. Med.* **4**, 745–53.

Franklin, G. F., Powell, J. D., and Emami-Naeini, A. (1994). *Feedback Control of Dynamic Systems, 3rd edition.* Reading, MA: Addison-Wesley.

Gatewood, L. C., Ackerman, E., Rosevear, J. W., and Molnar, G. D. (1968). Simulation studies of blood-glucose regulation: Effect of intestinal glucose absorption. *Comput. Biomed. Res.* **2**, 15–27.

Gause, G. F. (1932). Experimental studies on the struggle for existence. I. Mixed populations of two species of yeast. *J. Exp. Biol.* **9**, 389–42.

Gelb, A., ed. and the Technical Staff of the Analytic Sciences Corporation (1974). *Applied Optimal Estimation.* Cambridge, MA: MIT Press.

Gerhardt, M., Schuster, H., and Tyson, J. J. (1990). A cellular automaton model of excitable media including curvature and dispersion. *Science* **247**, 1563–66.

Glantz, S. A. (1979). *Mathematics for Biomedical Applications.* Berkeley and Los Angeles: University of California Press.

Glass, L. (1969). Moiré effect from random dots. *Nature* **223**, 578–80.

Glass, L. (1975). Combinatorial and topological methods in nonlinear chemical kinetics. *J. Chem. Phys.* **63**, 1325–35.

Glass, L., and Mackey, M. C. (1979). Pathological conditions resulting from instabilities in physiological control systems. *Ann. N. Y. Acad. Sci.* **316**, 214–35.

Glass L., and Mackey, M. C. (1988). *From Clocks to Chaos: The Rhythms of Life.* Princeton, NJ: Princeton University Press.

Glass, L., and Pasternack, J. S. (1978). Stable oscillations in mathematical models of biological control systems. *J. Math. Biol.* **6**, 207–23.

Glass, L., and Perez, R. (1973). Perception of random dot interference patterns. *Nature* **246**, 360–62.

Glass, L., and Perez, R. (1982). Fine structure of phase locking. *Phys. Rev. Lett.* **48**, 1772–75.

Glass, L., and Young, R. (1979). Structure and dynamics of neural network oscillators. *Brain Res.* **179**, 207–18.

Glass, L., Goldberger, A., and Bélair, J. (1986). Dynamics of pure parasystole. *Am. J. Physiol.* **251**. (*Heart Circ. Physiol.* **20**), H841–H847.

Glass, L., Guevara, M. R., Bélair, J., and Shrier, A. (1984). Global bifurcations of a periodically forced biological oscillator. *Phys. Rev. A* **29**, 1348–57.

Gleick, J. (1987). *Chaos: The Making of a New Science.* New York: Viking.

Grassberger, P., Schreiber, T., and Scharrrath, C. (1991). Nonlinear time sequence analysis, *Int. J. Bifurcat. Chaos* **1**, 521–47.

Grassberger, P., and Procaccia I. (1983). Characterization of strange attractors. *Phys. Rev. Lett.* **50**, 346–49.

Grodins, F. S. (1963). *Control Theory and Biological Systems.* New York: Columbia University Press.

Guckenhiemer, J., and Holmes, P. (1983). *Nonlinear Oscillations, Dynamical Systems, and Bifurcations of Vector Fields.* New York: Springer-Verlag.

Guevara, M. R., Glass, L., and Shrier, A. (1981). Phase locking, period-doubling bifurcations and irregular dynamics in periodically stimulated cardiac cells. *Science* **214**, 1350–53.

Guillemin, V., and Pollack, A. (1974). *Differential Topology.* Englewood Cliffs, NJ: Prentice-Hall.

Gurney, W. S. C., Blythe, S. P., and Nisbet, R. M. (1980). Nicholson's blowflies revisited. *Nature* **287**, 17–21.

Hao, B.-L. (1984). *Chaos.* Singapore: World Scientific.

Hirsch, M. W., and Smale, S. (1974). *Differential Equations, Dynamical Systems, and Linear Algebra.* New York: Academic Press.

Hodgkin, A. L., and Huxley, A. F. (1952). A quantitative description of the membrane current and its application to conduction and excitation in nerve. *J. Physiol.* **117**, 500–44.

Hohn, F. E. (1966). *Applied Boolean Algebra, 2nd edition.* New York: Macmillan.

Holden, A. V. (1986). *Chaos.* Manchester, UK: Manchester University Press.

Holland, J. H. (1975). *Adaptation in Natural and Artificial Systems, 2nd edition.* Cambridge, MA: MIT Press.

Hunter, F. N., Jr. (1992). Application of nonlinear time-series models to driven systems. In: Casdagli, M., and Eubank, S., eds. *Nonlinear Modeling and Forecasting, SFI Stud. Sci. Complexity, Proc. Vol. XII.* Reading, MA: Addison-Wesley.

Isidori, A. (1989). *Nonlinear Control Systems: An Introduction, 2nd edition.* New York: Springer-Verlag.

Jacob, F., and Monod, J. (1961). General conclusions: Teleonomic mechanisms in cellular metabolism, growth, and differentiation. *Cold Spring Harbor Symp. Quant. Bio.* **26**, 389–401.

Jenkins, G. M., and Watts, D. G. (1968). Spectral analysis and its applications. San Francisco: Holden-Day.

Jordon, D. W., and Smith, P. (1987). *Nonlinear Ordinary Differential Equations, 2nd edition.* Oxford: Clarendon Press.

Kailath, T. (1980). *Linear Systems.* Englewood Cliffs, NJ: Prentice-Hall.

Kaplan, D. T., and Cohen, R. J. (1990). Is fibrillation chaos? *Circ. Res.* **67**, 886–92.

Kaplan, D. T., and Glass L. (1992). Direct test for determinism in a time series. *Phys. Rev. Lett.* **68**, 427–30.

Kaplan, D. T., and Glass L. (1993). Coarse-grained embeddings of time series: random walks, gaussian random processes, and deterministic chaos. *Physica D* **64**, 431–54

Kaplan, D. T. (1994). Exceptional events as evidence for determinism, *Physica D* **73**, 38–48.

Katz, B., and Miledi, R. (1965). The measurement of the synaptic delay, and the time course of acetylcholine release at the neuromuscular junction. *Proc. Roy. Soc. B* **161**, 483–95.

Kauffman, S. A. (1969). Metabolic stability and epigenesis in randomly constructed genetic nets. *J. Theor. Biol.* **22**, 437–67.

Kauffman, S. A. (1993). *Origins of Order.* Oxford: Oxford University Press.

Kennel, M. B., Brown, R., Abarbanel, H. D. I. (1992). Determining minimum embedding dimension using a geometrical construct. *Phys. Rev. A* **45**, 3403–11.

Klein, G., and Révész, L. (1953). Quantitative studies on the multiplication of neoplastic cells. In vivo: I. Growth curves of the Ehrlich and MCIM ascites tumors. *J. Nat. Cancer Inst.* **14**, 229–77.

Kóvacs, I., and Julesz, B. (1992). Depth, motion and static-flow perception at metaisoluminant color contrast. *Proc. Natl. Acad. Sci.* **89**, 10390–94.

Lacker, H. M. (1981). Regulation of ovulation number in mammals. A follicle interaction law that controls maturation. *Biophys. J.* **35**, 433–54.

Laird, A. K. (1964). Dynamics of tumor growth. *Brit. J. Cancer* **18**, 490–502.

Lechleiter, J., Girard, S., Peralta, F., and Clapham, D. (1991). Spiral calcium wave propagation and annihilation in *Xenopis laevis* oocytes. *Science* **252**, 123–26.

Lewin, R. (1992). *Complexity: Life at the Edge of Chaos.* New York: Macmillan.

Li, T.-Y., and Yorke, J. (1975). Period three implies chaos. *Am. Math. Monthly* **82**, 985–92.

Liotta, L., and DeLisi, C. (1977). Method for quantitating tumor cell removal and tumor cell-invasive capacity in experimental metastases. *Cancer Res.* **37**, 4003–08.

Lorenz, E. N. (1964a). The problem of deducing the climate from the governing equations. *Tellus* **16**, 1–11.

Lorenz, E. N. (1964b). Deterministic nonperiodic flow. *J. Atmos. Sci.* **20**, 130–41.

Lotka, A. J. (1956). *Elements of Mathematical Biology.* New York: Dover Publications. (This is a reprint of the 1924 classic, *Elements of Mathematical Biology*, by Lotka, A. J., originally published by The Williams and Wilkins Co.)

Mackey, M. C., and Glass, L. (1977). Oscillation and chaos in physiological control systems. *Science* **197**, 287–89.

Mandelbrot, B. (1977). *Fractals: Form, Chance, and Dimension.* San Francisco: Freeman.

Mandelbrot, B. (1982). *The Fractal Geometry of Nature.* San Francisco: Freeman.

Mann, J. M., Chin, J., Piot, P., and Quinn, T. (1988). The international epidemiology of AIDS. *Scientific American* **259**, 82–89.

Marr, D. (1982). *Vision: A Computational Investigation into the Human Representation and Processing of Visual Information.* San Francisco: Freeman.

Martinez-Mekler, G.C., Mondragón, R., and Pérez, R. (1986). Basin-structure invariance of circle maps with bistable dynamics. *Phys. Rev. A* **33**, 2143–45.

Matsuura, S., and Miyazama, S. (1993). Colony of the fungus *Aspergillus oryzae* and self-affine fractal geometry of growth fronts. *Fractals* **1**, 11–19.

May, R. M. (1976). Simple mathematical models with very complicated dynamical behavior. *Nature* **261**, 459–67.

May, R. M. (1977). Thresholds and breakpoints in ecosystems with a multiplicity of stable states. *Nature* **269**, 471–77.

Meakin, P. (1988). Simple models for colloidal aggregation, dielectric breakdown and mechanical breakdown patterns. In: Stanley, H. E. and Ostrowsky, N., eds. *Random Fluctuations and Pattern Growth: Experiments and Models.* Dordrecht: Kluwer, 174–91.

Metropolis, N., Stein, M. L., and Stein, P. R. (1973). On finite limit sets for transformations on the unit interval. *J. Comb. Theory* **15**, 25–44.

Milhorn, H. T. (1966). *The Application of Control Theory to Physiological Systems.* Philadelphia: Saunders.

Milton, J. G., and Bélair, J. (1990). Chaos, noise and extinction in models of population growth. *Theor. Pop. Biol.* **37**, 273–90.

Mitchell, M., Hraber, P. T., and Crutchfield, J. P. (1993). Revisiting the edge of chaos: Evolving cellular automata to perform computations. *Complex Systems* **7**, 89–130.

Monod, J., Wyman, J., and Changeux, J. P. (1965). On the nature of allosteric transitions: A plausible model. *J. Mol. Biol.* **12**, 88–118.

Moon, F. (1992). *Chaotic and Fractal Dynamics: An Introduction for Scientists and Engineers.* New York: Wiley.

Murray, J. D. (1989). *Mathematical Biology.* Berlin: Springer-Verlag.

Nelson, E. (1967). *Dynamical Theories of Brownian Motion.* Princeton, NJ: Princeton University Press.

Nicholson, A. J. (1954). An outline of the dynamics of animal populations. *Austral. J. Zool.* **2**, 9–65.

Noble, D., and Tsien, R. W. (1969). Outward membrane currents activated in the plateau range of potentials in cardiac Purkinje fibres. *J. Physiol.* **200**, 205–31.

Oppenheim, A. V., and Schafer, R. W., (1989). *Discrete-time Signal Processing.* Englewood Cliffs, NJ: Prentice-Hall.

Packard, N. H., Crutchfield, J. P., Farmer, J. D., and Shaw, R. S. (1980). Geometry from a time series. *Phys. Rev. Lett.* **459**, 712-16

Packard, N. H. (1988). Adaptation toward the edge of chaos. In. Kelso, J. A. S, Mandell, A. J., and Shlesinger, M. F., eds. *Dynamic Patterns in Complex Systems.* Singapore: World Scientific, 293–301.

Peak, D. and Frame, M. (1994). *Chaos Under Control: The Art and Science of Complexity.* New York: W. H. Freeman.

Peebles, P. Z., Jr., (1987). *Probability, Random Variables, and Random Signal Principles.* McGraw-Hill.

Peitgen, H.-O., and Richter, P. H. (1986). *The Beauty of Fractals.* Berlin: Springer-Verlag.

Peitgen, H.-O., Jürgens, H., and Saupe, D. (1992). *Chaos and Fractals: New Frontiers in Science.* New York: Springer-Verlag.

Phang, J. M., Finerman, G. A. M., Singh, B., Rosenberg, L. E., and Berman, M. (1971). Compartmental analysis of collagen synthesis in fetal rat calvaria. I. Perturbations of proline transport. *Biochim. Biophys. Acta* **230**, 146–59.

Poincaré, H. (1954). *Oeuvres.* Paris: Gauthier-Villars.

Press, W. H., Teukolsky, S. A., Vetterline, W. T., and Flannery, B. R. (1992). *Numerical Recipes in C: The Art of Scientific Computing, 2nd edition.* Cambridge University Press.

Procaccia, I., and Schuster, H. G. (1983). Functional renormalization group theory of universal $1/f$-noise in dynamical systems. *Phys. Rev.* **28 A**, 1210–12.

Proctor, J. W., Auclair, B. G., and Rudenstam, C. M. (1976). The distribution and fate of blood-borne [125]IUdR-labelled tumour cells in immune syngeneic rats. *Int. J. Cancer* **18**, 255–62.

Ptashne, M. (1986). *A Genetic Switch: Gene Control and Phage λ.* Palo Alto, CA: Cell Press and Blackwell Scientific Publishers.

Rabiner, L. R., and Gold, B., (1975). *Theory and Application of Digital Signal Processing.* Englewood Cliffs, NJ: Prentice-Hall.

Rinzel, J. (1977). Repetitive nerve impulse propagation: Numerical results and methods. In: Fitzgibbon, W. E. (III) and Walker, H. R., eds. *Research Notes in Mathemtatics. Nonlinear Diffusion.* London: Pitman Publishing Ltd.

Rossler, O. E. (1976). An equation for continuous chaos. *Phys. Lett.* **57 A**, 397–98.

Sakmann, B., Noma, A., and Trautwein, W. (1983). Acetylcholine activation of single mauscarinic K^+ channels in isolated pacemaker cells of the mammalian heart. *Nature* **303**, 250–53.

Sauer, T. Yorke, J. A., Casdagli, M. (1991). Embedology. *J. Stat. Phys.* **65**, 579–616.

Shlesinger, M. F., Zaslavsky, G. M., and Klafter, J. (1993). Strange kinetics. *Nature* **363**, 31–37.

Simmons, G. F. (1991). *Differential Equations with Applications and Historical Notes.* New York: McGraw-Hill.

Simson, M. B., Spear, J. F., and Moore, E. N. (1981). Stability of an experimental atrioventricular reentrant tachycardia in dogs. *Am. J. Physiol.* **240** (*Heart Circ. Physiol.* **9**), H947–H953.

Snedecor, G. W., and Cochran, W. G. (1989). *Statistical Methods.* Iowa State University (Ames).

Sugihara, G., and May, R. M. (1990). Nonlinear forecasting as a way of distinguising chaos from measurement error in time series. *Nature* **344**, 734–41.

Stanley, H. E., and Ostrowsky, N., eds. (1988). *Random Fluctuations and Pattern Growth: Experiments and Models.* Dordrecht: Kluwer Academic.

Solomon, T. H., Weeks, E. R., and Swinney, H. (1993). Observation of anomalous diffusion and Lévy flights in a two-dimensionsal rotating flow. *Phys. Rev. Lett.* **71**, 3975–78.

Székely, G. (1965). Logical network for controlling limb movements in Urodela. *Acta Physiol. Hung.* **27**, 285–89.

Takens, F. (1981). Detecting strange attractors in turbulence. In: Rand, D. A., and Young, L. S., eds. *Dynamical Systems and Turbulence. Lect. Notes Math.* **898**. Berlin: Springer-Verlag, 336–81.

Theiler, J., Eubank, S., Longtin, A., Galdrikian, B., and Farmer, J. D. (1992). Testing for nonlinearity in time series: the method of surrogate data. *Physica D* **58**, 77–94.

Theiler, J., and Lookman, T. (1993). Statistical error in a chord estimator of the correlation dimension: the 'rule of five'. *Int. J. Bifurcat. Chaos* **3**, 765–71.

Thieffry, D., and Thomas, R. (1994). Dynamical behavior of biological regulatory networks. II. Immunity control in bacteriophage lambda. *Bull. Math. Biol.* (In Press.)

Thomas, R., Gathoye, A. M., and Lambert, L. (1976). A complex control circuit: Regulation of immunity in temperate bacteriophages. *Eur. J. Biochem.* **71**, 211–27.

Thomas, R., and D'Ari, R. (1990). *Biological Feedback.* Boca Raton, FL: CRC Press.

Tont, S. A. (1986). W. E. Allen's 20 year phytoplankton collection. Volume 1—Diatoms. IMR Reference No. 86–3. Scripps Institution of Oceanography.

Tyson, J. (1979). Periodic enzyme synthesis: Reconsideration of the theory of oscillatory repression. *J. Theor. Biol.* **80**, 27–38.

Vicsek, T., Cserző, M., and Horváth, V. K. (1990). Self-affine growth of bacterial colonies. *Physica A* **167**, 315–21.

Voss, R. F., and Clarke, J. (1975). $1/f$ noise in music and speech. *Nature* **258**, 317–18.

Waldrop, M. M. (1992). *Complexity: The Emerging Science at the Edge of Order and Chaos.* New York: Simon & Schuster.

Winfree, A. T. (1972). Spiral waves of chemical activity. *Science* **175**, 634–36.

Winfree, A. T. (1980). *The Geometry of Biological Time.* New York: Springer-Verlag.

Winfree, A. T. (1987). *When Time Breaks Down: The Three-Dimensional Dynamics of Electrochemical Waves and Cardiac Arrhythmias.* Princeton, NJ: Princeton University Press.

Witten, T. A., and Sander, L. M. (1981). Diffusion limited aggregation: A kinetic critical phenomenon. *Phys. Rev. Lett.* **47**, 1400–03.

Wolf, D. (1978). *Noise in Physical Systems. Series in Electrophysics 2.* Heidelberg: Springer-Verlag.

Wolfram, S. (1983). Statistical mechanics of cellular automata. *Rev. Mod. Phys.* **55**, 601–44.

Wolfram, S. (1984). Universality and complexity in cellular automata. *Physica D* **10**, 1–35.

Yagil, G., and Yagil, E. (1971). On the relation between effector concentration and the rate of induced enzyme synthesis. *Biophys. J.* **11**, 11–27.

Index